Palliative Care for Older People
A public health perspective

Palliative Care for Older People
A public health perspective

Edited by

Lieve Van den Block

Gwenda Albers

Sandra Martins Pereira

Bregje Onwuteaka-Philipsen

Roeline Pasman

and

Luc Deliens

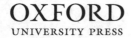

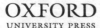

OXFORD
UNIVERSITY PRESS

Great Clarendon Street, Oxford, OX2 6DP,
United Kingdom

Oxford University Press is a department of the University of Oxford.
It furthers the University's objective of excellence in research, scholarship,
and education by publishing worldwide. Oxford is a registered trade mark of
Oxford University Press in the UK and in certain other countries

First Edition published in 2015

Impression: 1

Published in the United States of America by Oxford University Press
198 Madison Avenue, New York, NY 10016, United States of America

British Library Cataloguing in Publication Data

Data available

Library of Congress Control Number: 2015930600

ISBN 978–0–19–871761–4

Printed in Great Britain by
Clays Ltd, St Ives plc

Foreword

Society is facing one of the largest public health challenges in its history — the growth of the population of older adults. For most, the years after age 65 are a time of good health, independence, and integration of a life's work and experience. Eventually, however, most adults will develop one or more serious illnesses with which they may live for many years before they die. Over three-quarters of deaths are now the result of chronic diseases of the heart, lungs, brain, and other vital organs. For a minority of patients with serious illness (e.g., metastatic cancer), the time following diagnosis is characterized by a stable period of relatively good functional and cognitive performance followed by a predictable and short period of functional and clinical decline. However, most persons with serious illness face months to years of physical and psychological symptom distress; progressive functional dependence and frailty; often cognitive impairment; high family support needs; and escalating health care resource use. Indeed, over the next decades, our health care systems and providers will be caring for predominantly seriously ill older people with multiple comorbidities, lengthy durations of illness, and intermittent acute disease exacerbations interspersed with periods of relative stability.

Palliative care focuses on improving quality of life for persons living with serious illness and their families and offers a key solution to the growing population of the seriously ill. By addressing pain and other physical symptoms, emotional and spiritual distress, and family needs, palliative care provides an added layer of support to patients, their families and caregivers, and their health care providers. By providing this extra layer of support, palliative care not only improves health care quality but reduces health care costs as well. Whereas much has been written about palliative care, few articles, and even fewer books, have focused on the specific needs of seriously ill older adults — the fastest growing segment of the population in industrialized nations.

The nature and trajectory of serious illness experienced by older people requires that palliative care for this section of the population differs from what is usually appropriate for younger persons. The extended duration of most serious illnesses in older people, the high prevalence of prolonged functional and cognitive impairment, and the need for long-term caregivers are rarely observed in younger populations. Palliative care for younger adults is typically focused on identification of acute symptoms associated with a specific terminal illness and its immediate manifestations, or on signs of grave prognosis or imminent death. In contrast, many of the characteristics of advanced old age (frailty, functional dependence, cognitive impairment, multiple comorbidities, symptom distress) are multifactorial in aetiology and present over many years. In frail older people, disease-specific treatments may ameliorate or lessen the burdens of frailty, dependence, and symptom distress but are unlikely to eliminate them. Thus, palliative care in older people is centred on the identification and amelioration of functional and cognitive impairment; management of frailty leading to dependence on caregivers; treatment of symptom, emotional, and spiritual distress; and bereavement needs of adult children and elderly partners.

The chapters that follow in this important book address key health and policy issues facing ageing societies. What separates this book on palliative care from those that have gone before is its focus not only on the needs of older people and their families but, as essentially, on the needs of health systems. By demonstrating how palliative care addresses both the needs of individual patients and families and of society, the editors and authors have provided an invaluable road map to guide the future of health care for our public health officials, medical professionals, and policy makers.

Sean Morrison, MD
National Palliative Care Research Center, USA

Acknowledgements

The editors would like to thank Jane Ruthven for her editing work. They would also like to thank the advisory board: Paul Vanden Berghe, Nele Van Den Noortgate, Katherine Froggatt, and Sophie Pautex.

EURO IMPACT (**Euro**pean Intersectorial and **M**ultidisciplinary **Pa**lliative **C**are Research **T**raining) is funded by the European Union Seventh Framework Programme (FP7/2007–2013, under grant agreement no. 264697). EURO IMPACT aims to develop a multidisciplinary, multi-professional, and inter-sectorial educational and research training framework for palliative care research in Europe.

Contents

Contributors

Gwenda Albers
End-of-Life Care Research Group
Vrije Universiteit Brussel
and Ghent University
Brussels, Belgium

Bárbara Antunes
Department of Palliative Care, Policy,
and Rehabilitation
Cicely Saunders Institute
King's College London
London, UK

Margaret P. Battin
Department of Philosophy
Division of Medical Ethics and Humanities
University of Utah
Utah, USA

Noorhazlina Binte Ali
Department of Geriatric Medicine
Tan Tock Seng Hospital
Singapore

Liesbeth Borgermans
Department of Family Medicine
Vrije Universiteit Brussel
Brussels, Belgium

José Miguel Carrasco
Institute for Culture and Society
ATLANTES Program
University of Navarra
Pamplona, Spain

Thomas M. Carroll
Department of Medicine, Division of
General Medicine University of Rochester
Medical Center
New York, USA

Carlos Centeno
Faculty of Medicine and Institute
for Culture and Society
ATLANTES Program
University of Navarra
Pamplona, Spain

Kenneth Chambaere
End-of-Life Care Research Group
Vrije Universiteit Brussel
and Ghent University
Brussels, Belgium

Noreen Chan
Department of Haematology-Oncology
National University Cancer Institute
Singapore

Joachim Cohen
End-of-Life Care Research Group
Vrije Universiteit Brussel
and Ghent University
Brussels, Belgium

David Currow
Discipline, Palliative and Supportive
Services, Flinders University, Adelaide,
Australia

Liliana De Lima
International Association for Hospice
and Palliative Care
Houston, Texas, USA

Luc Deliens
End-of-Life Care Research Group
Vrije Universiteit Brussel and Ghent
University
Brussels and Ghent, Belgium

Karen Detering
Austin Health
Australia

Katherine Froggatt
International Observatory on End
of Life Care
Lancaster University
Lancaster, UK

Clare Gardiner
School of Nursing
The University of Auckland
Auckland, New Zealand

Eduardo Garralda
Institute for Culture and Society
ATLANTES Program
University of Navarra
Pamplona, Spain

Marie-Jose H.E. Gijsberts
Department of Nursing Home
Medicine and Department of Public
and Occupational Health
EMGO Institute for Health
and Care Research
VU University Medical Center
Amsterdam, the Netherlands

Cynthia Ruth Goh
Duke-NUS Graduate Medical School
Singapore
Department of Palliative Medicine
National Cancer Center
Singapore
National University of Singapore
Singapore

Merryn Gott
School of Nursing
The University of Auckland
New Zealand

Liz Gwyther
Hospice Palliative Care Association
South Africa
Cape Town, South Africa

Marjolein Gysels
Centre for Social Science and Global
Health
University of Amsterdam
The Netherlands and
Department of Palliative Care, Policy,
and Rehabilitation
Cicely Saunders Institute
King's College London
London, UK

Richard Harding
Department of Palliative Care, Policy,
and Rehabilitation
Cicely Saunders Institute
King's College London
London, UK

Agnes van der Heide
Department of Public Health
Erasmus University
Rotterdam, the Netherlands

Lilian Hidalgo
OncoSalud
Lima, Peru

Irene J Higginson
Department of Palliative Care, Policy,
and Rehabilitation
Cicely Saunders Institute
King's College London
London, UK

Christine Ingleton
School of Nursing and Midwifery
University of Sheffield
Sheffield, UK

Allan Kellehear
Faculty of Health Studies
University of Bradford
Bradford, UK

Diane Meier
Center to Advance Palliative Care
Icahn School of Medicine at Mount Sinai
New York, USA

Sumytra Menon
Lien Centre for Palliative Care
Duke-National University of Singapore
Graduate Medical School
Singapore

Rocio Morante
SaludExpertos
Lima, Peru

Hazel Morbey
Division of Health Research
Lancaster University
Lancaster, UK

Zeynep Güldem Ökem
TOBB University of Economics and
Technology
Ankara, Turkey

Bregje Onwuteaka-Philipsen
Department of Public and Occupational
Health
EMGO Institute for Health and Care
Research
Expertise Center for Palliative Care
VU University Medical Center
Amsterdam, the Netherlands

Katherine Ornstein
Icahn School of Medicine at Mount Sinai
New York, USA

Anne-Sophie Parent
AGE Platform Europe
Brussels, Belgium

Jose Parodi
Universidad de San Martin de Porres
Peru

Roeline Pasman
Department of Public and Occupational
Health
EMGO Institute for Health and Care
Research
Expertise Center for Palliative Care
VU University Medical Center
Amsterdam, the Netherlands

Sheila Payne
International Observatory on End
of Life Care
Lancaster University
Lancaster, UK

Sandra Martins Pereira
Department of Public and Occupational
Health
EMGO Institute for Health and Care
Research
Expertise Center for Palliative Care
VU University Medical Center
Amsterdam, the Netherlands

Jane Phillips
Centre for Cardiovascular and Chronic
Care, University of Technology Sydney,
Australia

Ruth Piers
Department of Geriatric Medicine
Ghent University Hospital
Ghent, Belgium

Kristian Pollock
School of Health Sciences
University of Nottingham
Queen's Medical Centre
Nottingham, UK

Richard A. Powell
Formerly Director of Research and
Learning
African Palliative Care Association
Kampala, Uganda
Presently Global Health Researcher
Nairobi, Kenya

Timothy Quill
Palliative Care Program, Department
of Medicine
University of Rochester School of Medicine
New York, USA

Tony Ryan
School of Nursing and Midwifery
University of Sheffield
Sheffield, UK

Jane Seymour
School of Health Sciences
University of Nottingham
Nottingham, UK

Jennifer S. Shaw
Department of Internal Medicine
Division of Oncology/Palliative Care
Huntsman Cancer Institute
University of Utah
Utah, USA

William Silvester
Respecting Patient Choices Programme
and Austin Health
Victoria, Australia

Joyce Simard
School of Nursing and Midwifery
University of West Sydney
Sydney, Australia

Lieve Van den Block
End-of-Life Care Research Group
Vrije Universiteit Brussel and Ghent
University
Brussels, Belgium

Nele Van Den Noortgate
Department of Geriatric Medicine
Ghent University Hospital
Ghent, Belgium

Liesbeth Van Vliet
Department of Palliative Care, Policy,
and Rehabilitation
Cicely Saunders Institute
King's College London
London, UK

Ladislav Volicer
School of Ageing Studies
University of South Florida
Florida, USA

Hubertus J.M. Vrijhoef
Saw Swee Hock School of Public Health
National University of Singapore
Singapore

Andre Vyt
Artevelde University College and
University of Ghent
Ghent, Belgium

Kathrin Woitha
Institute for Culture and Society
ATLANTES Program
University of Navarra
Pamplona, Spain

Part I

Palliative care for older people: an introduction

Chapter 1

A public health perspective on palliative care for older people: an introduction

Gwenda Albers, Sandra Martins Pereira, Bregje Onwuteaka-Philipsen, Luc Deliens, Roeline Pasman, and Lieve Van den Block

Introduction to a public health perspective on palliative care for older people

Populations around the world are ageing rapidly. More people survive to older ages, suffer from multiple chronic conditions, and will need some form of advanced care towards the end of life. Caring for this growing number of older people and meeting their care needs have huge implications for the organization and provision of health and social care. This is a growing public health issue that poses important social and economic challenges to individuals, families, and societies (1–3). Many public health and health care policy makers all over the world are concerned about how to plan, organize, and provide appropriate care towards the end of life for the increasing number of older people.

In this book, we aim to provide a worldwide public health perspective on the development and organization of palliative care for older people. Knowledge and expertise concerning the organization, availability, and quality of palliative care for older people are scattered over different disciplines, various settings, and different countries, and are not easily accessible. We focus on bringing together policies, evidence-based knowledge, and good practice initiatives and presenting this in an accessible way for all those stakeholders who can potentially bring change to this area, such as policy and decision-makers in health and social welfare, commissioners of services, academics, educators, managers, and senior practitioners.

In this introductory chapter, we first describe the challenges of an ageing population including the global trends and future projections regarding epidemiology and socio-demographics, and the needs of older people in the last years of their lives. Subsequently, we outline the existing definitions of palliative care and discuss the definitions of palliative care for older people by highlighting how they relate to and diverge from the definitions of palliative care in general. Then, we will describe the concept of public health and explain how a public health perspective on palliative care can help us move forward in planning for a future in which we need to face the consequences of ageing populations worldwide and the increasing number of people dying in old age. An overview of the content of the rest of the book is provided at the end of this chapter.

The challenges of an ageing population

Ageing of populations is a global phenomenon happening in all regions and in countries at various levels of development. Important demographic, epidemiologic, and social changes have been occurring worldwide. Hence, the emerging needs of people living and dying in old age have been steadily increasing.

Demographic and epidemiologic trends

Populations around the world are ageing. The changing age structure can be considered as a global phenomenon arising from decreasing fertility together with increasing life expectancy. More people will survive into old age, and those people surviving into old age will tend to live longer. Mortality declines, especially at older ages, and therefore gains in life expectancy are expected to be relatively higher in the older age groups (4).

Currently, in almost all industrialized countries, the total fertility rate is below the replacement level. Although the fertility decline started later and is in an earlier stage in less developed countries, the demographic transition process is occurring there as well. In the more developed regions, life expectancy is expected to have risen to 82 years, compared to 75 years in less developed regions (4).

The World Health Organization stated that between 2000 and 2050, the proportion of the world's population over 60 years will double from about 11% to 22%. The absolute number of people aged 60 years and over is expected to rise from 605 million to 2 billion over the same period (5). In particular, the number of people aged 80 years or over is growing significantly in most nations, regardless of the state of development and geographical location. The absolute number of people aged 80 years or over is projected to increase by almost fourfold from 2000 to 2050 (4), with women outnumbering men (Figure 1.1).

In terms of continents, the majority of the world's older people reside in Asia, while Europe has the next largest share. However, the pace of increase in the ageing population is more rapid in less developed countries such as Brazil, Indonesia, the Republic of Korea, and Tunisia (6).

Together with the shift in the distribution of populations towards older ages and increasing numbers of deaths at an older age, the leading causes of death are changing. Data regarding health and time trends among older people are still scarce (7). However, it is undeniable that chronic health problems have replaced infectious diseases as the leading health care burden. Chronic diseases such as heart and cardiovascular diseases, cerebrovascular diseases, diabetes, arthritis, osteoporosis, and cognitive disorders become more common with age, being, together with Alzheimer's disease, Parkinson's disease, and cancer, the major causes of death among people older than 60 years (8). Dementia, one

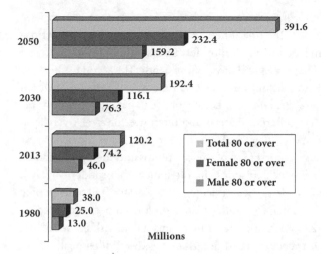

Figure 1.1 Estimated world population aged 80 or over
United Nations, Profiles of Ageing 2013.

of the cognitive disorders closely related to older age, is becoming a serious public health concern itself. There will be a dramatic increase in the number of people with dementia worldwide, with an expected 25–30% of people aged 85 or older having some degree of cognitive decline (5).

The prevalence of multi-morbidity, the coexistence of multiple chronic diseases in one person, ranges from 55% to 98% (7). In addition to older age, female gender and low socio-economic status are factors associated with multi-morbidity (7). Accordingly, distinct epidemiological trends can be identified between different socio-economic groups and between geographical areas (e.g. rural and urban or rich and poor regions). Most developing countries are experiencing similar trends regarding demographics, illness, and cause of death. The World Health Organization projected in 1998 that, by 2020, three-quarters of all deaths in developing countries will be related to old age and mainly caused by diseases of the circulatory system, cancer, hypertension, and diabetes (9).

The needs of people living and dying in old age

Population ageing and its consequences have a major impact on the care needs of populations. More people are living longer but increasing life expectancy does not necessarily mean that the added years of life are spent in good health.

Chronic diseases such as dementia, cancer, chronic respiratory diseases, heart, cardio, and cerebrovascular diseases become more common with age (3, 10, 11) and most older people experience some chronic conditions. Many older people are suffering long periods of illness and are confronted with disabilities, frailty, or other physical or mental health problems. However, many of those chronically ill older people have ambiguous medical prognoses; they may be ill enough to die from their old age and/or complications due to end-stage chronic diseases but could also live for many years (12).

Three different illness trajectories have been described for people with progressive chronic illnesses (Figure 1.2) (12–17). The first illness trajectory describes how most patients with cancer maintain comfort and functioning for a substantial period, followed by relatively rapid decline in the final weeks and days before death. The second trajectory describes long-term limitations with intermittent exacerbations and sudden dying which can be associated with organ failure. Patients in this category (e.g. patients with respiratory and heart failure) follow a very different pattern and often live for a relatively long time with only minor limitations in everyday life. From time to time, physiological stress overwhelms the body reserves causing worsening of the symptoms and the overall condition of the patient. They survive a few such episodes and often die rather suddenly from a complication or exacerbation (18). The last illness trajectory is typical for frail older people or people, especially those with dementia, who suffer from a prolonged period of gradual decline. A study in the United States analysing Medicare claims data classified decedents into groups representing the three trajectories just described besides sudden death. They found that most people who died after a distinct terminal phase of illness were younger, 40% under the age of 75, whereas most decedents in the organ system failure group died between the age of 75 and 84, and 66% of those in the frailty group were aged 80 or older when they died (17).

Although the trajectories may help to prognosticate and further plan care, older people cannot be clearly categorized into one of these trajectories due to multi-morbidity. Moreover, a combination of these trajectories may occur as older people often suffer from cancer, chronic diseases, and frailty simultaneously. Older people often experience several medical problems and co-morbidities simultaneously over an extended period of time. Not much research has studied the illness trajectories and care needs of older people. Nevertheless, older people clearly have special needs. The problems older people are confronted with are different and often more complex compared with those of younger people (2). The cumulative effect may be much greater than the effect of any single disease and often leads to greater impairment, dependency, and need for care; and minor problems may have greater cumulative psychological impact in older people. Moreover, older people are at greater risk of drug side-effects and iatrogenic diseases. Problems of acute illness may be superimposed on physical or mental impairment, financial problems, and social depletion and isolation (1, 2).

According to the World Health Organization, 'older people suffer unnecessarily, owing to widespread underassessment and under-treatment of their problems and lack of access to palliative care' (2). The prevalence of cognitive impairment and dementia among older people increases the complexity and challenges of care provision. A progressive deterioration in ability and awareness raises many ethical issues as people with dementia are unable to communicate their wishes and preferences for care (2). Older people and especially those with dementia have been found to be at risk of poor pain control due to communication problems which make them less able to report pain and it may be more difficult for care professionals as well as for family members to assess it properly (19). Older people tend to underreport their symptoms and doctors tend to

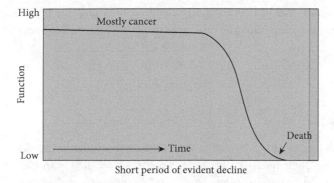

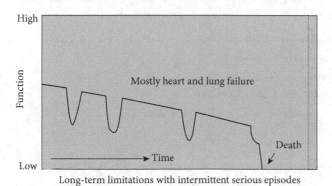

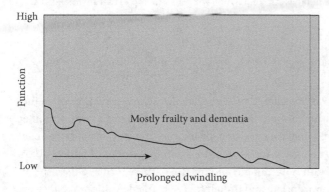

Figure 1.2 Chronic illness trajectories
Adapted from J Lynn and DM Adamson, Living Well at the End of Life: Adapting Health Care to Serious Chronic Illness in Old Age, White Paper; WP-137, p. 8, figure 3, Copyright © 2003, RAND Corporation. Reprinted with permission of RAND Corporation, Santa Monica, CA.

undertreat pain. Research has shown consistently that patients with dementia are undertreated for pain (20–23).

This all can also create difficult situations for family members who might take the role of informal caregivers. Being an informal caregiver for older seriously ill people can have a major impact on the individual, which may cause social problems and problems in health and well-being. Physical and emotional burden in family caregivers—whose age is also rising along with the trend of the ageing population—create needs for care and support among family carers too (24).

Palliative care

Defining palliative care

According to the World Health Organization, palliative care is 'an approach that improves the quality of life of patients and their families facing the problems associated with life-threatening illness, through the prevention and relief of suffering by means of early identification and treatment of other problems, physical, psychosocial and spiritual' (25). Moreover, the World Health Organization defined the following core principles of palliative care:

◆ provides relief from pain and other distressing symptoms;

◆ affirms life and considers dying as a normal process;

◆ intends to neither hasten nor postpone death;

◆ integrates the psychological and spiritual aspects of patient care;

◆ offers a support system to help patients live as actively as possible until death;

◆ offers a support system to help the family cope during the patients' illness and in their own bereavement;

◆ uses a team approach to address the needs of patients and their families, including bereavement counselling, if indicated;

◆ will enhance quality of life, and may also positively influence the course of illness;

◆ is applicable early in the course of illness, in conjunction with other therapies that are intended to prolong life and includes those investigations needed to better understand and manage distressing clinical complications (25).

Reproduced from *WHO Definition of Palliative Care* © WHO, 2014. <http://www.who.int/cancer/palliative/definition/en/>

Traditionally, palliative care was considered to be applicable exclusively at the end of life. This is also why the term 'palliative care' is sometimes used interchangeably with terminal or end-of-life care. Although terminal care and end-of-life care can be considered as part of the continuum of palliative care, these terms refer to the management of patients during the terminal period when death is imminent, and the use of these terms to describe all elements of palliative care is inappropriate and unhelpful (26). The definition of palliative care has evolved over the years and it is now increasingly recognized that palliative care has much to offer at a much earlier stage in the course of progressive disease. Nowadays, palliative care is not only for dying people or people with cancer. Palliative care is defined not by reference to organ, age, disease type, or pathology but, rather, by an assessment of the specific needs of an individual patient and his/her family (26). This means that palliative care can be provided to any patient without restriction to disease or prognosis, and alongside curative or life-prolonging treatments.

Throughout this book, the term 'palliative care' refers to the care focusing on relieving and preventing suffering to improve the quality of life of the patient with serious life-threatening illness and his or her family, using a multidisciplinary approach to address physical, emotional, spiritual, and social concerns as defined by the World Health Organization.

Palliative care for older people

The expansion of the definition of palliative care just described means that palliative care is applicable early in the course of an illness, alongside therapies intended to prolong life, and that it is about living well with a life-threatening or life-limiting illness rather than just about dying.

Current research in palliative care has shown the potential benefits of an early palliative care approach, not only in terms of symptom assessment and treatment (27), but also in terms of improving the quality of life and quality of care, meeting patients' wishes and preferences, and avoiding unnecessary and burdensome life-prolonging treatments and hospitalizations, thus allowing a more peaceful death (2, 27–29). Although most research has been conducted in cancer patients and not explored in full, a potential added value of palliative care for older people can be presumed and will be further elaborated in this book.

Older people often suffer from more than one chronic condition towards the end of life. Multi-morbidity causes a wide range of physical, psychological, and social problems and leads to complex needs for care and support. Providing care to older people therefore needs a multidisciplinary team approach dealing with the different dimensions of suffering and the coordination and continuity of care as well—which is consistent with palliative care. This care approach not only intends to improve the quality of life of the patient, but also considers and includes the family as part of the process of care and as the beneficiaries of care. Geriatric medicine, a sub-specialty of internal medicine and family medicine, that focuses on health care of older people, is closely related to palliative care (30). Palliative care, geriatric medicine, as well as family medicine aim to provide patient-centred family-focused care and work from a holistic and multidisciplinary approach. The overlap between these disciplines can be considered as having the potential for synergy which also relates to other medical specialties and groups of health professionals (such as neurologists, internal medicine specialists, cardiologists, psychologists, nurses, occupational health practitioners, and social and spiritual caregivers) being involved in providing care for older people. To a greater or lesser extent, they all seek to address the older person's needs and are dealing with the common problem of care fragmentation for older people suffering from any chronic condition, promoting integrated care, and advocating interdisciplinary care and coordination from a patient perspective (30, 31).

Nonetheless, no clear or commonly accepted definition of palliative care for older people exists. The European Union Geriatric Medical Society (EUGMS) recently defined 'geriatric palliative medicine' as: 'the medical care and management of older patients with health-related problems and progressive, advanced disease for which the prognosis is limited and the focus of care is quality of life' (30). Hence, this definition of 'geriatric palliative medicine' seems to refer mainly to end-of-life care, while the World Health Organization states that palliative care is for all people with life-threatening illness, regardless of the diagnosis and prognosis. Regardless of the exact definitions used, the core values of palliative care concern the holistic approach towards the patient and his or her family, the focus on quality of life and dignity, patient autonomy, the provision of needs-based rather than diagnosis-based care, and coordination and continuity of care. These values are also of great importance for frail older people and people with dementia, whether or not they are at the very end of life.

Public health

Defining public health

Public health has early roots in ancient times when it was recognized that polluted water and a lack of proper waste disposal spread communicable diseases and public health legislation and sanitary reform were introduced. In the late nineteenth and the twentieth century, public health achievements such as vaccination programmes controlling many infectious diseases, effective health and safety policies concerning road traffic, family planning, and tobacco control contributed to a further increase in the average life span. When the prevalence of infectious diseases decreased and with the onset of the epidemiological changes, public health began to put more focus on chronic diseases such as cancer and heart disease.

Public health can be defined as all organized activities to prevent disease, promote health, and prolong life among the population as a whole. According to the World Health Organization (31), the three main public health functions are:

♦ The assessment and monitoring of the health of communities and populations at risk to identify health problems and priorities.

♦ The formulation of public policies designed to solve identified local and national health problems and priorities.

♦ To assure that all populations have access to appropriate and cost-effective care, including health promotion and disease prevention services.

Reproduced from *Public Health* © WHO, 2014. <http://www.who.int/trade/glossary/ story076/en/>

The concept of health plays an important role in this definition, as it does not only refer to the absence of illness and disability (32). As a subjective concept, health is highly determined by the diversity of human experience, socio-cultural influences, self-perceptions, and beliefs. *Being healthy* (as the absence of a disease) and *feeling healthy* (as the absence of burdensome symptoms and having capacity to experience meaningful life events and quality of life) are, therefore, inter-related floating concepts that evolve over time due to the influence of circumstances and life events. A public health approach implies a view at population level much broader than a strictly medical or paramedical focus on clinical interventions or aspects of individual quality of life.

A public health perspective on palliative care for older people

Death is both inevitable and universal. In developed and less developed societies, everyone is confronted with death and dying (either directly or indirectly in the case of a dying relative) and it impacts on several aspects of health and well-being. The quality of dying, and maintaining quality of life for those who are dying and those caring for them, can be considered a public health issue equal to all other public health issues (33–39).

According to the *Global Atlas of Palliative Care at the End of Life* published in 2014, worldwide, over 29 million people died in 2011 from diseases requiring palliative care (3). Among those, 94% are adults and 69% of them are aged above 60 (3). With the trend of the ageing population worldwide, it is foreseen that more people will die at older ages and the number of old frail people will also rise in the following decades. To best meet the needs of their populations living and dying in old age, societies need to prepare for an ageing world and put the right policies and national health strategies in place. In order to improve circumstances for those living and dying in old age and to integrate palliative care throughout health care systems, a public health perspective helps to focus on the health of the population rather than the health and health care needs of the individual.

A public health perspective is used in this book to address the challenges of providing appropriate care for older people on the health care organization, community, and policy level (meso and macro level) rather than the micro (referring to health care professional and patient interaction) level. In order to develop proper public health strategies to promote and improve palliative care for older people, societies must consider the organization of their health care systems, monitor the quality as well as access to palliative care, and take into account the socio-cultural and clinical context of those living and dying in old age. Hence, in this book we intend to show and reflect on the need for and importance of a public health perspective and approach towards people living and dying in old age and the challenges posed by an ageing population.

Outline of the book

With this book, we hope to stimulate reflection and debate on palliative care for older people from a public health perspective. To achieve this, we have divided this book into six parts. Part I is the present introduction (Chapter 1) in which we provide the reader with the rationale behind developing a public health perspective on palliative care for older people.

Part II will start with a more conceptual approach to long-term care and integrated, person-centred care. Hence, while Chapter 2 will present, define, and explore the overall organization of long-term care, Chapter 3 will reflect more on the state and potential for development of palliative care within long-term care, providing information on possible key drivers for change at this level. Chapter 4 will describe integrated and person-centred care, exploring why, and to what extent, older people requiring palliative care may benefit from this approach and future developments considered necessary to develop, evaluate, and implement integrated and person-centred palliative care. These three chapters will set up the scenario for a set of chapters (Chapters 5 to 10) in which policies on palliative care for older people all over the world will be explored. These chapters, written by authors from several countries, will provide a culturally sensitive overview of the palliative care needs and specificities within each context and will reflect on the future developments needed in this field worldwide.

The social, cultural, and clinical contexts of living and dying in old age will be explored in Part III, beginning with Chapter 11 describing where older people die in different countries and how age influences place of death. Cross-cultural and sociological differences will be explored when comparing preferred and actual place of death, discussing the impact of different national policies on this matter. Understanding where and how older people die, and mapping the circumstances of dying in older age groups have relevance from a public health perspective. Hence, Chapter 12 will describe such circumstances, providing information on the quality of care and dying, and pointing out possible strategies that can be implemented to improve palliative care for older people.

Within the context of the ageing population and the growing tension between, on the one hand, the variety of medical-therapeutic possibilities and, on the other, the demands for quality of life and patient-centred care, there is the need to explore topics related to end-of-life decision-making. Medical decision-making in older people is often about setting limits to life support in favour of the patient's quality of life and dignity. In Chapter 13, end-of-life decisions will be defined and information provided on how often these decisions are made in older people, and there will be a reflection on the limited decision-making capacity in many older people and dementia that can hinder decision-making at the end of life.

In the context of the ethical dimensions of palliative care provision for older people and the ethical principles that emerge in this field, Chapter 14 will explore the ethical issues involved in palliative care for older people and the similarities and differences between providing palliative care for older and younger people and the ethical debates in this field. The ethical vocabulary is thus revisited with an emphasis on attempts to construct patient-specific ethical narratives.

A public health perspective on palliative care for older people would not be complete without including some cultural reflections and insights. Culture, including knowledge, beliefs, morality, law, and tradition, is a fundamental ingredient of the individual and of society and influences how palliative care is perceived, conceived, and organized. Chapter 15 will discuss cultural aspects surrounding dying and death in older age and how culture may influence attitudes. Finally, the last chapter in Part III (Chapter 16) will reflect on the multiple dimensions of the concept of 'spirituality' and how to measure and include it in palliative care for older people.

In Part IV of this book, we provide the reader with an overview of access to and use of palliative care by older people. Chapter 17 will address the distinction between specialist and palliative care, reflecting on how both levels of and approaches to palliative care can be utilized to provide high-value quality care to older adults. In this chapter, the evolution of palliative care will be considered and a framework proposed for ensuring its efficient and effective provision for all patients in need. The need for compassionate communities and societies caring for older people towards the end of life will be explored in Chapter 18 which will examine issues concerning death and loss from a public health viewpoint.

Chapter 19 will reflect on the applicability and added value of palliative care for older people with dementia including discussion of maintaining and improving quality of life, the avoidance of aggressive and burdensome treatments, and the difficulties of prognostication, together with the challenges of improving the knowledge and skills of health professionals in order to meet the needs of people with dementia.

The involvement of family members caring for older people will be covered in Chapter 20. The complexity of family carer experiences and needs and their roles, tasks, and experiences in the context of an ageing demographic will be explored. This chapter will also suggest strategies to help family caregivers and to minimize the burden of caring for an older person. Following this, Chapter 21 will explore how collaboration between professionals can be enhanced to meet older people's needs by means of improving intra- and inter-professional communication. The relevant skills, attitudes, and professional competences will be covered and strategies to prevent burnout, compassion fatigue, and other associated problems will be suggested.

The last chapter of this part, Chapter 22, will focus on communication and advance care planning—an essential dimension of palliative care. It will start with a definition of communication and advance care planning in palliative care for older people and give an overview of the latest empirical findings.

Part V of this book will describe a set of innovative practices and interventions in palliative care for older people worldwide. Chapter 23 will present some initiatives from inside the European Union—AGE Platform Europe, EUSTACEA project, and the WeDO project—developed to improve the quality of life of older people. In Chapter 24, different programmes referring to various care pathways (e.g. Gold Standards Framework, Liverpool Care Pathway, and Route-to-Success) for older people in need of palliative care will be discussed. Chapter 25 will present the Australian programme of advance care planning—Respecting Patient Choices; the background, goals, and objectives of the programme will be described together with evidence reflecting its effect on palliative care provision for older people.

In the final part and chapter of this book (Part VI, Chapter 26), we will elaborate on the growing evidence supporting a public health approach to palliative care for older people and build on some of the WHO recommendations using the contributions of the different authors brought together in this book. We first reflect on what and how palliative care might complement care for older people, and the policy developments in palliative care, before we formulate specific recommendations for academics and health care managers and staff as well as policy- and decision-makers at international and national level in the field of palliative care for older people.

References

1 Davies E, Higginson IJ. *Better palliative care for older people.* Copenhagen: World Health Organization; 2004.

2 Hall S, Petkova H, Tsouros AD, Costantini M, Higginson IJ. *Palliative care for older people: better practices.* Copenhagen: World Health Organization; 2011.

3 World Health Organization. *How many people are in need of palliative care worldwide? Global atlas of palliative care at the end of life.* Geneva: World Health Organization and Worldwide Palliative Care Alliance; 2014.

4 United Nations. *World population aging: 1950–2050.* New York: Department of Economic and Social Affairs, Population Division, United Nations; 2011.

5 World Health Organization. 'Interesting facts about ageing'. Available at: <http://www.who.int/ageing/about/facts/en/> (Accessed April 2014). Ref. type: online source.

6 Mirkin B, Weinberger M. *The demography of population ageing.* New York: Department of Economic and Social Affairs, Population Division, United Nations; 2000.

7 Marengoni A, Angleman S, Melis R, Mangialasche F, Karp A, Garmen A, et al. Aging with multimorbidity: a systematic review of the literature. *Ageing Res Rev* 2011; **10**(4):430–9.

8 World Health Organization. *Strengthening of palliative care as a component of integrated treatment throughout the life course.* EB134/28. 134th session; 2013.

9 World Health Organization. *The world health report. Life in the 21st century: a vision for all.* Geneva: World Health Organization; 1998.

10 Matzo ML. Palliative care: prognostication and the chronically ill: methods you need to know as chronic disease progresses in older adults. *Am J Nurs* 2004; **104**(9):40–9.

11 Lafortune G, Balestat G. *Trends in severe disability among elderly people: assessing the evidence in 12 OECD countries and the future implications.* Organisation for Economic Co-operation and Development Health Working Papers, No. 26; 2007.

12 Lynn J, Adamson D. *Adapting health care to serious chronic illness in old age.* Rand Health White Paper WP-137; 2003.

13 Glare PA, Christakis NA. Predicting survival in patients with advanced disease. In: Doyle D, Hanks G, Cherny N, Calman K (eds). *Oxford textbook of palliative medicine.* Oxford: Oxford University Press; 2004, 81–110.

14 Lehman R. How long can I go on like this? Dying from cardiorespiratory disease. *Br J Gen Pract* 2004; **54**(509):892–3.

15 Lunney JR, Lynn J, Foley DJ, Lipson S, Guralnik JM. Patterns of functional decline at the end of life. *JAMA* 2003; **289**(18):2387–92.

16 Murtagh FE, Preston M, Higginson I. Patterns of dying: palliative care for non-malignant disease. *Clin Med* 2004; **4**(1):39–44.

17 Lunney JR, Lynn J, Hogan C. Profiles of older medicare decedents. *J Am Geriatr Soc* 2002; **50**(6):1108–12.

18 Lynn J, Forlini JH. 'Serious and complex illness' in quality improvement and policy reform for end-of-life care. *J Gen Intern Med* 2001; **16**(5):315–9.

19 Frampton M. Experience assessment and management of pain in people with dementia. *Age Ageing* 2003; **32**(3):248–51.

20 Nygaard HA, Jarland M. Are nursing home patients with dementia diagnosis at increased risk for inadequate pain treatment? *Int J Geriatr Psychiatry* 2005; **20**(8):730–7.

21 Scherder E, van Manen F. Pain in Alzheimer's disease: nursing assistants' and patients' evaluations. *J Adv Nurs* 2005; **52**(2):151–8.

22 Tait RC, Chibnall JT. Under-treatment of pain in dementia: assessment is key. *JAMDA* 2008; **9**(6):372–4.

23 Payne S. White Paper on improving support for family carers in palliative care. *Eur J Pall Care* 2010; **17**(5):238–45.

24 World Health Organization. *National cancer control programmes: policies and managerial guidelines.* Geneva: World Health Organization; 2002.

25 Council of Europe (2003) Recommendation Rec (2003) 24 of the Committee of Ministers to member states on the organisation of palliative care.

26 Bakitas M, Lyons KD, Hegel MT, Balan S, Brokaw FC, Seville J, et al. Effects of a palliative care intervention on clinical outcomes in patients with advanced cancer: the Project ENABLE II randomized controlled trial. *JAMA* 2009; **302**(7):741–9.

27 Temel JS, Greer JA, Muzikansky A, Gallagher ER, Admane S, Jackson VA, et al. Early palliative care for patients with metastatic non-small-cell lung cancer. *NEJM* 2010; **363**(8):733–42.

28 Hall S, Kolliakou A, Petkova H, Froggatt K, Higginson IJ. Interventions for improving palliative care for older people living in nursing care homes. *Cochrane Database Syst Rev* 2011; **3**:CD007132.

29 Pautex S, Curiale V, Pfisterer M, Rexach L, Ribbe M, Van Den Noortgate N. A common definition of geriatric palliative medicine. *JAGS* 2010; **58**(4):790–1.

30 McCormick WC, on behalf of American Geriatrics Society, American Association for Hospice and Palliative Medicine, and John A Hartford Foundation. Report of the Geriatrics-Hospice and Palliative Medicine Work Group: American Geriatrics Society and American Academy of Hospice and Palliative Medicine leadership collaboration. *JAGS* 2012; **60**(3):583–7.

31 World Health Organization. 'Public health'. Available at: <http://www.who.int/trade/glossary/story076/en/> (Accessed April 2014). Ref. type: online source.

32 Baum NM, DesRoches C, Campbell EG, Goold SD. Resource allocation in public health practice: a national survey of local public health officials. *J Public Health Manag Pract* 2011; **17**(3):265–74.

33 Cohen J, Deliens L. *A public health perspective on end of life care.* Oxford University Press, Oxford; 2012.

34 Stjernsward J, Foley KM, Ferris FD. The public health strategy for palliative care. *J Pain Symptom Manage* 2007; **33**(5):486–93.

35 Palliative care—an urgent but neglected public health priority. *World Health Forum* 1991; **12**(4):399.

36 Behmann M, Luckmann SL, Schneider N. Palliative care in Germany from a public health perspective: qualitative expert interviews. *BMC Res Notes* 2009; **2**:116.

37 Webster R, Lacey J, Quine S. Palliative care: a public health priority in developing countries. *J Public Health Policy* 2007; **28**(1):28–39.

38 Ela S, Espinosa J, Martinez-Munoz M, Lasmarias C, Beas E, Mateo-Ortega D, et al. The WHO Collaborating Centre for Public Health Palliative Care Programs: an innovative approach of palliative care development. *J Palliat Med* 2014; **17**(4):385–92.

39 Wiener JM, Tilly J. Population ageing in the United States of America: implications for public programmes. *Int J Epidemiol* 2002; **31**(4):776–81.

Part II

Organization of and policies for palliative care for older people

Chapter 2

Long-term care systems

Zeynep Güldem Ökem

Introduction to long-term care systems

Demographic changes create challenges for health and social systems, necessitating them to adjust both the size and the scope of the services provided. In most developed countries, the ageing population has increased the financial burden on the public sector of providing health and long-term care services, threatening the sustainability of health and social systems.

Health and long-term care systems are usually treated separately within social security policies in most advanced countries. Long-term care encompasses care provided through a complex network of systems involving different public programmes and bringing various sectors and private initiatives together. This chapter provides a general introduction to the analysis of the long-term care system in a country through showing various implementations in EU countries as well as others. After explaining basic concepts in long-term care, including its objectives, target groups, and services—while emphasizing differences between health and long-term care systems, the assessment of need for long-term care, coverage, provision—types of services, long-term care expenditures, and financing methods are explained. The last part focuses on key policy issues in long-term care.

The characteristics of long-term care systems

The term 'long-term care' includes a range of services for people who cannot function independently in the activities of daily living due to loss or impairment in their physical, functional, or cognitive capacity. The impairment or loss in activity usually occurs due to ageing or chronic conditions of physical or mental disability. The objective of long-term care services is to improve the quality of life while reducing the negative consequences of old age or disability. A wide range of services are provided including medical services, nursing care, prevention, rehabilitation, and palliative care, along with home care for sustaining daily and social life (1, 2). Hence, the scope of services is wider than that of the health services and encompasses both care and cure and entails both health and social issues. The responsibility for long-term care lies between the health care and the social care systems (3).

The target group is the older one usually defined as 65 years of age and older, disabled persons, or people with chronic diseases. The need for long-term care usually occurs towards the end of life. One out of every three people needs long-term care but some do not need it at all (4). Unlike the health system, where the need for health care usually occurs due to acute conditions and people enter the system and leave after some time, the need for care and support is continuous in long-term care. The main objective of the health system is to prevent diseases and cure the patient. Due to continuity in need, improving the quality of life of the target group and their families is a more prominent objective in long-term care. Physical adaptation of the home or the infrastructure of facilities (e.g. ramps and hand rails) to ensure safety for old or disabled people is also often needed (5).

An interdisciplinary team of professionals involved in long-term care services includes physicians, geriatric specialists, geriatric/long-term care nurses, pharmacists, social workers, dieticians, physical therapists, occupational therapists, speech language pathologists, case managers, respiratory therapists, physician assistants, and other members working in the long-term care setting. Long-term care is labour intensive, though usually involves lower levels of specialization and less skilled workers than do health services. High care, necessitating higher nursing skills, is needed for people affected by dementia or with multiple chronic conditions. A geriatric or long-term care nurse is a key person, caring for patients who require an extended level of care due to chronic conditions and long-term disabilities. Geriatric nurses manage patient care, perform various nursing skills, address changes in condition, and provide interventions. They also give physical and psychosocial support and educate residents and their families. The geriatric nurse assists care recipients or residents with activities of daily living such as grooming, feeding, dressing, toileting, and bathing. They are also capable of applying adaptive equipment. In some countries, nurses or nurse case managers, allied health professionals, and health technicians are appointed for the management of long-term care for chronically ill patients. But most of the work of long-term care requires a relatively low level of skills (6). The service is usually provided by family members, friends, or immigrant carers. Two-thirds of the services are provided by women (7). Resources are less complex and medical devices are less costly (e.g. assistive devices, canes and walkers) than those employed in health services. However, sometimes more advanced technologies may be required (e.g. emergency alert systems and computerized medication reminders) (8).

The need for long-term care

The levels of disability and dependence accepted as primary determinants of the need for long-term care increase with age (9). Half of all long-term care users are above 80 years of age across OECD countries (10). Long-term care is also targeted at the disabled and people with chronic illnesses. Patients who suffer from progressive diseases such as osteoporosis, dementia, Lou Gehrig's disease, Alzheimer's disease, Parkinson's disease, AIDS wasting complex, rheumatoid arthritis, and multiple sclerosis may need long-term care services, as may many individuals who have chronic diseases such as hypothyroidism, hypertension, congestive heart failure, coronary artery disease, diabetes mellitus, peripheral vascular disease, chronic kidney disease, and chronic obstructive pulmonary disease (11).

In order to determine the level of disability and eligibility for long-term care, countries use needs assessment methods—tools that measure the physical, functional, and cognitive capacities of the target group and their development. Limitations in activities, including activities of daily living (ADL) and instrumental activities of daily living (IADL) are measured and impairments are ranked in scales (12). Canada, Finland, Iceland, Italy, the United States, and Spain use the Resident Assessment Instrument; France uses the AGGIR (Autonomie, Gérontologie, Groupe Iso-Ressources) scale; Belgium uses KATS and the Residents Assessment Instrument. Questionnaires and medical evidence are used in England. Needs assessment is done by a general practitioner, a qualified nurse, or a social worker; a group of professionals are involved in the assessment in Belgium, Canada, France, Germany, Ireland, Portugal, and Japan (13). Detailed guidelines are used for assessment procedures and standards in Germany (14).

Needs assessment helps governments to plan better and to improve the capacity of long-term care systems in meeting care and cure needs. It also helps coordination of care across different settings. In most European countries, people are entitled to long-term care services and the level of benefit depends on the care level needed. But, in some countries (England, Italy, Spain, Poland, and the United States), means testing is used to differentiate the level of benefits and to exclude people with high incomes. An important flaw in means testing is that it restricts access to publicly financed services and involves a heavy administrative burden (15). Needs assessment is also used in making tailored care plans in Canada, Spain, the United States, and Japan (13).

The provision and utilization of long-term care

Long-term care services have two components that entail both care and cure. The services that are provided involve personal care, which are mostly health care services (e.g. medical services, nursing care, prevention, rehabilitation or palliative care) and care related to help with (instrumental) activities of daily living and/or life management (e.g. walking, bathing, dressing, eating, cooking, driving, shopping, managing medication). These services are provided in different settings. Long-term care is provided either in an institution or at home.

Institutional care

Long-term care institutions exist in various forms such as nursing homes, group homes, nursing and rehabilitation centres, long-term acute care hospitals, assisted living facilities, independent living complexes, adult day care centres, skilled nursing facilities, and retirement communities.

In general, institutional care can be provided in nursing homes or in assisted living facilities. Residents of nursing homes need extensive medical services, nursing, and personal care because they are unable to live independently due to their advanced age, illness, or physical infirmity. In general, nursing homes provide a greater range of health care services than assisted living facilities. An assisted living facility provides housing, meals, and personal services for extended periods of time, in a residential setting, for individuals. Individuals using assisted living facilities need limited health care monitoring, but cannot live independently.

The level of disability and need is the main determinant of using an institution. Having a physical health problem, dementia, stroke, other neurodegenerative disease, and/or mental health problems is associated with utilization of institutional care. Proximity to death is also a factor affecting institutional care use but availability of informal support from family members or informal care workers reduces this need (16).

Utilization of institutional care is also stimulated by the availability of long-term care settings, the level of coverage or eligibility regimes (i.e. whether people are entitled to long-term care services or there is means testing), and socio-economic factors (e.g. marital status, household composition, financial status) (16). In most European countries, people who fulfil the eligibility criteria must be granted entitlement to services. On the other hand, means testing excludes people with high incomes or varies provision according to income level. It has been reported that access to institutional care is difficult in England due to means testing (17), resulting in cost sharing, usually in the form of an accommodation charge and linked to retirement income (15).

Home care

Usually, care recipients would prefer to stay in their own homes. Personal care that includes assistance with activities of daily living, care services that help with the instrumental activities of daily living, and home help are provided by home care (18). The majority of EU long-term care systems (except in Finland) offer a choice between institutional and home care. In the United States, more than 85% of preferred care is outside nursing homes (19). Considering the cost of home care is much less than that of institutional care and people prefer it, improving home care services will be of benefit to society (20, 21).

Personal care and home help can be supplied in a formal or informal setting. Home care is mostly provided by family members, relatives, friends, neighbours, or migrant workers. This raises the issue of distinguishing informal from formal care. Kraus et al. (15) defined formal care as services provided under a contractual relationship either by the employees of any organization or by self-employed carers. Formal care is provided by professionally trained assistants, nurses, or untrained care assistants, either in institutions (like nursing homes) or at home and is public or private. Informal care is provided in a non-contractual relationship by caregivers who are family members, relatives, friends, or neighbours. The caregivers are usually unpaid or paid out-of-pocket by the families of the person in need. As there is no third party involved in the financing of informal care, it functions to fill the gaps in meeting need in the provision of formal care. An important role played by informal care may also indicate a preference for this type of care. For example, both formal and informal care use is high in Belgium where people prefer care at home as well as in institutions. Informal care use is highest in Austria, followed by France, England, Germany, and Spain. This may indicate there could be an unmet need for formal care in these countries.

In contrast, there is a very small role for informal care in Denmark and the Netherlands and the use of formal care is high (15).

In OECD countries, more than one in ten adults provides informal care. Italy and Spain have the highest shares of people providing informal care. There are also many new migrant long-term care workers in Italy, Israel, and the United States. Formal and informal care are mostly provided by women. Sweden and Norway have the highest density of formal workforce—over 40 long-term care workers per 100 people older than 80 years of age (10).

Support to caregivers

The responsibility for providing care puts a heavy pressure on family members—psychologically, physically, and economically. Depending on the duration and severity of the illness, the amount of stress from providing care varies. The caregiver might feel that providing care interferes with his/her ability to maintain their personal and professional life. Due to the heavy involvement of family members and the need for continuity in care, support for informal caregivers constitutes an important dimension in long-term care provision. Cash benefits, income support, and support services can be provided. Cash benefits improve choice of care and make up for loss in family income (22) and are provided in most European countries except Bulgaria, Denmark, Hungary, Romania, and Sweden, and are relatively high in Spain, Italy, Estonia, the Netherlands, and Austria (15).

Caregivers need support services such as training, counselling, and respite care (i.e. a break from duties). Counselling and training are mostly provided by local and voluntary initiatives. *Caring for Carers* (a training course in Ireland) and preventive counselling in the Netherlands are two successful programmes. Information and coordination centres also have important roles in helping informal caregivers. Some countries also provide respite care (e.g. up to four weeks' duration in Austria and Germany; at least three days per month in Finland). However, respite care requires an adequate supply of institutional settings and a trained long-term care workforce, as well as involving a high level of coordination. Due to this, waiting lists occur in some countries such as France (10).

Family caregivers have difficulty in participating in the formal workforce and have a higher risk of poverty due to the responsibilities of intensive caregiving. They need some support in entering and continuing in work. Some countries provide the opportunity of paid and/or unpaid care leave. Belgium provides the longest publicly paid leave, up to 12 months. The duration of paid leave is six months in Germany and three months in the Netherlands. Austria allows paid leave up to six months for people if the care recipient is terminally ill. Unpaid leave is provided in Belgium, France, Spain, and Ireland. A strict criterion for paid leave is applied in France, where in order to obtain this leave the care beneficiary should have up to 80% loss of autonomy. There are some measures to increase the value of informal care in France, such as the specific status of the informal caregiver as defined by law. Additionally, the 'informal caregivers' notebook' provides information to caregivers about their rights and there is also a possibility for informal caregivers to be paid (23).

The United Kingdom, Australia, and the United States enable flexible work conditions that may lessen the risk of loss of working hours due to caring responsibility. Tax advantages and social security rights are given in Belgium and France. Carers are considered as remuneration in Denmark, Finland, Norway, and Sweden and they are usually employed by municipalities (10).

Spending on and financing of long-term care

Long-term care expenditure accounts on average for 1.6% of Gross Domestic Product (GDP) across OECD countries and is expected to double by 2050 (13). Sweden (3.58% of GDP in 2010) and the Netherlands (3.7% of GDP in 2010) are the highest spenders. Japan is shown as successful in containing long-term care spending at 1.2% of GDP in 2010 despite having the highest projected share of the population aged over 80 years in the world for 2050 (13).

Long-term care expenditure is financed through public sources (taxes), social insurance (either compulsory or not), and private funding (private insurance and/or out-of- pocket payments). One third of the OECD countries have universal coverage. The long-term care system is part of the social system in Nordic countries (Norway, Sweden, Denmark, and Finland); usually known as 'generous', it is funded by taxes. The United Kingdom also has a tax-funded system but the long-term care costs are means-tested. There is a social insurance scheme in Germany, Japan, Korea, the Netherlands, and Luxembourg. The long-term care system is part of the health care system in Belgium where there is compulsory health insurance. In France, a tax-funded and insurance-based system exists, with large family contributions. France has the largest private insurance market along with the United States. Medicare, the federal programme for older and disabled people, covers many of the costs of acute medical care, but care and support falls outside its scope. Medicaid is health insurance for the poor that functions as a safety net for long-term care financing. The private insurance market in health and long-term care is well developed in the United States, although due to prolongation of life, the costs of long-term care insurance have been rising and coverage is limited. This imposes a heavy burden on families, specially those caring for their older members.

Cost-sharing is required for institutional care and private funding usually becomes unaffordable for most people (1). Average long-term care expenditure accounts for almost 60% of disposable income for those in the bottom 80% of the income distribution. The private contributions are capped in Sweden (based on disposable income) and Norway; there is a flat fee (11% of long-term care costs) in Korea (10). However, such measures are not common in all countries. Therefore, due to the continuity and uncertainty involved in the need for long-term care services, universal coverage is more appropriate than relying on private sources.

Key policy issues in long-term care

In Europe, the proportion of people aged over 65 in the population will rise from 18% in 2010 to 30% in 2060 (24). The proportion of these aged over 80 will rise from 4.7%

to 11.3% across Europe and from 3.9% in 2010 to 10% across OECD countries by 2050 (13). The highest share of very old people is found in Japan (about 17%) and in Germany (about 15%).

Higher life expectancy may bring more bad health. The causes of disability shift from fatal to non-fatal diseases as people age. Hence, the need for long-term care and health care rises with ageing. People aged 65 and older use health services four times more than other age groups (10). Disease patterns are also changing due to ageing. Alzheimer's disease, dementia, cardiovascular diseases, and other chronic diseases are mostly related to ageing. Moreover, chronic disease may create a risk factor for other diseases. This creates more need for long-term care services and especially for such medical components as medication, health monitoring, pain management, prevention, rehabilitation, or palliative care. Age-related public spending will reach 4.3% of GDP by 2060, mainly due to expenditure on health care and long-term care, raising both by 1.7% of GDP (25). Health spending per capita in total long-term care has increased 7%, while there has been a 4% rise in real per capita health spending across 22 OECD countries. Public long-term care expenditure across the OECD is expected to double by 2050 from the level of 1.5% of GDP in 2010 (10). In addition to a rise in public spending, there will be a reduction of the working-age population which will put more burden on social systems and threaten their sustainability.

Integration of LTC services

Due to the increase of old and very old people and to social changes (higher female labour force participation and changing family structure), there will be more need for formal care provision which may lead to problems in access to long-term care services. Planning has to be done according to changing needs, which also raises the question of how to attain better value for money in long-term care services. The wide range of services provided in long-term care requires effective integration between care and cure and coordination among service providers. The needs for care and/or cure of older, chronically ill, or disabled people may alter during their lifetimes; their health status and degree of disability may change or they may develop co-morbidities. Improved coordination between health and long-term care services has been accepted as a key factor for efficiency improvements and for obtaining better value for money (6). The lack of coordination among multiple service providers in both the public and private sphere may lead to inadequacy of and discontinuity of services. Better coordination will bring a superior mix of preventive, acute, rehabilitative, palliative, and long-term care services for the service user. Care managers or assessment teams are assigned to plan and coordinate long-term care for a care recipient with multiple needs and also to enable better monitoring and assessment of quality (10).

Some evidence has shown that acute and long-term care services can be substitutes for others; for example, in the UK, the availability of residential and informal care reduces utilization of acute care. In Sweden, in 1990s, reducing acute care beds led to higher demand for long-term care. Accordingly, demand for informal care and home care increased, despite the rise in the number of beds in nursing homes (16). Such measures may help to reduce public health and long-term care expenditures, but their effects on quality and accessibility of long-term care services should be considered. Further research should focus on the substitutability between hospital/acute care and long-term care, and formal institutional care and informal/home care. Substitution may improve efficiency but should entail meeting the care needs of older people without sacrificing quality.

Quality of LTC

Quality in long-term care—including effectiveness of care, patient safety, responsiveness or patient centredness, and coordination of care—is multidimensional (26–28). Almost all countries apply regulatory measures that ensure minimum standards on inputs and infrastructure (such as the ratio of skilled worker to long-term care user, standards for infrastructure in nursing homes). Accreditation or minimum standards require that long-term care facilities meet certain criteria to operate. These standards are mostly classified as input indicators for quality. Some countries, such as Austria, England, Germany, Ireland, Portugal, Spain, and the United States stipulate these standards as a basis for reimbursement and contracting. Accreditation of home and community-based services is not commonly used except in France, Portugal, Spain, and the United States. Legislation about protection from clinical abuse, or ensuring adequate and safe care, exists in all countries. Although difficult to detect, reporting for neglect or improper care is compulsory in Israel, Ireland, Canada, Germany, Japan, Korea, and Norway (6). Despite these standards and legislation, clinical effectiveness, patient safety, and quality of life may not be assured. Clinical quality indicators such as measures of falls, bed sores, medication use, and weight loss are more informative about the quality of long-term care than input indicators. Patient and user experience are related to outcomes of long-term care quality. Depression and quality of life are difficult to measure, but these indicators are applied in Denmark, England, Spain, and the Netherlands (6).

Apart from clinical quality, the responsiveness of a long-term care system is accepted as a second dimension of quality. It is usually measured by waiting times for admission to a nursing home, duration of waiting to receive formal help, or delay in transfer to a long-term care facility from a hospital. Due to existence of multidimensional services and various providers with different degrees of responsibilities involved in long-term care, co-ordinated care is an essential element for quality (27, 28). Avoidable hospital admissions for old patients with chronic diseases demonstrate better coordination between primary and long-term care systems (6).

Use of information and communication technologies supports integration and coordination among services, providers, and patients, facilitates information sharing, and improves standardization of care processes. Integrated information systems enable the transferability of patient data across health and care settings. In addition, remote monitoring of care, through use of information and communication technologies, improves clinical outcomes, prevents patient abuse, and helps empowerment of patients (8). Further research on analysing best practices will guide better implementation.

Use of clinical guidelines is an important means of improving efficiency, standardizing care practices, and providing best evidence of care and cure in health services. But their application is more difficult in long-term care than in health care. Guidelines combining both care and cure are limited. Including older people in experimental studies or clinical trials for guideline development is difficult. However, clinical guidelines on dementia have been applied recently under national dementia strategies in several countries (6).

Monitoring and reporting quality measures to the public and linking reimbursement and contracting with quality indicators are effective implementations to improve quality as well as efficiency. Quality assessments are publicly available in Germany, England, the United States, the Netherlands, and Sweden. Providers are also ranked according to their grading in the United States and Germany. This will improve consumers' and social insurance funds' (either private or public) choice of better quality services. Hence, the reporting and grading of quality indicators provides an incentive to the market for improving quality (27). Few countries have initiated performance-related payments. Value-based purchasing of services from nursing homes has recently begun in the United States, but value-based purchasing of long-term care is a relatively new method and, therefore, its effects on quality and efficiency need to be explored by further research (6).

More emphasis to caregivers

Since home care is preferred by individuals, governments support home care. Most long-term care services are being provided informally, through families or relatives. Due to continuity and uncertainty of need and family responsibilities in caregiving, the target group of a long-term care system is not only older, chronically ill, or disabled people but also the families of care recipients. There could be a catastrophic burden on patients and their families. Hence, the long-term care systems should support caregivers as well as care recipients. Increased demand for long-term care will create demand for long-term care workers. An OECD study estimated that such a demand will roughly double by 2050 (10). Supporting and improving the conditions of informal caregivers must be given more attention, and governments should enhance their pay and work conditions. Giving tax advantages and social security rights, as applied in Belgium and France, and developing standard training programmes for informal long-term care workers will create a positive image for such work. These training programmes can be linked to formal job contracts and may attract more people to the sector. Such programmes for informal carers will also help to improve the quality of home care.

Healthy ageing

Encouraging healthy ageing is another important policy dimension that long-term care systems should focus on in pursuit of better value for money (10). Christensen et al. (29) observed that despite a reported increase in morbidities in older people, these morbidities are less likely to cause disability or limit the activities of daily living, especially for those aged below 85 years. They indicate that increased health knowledge and awareness, in addition to earlier diagnosis, advances in treatment of certain conditions, higher utilization of health services, and increased use of technological aids in the home, have contributed to this observation. Promoting healthy ageing will improve the quality of life and may lessen or retard the need for long-term care. Various programmes in Europe can guide long-term care systems in improving healthy ageing (30). Economic evaluations of such programmes will facilitate prioritization in allocating resources in service provision and the decision-making of long-term care planners.

Caring for the elderly with LTC systems

There is no standard system of long-term care. The structure of long-term care is associated with health care, social security, and welfare systems, which are policy preferences generally shaped by the political views, social values, and cultural traditions of a country. Accordingly, different patterns of provision and funding systems have developed. Some countries have a large proportion of formal care, mostly provided in institutional settings, and thus have high levels of public spending, while others support home care and rely on informal provision by family members. But in countries where there is limited public provision of formal care, people use health systems for their long-term care needs. Almost all industrialized countries have been experiencing a common problem i.e. how to provide assistance to their rapidly ageing populations. Whichever approach is followed, the long-term care system should be accessible, continuous, and designed to meet the changing needs of the population. These objectives can be maintained through constantly observing people's needs and preferences as well as the quality of long-term care provision.

References

1 Organisation for Economic Co-operation and Development. *Long-term Care for Older People*. Paris: OECD; 2005.

2 World Health Organization. *Lessons for LTC Policies. The Cross-Cluster Initiative on Long-Term Care: Non-communicable Diseases and Mental Health Cluster.* Geneva: World Health Organization and the WHO Collaborating Centre for Research on Health of the Elderly, JDC-Brookdale Institute; 2002.

3 Leichsenring K, Billings J and Nies H (eds.) *Long-term care in Europe, Improving policy and practice.* Basingstoke: Palgrave Macmillan; 2013.

4 Allen K, Bednárik R, Campbell L, et al. Governance and finance of long-term care across Europe, An overview report. Interlinks, health systems and long-term care for older people in Europe. Modelling the interfaces and links between prevention, rehabilitation, quality of services and informal care. Birmingham, Vienna; 2011. Available at: <http://www.birmingham.ac.uk/Documents/college-social-sciences/social-policy/HSMC/research/interlinks-wp6-final.pdf> (Accessed April 2014).

5 Institute of Medicine (IOM). *Improving the Quality of Long-Term Care, IOM Report*. Washington, D.C.:IOM; 2000.

6 Fujisawa R, Colombo F. *The Long-Term Care Workforce: Overview and Strategies to Adapt Supply to a Growing Demand*. OECD Health Working Papers, No. 44, OECD Publishing; 2009. Available at: <http://dx.doi.org/10.1787/225350638472> (Accessed April 2014). Ref. type: online source.

7 Geerts J. *The Long-Term Care Workforce: Description and Perspectives*. ENEPRI Research Report No. 93; 2011. Avaiable at: file:///C:/Users/guldem/Downloads/ENEPRI%20RR93%20_ANCIEN%20WP3%20(1).pdf. (Accessed April 2014)

8 Rossi-Mori A, Dandi R. *The Technological Solutions Potentially Influencing the Future of LTC Activities*. ENEPRI Research Report, No. 114; 2012. Available at: file:///C:/Users/guldem/Downloads/RR%20No%20114%20_ANCIEN%20WP4_%20Technological%20Solutions.pdf. (Accessed April 2014)

9 Schulz E. *Use of Health and Nursing Care by the Elderly*. ENEPRI Research Report; 2004. Available at: <http://aei.pitt.edu/9515/2/9515.pdf> (Accessed April 2014).

10 Colombo, F. et al. *Help Wanted? Providing and Paying for Long-Term Care*. OECD Publishing; 2011. Available at: <http://ec.europa.eu/health/reports/docs/oecd_helpwanted_en.pdf> (Accessed April 2014). Ref. type: online source.

11 *Geriatric/Long Term Care Nursing*; 2013. Available at: <http://allnurses.com/geriatric-nurses-ltc/geriatric-long-term-890471.html> (Accessed April 2014). Ref. type: online source.

12 Bonneux L, Van der Gaag N, Bijwaard G. *Demographic Epidemiologic Projections of Long-Term Care Needs in Selected European Countries: Germany, Spain, the Netherlands and Poland*. ENEPRI Research Report No. 112; 2012. Available at: file:///C:/Users/guldem/Downloads/RR%20No%20 112%20_ANCIEN%20WP2_%20Demographic%20Epidemiologic%20Projections_final.pdf (Accessed April 2014).

13 Organisation for Economic Co-operation and Development, European Commission. *A Good Life in Old Age? Monitoring and Improving Quality in Long-Term Care*. OECD Health Policy Studies, OECD Publishing; 2013.

14 Schulz E. *The Long-Term Care System for the Elderly in Germany*. ENEPRI Research Report No. 78; 2010. Available at: file:///C:/Users/guldem/Downloads/ENEPRI%20_ANCIEN_%20RR%20No%20 78%20Germany.pdf. (Accessed April 2014)

15 Kraus M, Riedel M, Mot E, Willemé P, Röhrling G, Czypionka T. *A Typology of Long-Term Care Systems in Europe*. ENEPRI Research Report No. 91; 2010. Available at: file:///C:/Users/guldem/ Downloads/ENEPRI%20RR%20No%2091%20Typology%20of%20LTC%20%20Systems%20in%20 Europe.pdf. (Accessed April 2014)

16 Wren M-A, Normand C, O'Reilly D, Cruise S M, Connolly S, Murphy C. *Towards the Development of a Predictive Model of Long-Term Care Demand For Northern Ireland and the Republic of Ireland*. Dublin: Centre for Health Policy and Management, Trinity College; 2012.

17 Comas-Herrera A, Pickard L, Wittenberg R, Malley J, King D. *The Long-Term Care System for the Elderly in England*. ENEPRI Research Report No. 74; 2010. Available at: file:///C:/Users/guldem/ Downloads/ENEPRI%20_ANCIEN_%20RR%20No.%2074%20England%20(2).pdf. (Accessed April 2014)

18 Organisation for Economic Co-operation and Development. *Conceptual Framework and Definition of Long-term Care Expenditure, Revision of the System of Health Accounts*. Paris: OECD; 2008.

19 Dugas C. New long-term care insurance policies offer more options. *USA Today*, 21 October 2013. Available at: <http://www.usatoday.com/story/money/personalfinance/2012/11/12/long-term-care-insurance/1677385/> (Accessed April 2014). Ref. type: online source.

20 Francis J, Fisher M, Rutter D. *Re-ablement: A Cost-effective Route to Better Outcomes?*;2011. Available at: <http://www.scie.org.uk/publications/briefings/files/briefing36.pdf> (Accessed January 2014). Ref. type: online source.

21 Glendinning C. et al. *Home Care Re-ablement Services: Investigating the Longer-term Impacts (Prospective Longitudinal Study)*; 2010. Available at: <http://www.york.ac.uk/inst/spru/research/pdf/ Reablement.pdf/> (Accessed January 2014). Ref. type: online source.

22 World Health Organization. Key policy issues in long-term care. Brodsky J, Habib J, Hirschfeld M (eds). *World Health Organization Collection on Long-Term Care*. Geneva; 2003. Available at: <http:// whqlibdoc.who.int/publications/2003/9241562250.pdf> (Accessed May 2014).

23 Joël M-E, Dufour-Kippelen S, Duchêne C, Marmier M. *The Long-Term Care System for the Elderly in France*. ENEPRI Research Report No. 77; 2010. Available at: file:///C:/Users/guldem/Downloads/ France.pdf/ (Accessed April 2014)

24 European Union. *The 2012 Ageing Report: Underlying Assumptions and Projection Methodologies*. Joint Report prepared by the European Commission (DG ECFIN) and the Economic Policy

Committee (AWG); 2011. Available at: <http://ec.europa.eu/economy_finance/publications/european_economy/2011/pdf/ee-2011-4_en.pdf> (Accessed February 2014).

25 European Commission Directorate-General for Economic and Financial Affairs. *Fiscal Sustainability Report 2012*. European Union; 2012. Available at: <http://ec.europa.eu/economy_finance/publications/european_economy/2012/pdf/ee-2012-8_en.pdf> (Accessed February 2014).

26 **Dandi R, Casanova G.** *Quality Assurance Indicators of Long-Term Care in European Countries.* ENEPRI Research Report No. 110; 2012. Available at: file:///C:/Users/guldem/Downloads/RR%20No%20110%20_ANCIEN%20WP5%20D5.2_%20LTC%20Quality%20Assurance%20Indicators%20in%20European%20Countries.pdf. (Accessed April 2014)

27 **Dandi R.** *Quality Assurance Policies and Indicators for Long-Term Care in the European Union.* ENEPRI Policy Brief No. 11; 2012. Available at: file:///C:/Users/guldem/Downloads/ENEPRI%20PB%20No%2011%20_ANCIEN_%20%20Quality%20Policies%20and%20Indicators%20for%20LTC%20(1).pdf. (Accessed April 2014).

28 **Dandi R, Casanova, Lillini R, Volpe M, Giulio De Belvis A, Avolio M, Pelone F.** *Long-Term Care Quality Assurance Policies in European Countries.* ENEPRI Research Report No. 111; 2012. Available at: file:///C:/Users/guldem/Downloads/Quality%20Assurance%20Policies%20for%20LTC%20in%20in%20the%20EU.pdf. (Accessed April 2014).

29 **Christensen K, Doblhammer G, Rau R, Vaupel JW.** Ageing populations: the challenges ahead. *Lancet* 2009; **374**:1196–208.

30 European Commission: Digital Agenda for Europe. *Excellent Innovation for Ageing—a European Guide: the Reference sites of the European Innovation Partnership on Active and Healthy Ageing.* Available at: <http://ec.europa.eu/digital-agenda/en/news/excellent-innovation-ageing-european-guide-reference-sites-european-innovation-partnership> (Accessed April 2014). Ref. type: online source.

Chapter 3

Development of palliative care in long-term care settings

Katherine Froggatt and Hazel Morbey

Introduction to development of palliative care in long-term care settings

With a global ageing population, the availability of different care options for older people is recognized as being important, and these range from domiciliary support to enable older people to remain living at home, supported housing and assisted living models, and residential and nursing care facilities. Across Europe, it is estimated that more than 100 million people per year would benefit from palliative care interventions. However, less than 8% of those in need have access to it (1). Providers of long-term care for older people increasingly recognize their role in supporting residents to live and die well. For some older people, changes in physical, psychological, and/or social circumstances will require a move into a long-term care setting as they can no longer be supported to live in their own homes. Of particular note is the increasing number of older people who live with dementia that this will apply to. Older people living in long-term care settings will go on to require palliative and end-of-life care, and they need to be supported by staff who work within, and who are external to, these organizations.

This chapter aims to critically describe the context and nature of palliative care provision in relation to long-term care settings across Europe and other developed countries. The complexity, challenge, and variability of long-term care organization and implementation is presented. Drawing on the work of the recently completed European Association for Palliative Care (EAPC) Taskforce on Palliative Care in Long-term Care Settings, the chapter presents a framework for understanding the advancement of palliative care through specific initiatives and intervention developments, and highlights key drivers for change at local, regional, and national levels.

The context of palliative care in long-term care settings

Calls are increasingly made for both improvements in palliative care for older people (2, 3) and, more specifically, for quality care of older people who live in long-term care settings (4–6). There is an imperative to bring these two significant areas of later life experience and need together when we consider global ageing demographics and projected requirements for palliative care in long-term care environments (1, 7). Recognizing the lack of a pan-European strategy of palliative care for older people, joint work at European level between the European Association for Palliative Care and the European Union Geriatric Medicine Society, since 2012, has aimed to influence policy makers and national level improvements in this sphere of provision, with the intention of establishing priority pointers for the palliative care and geriatric medicine disciplines (1).

While this chapter focuses primarily upon palliative care provision in long-term care settings, such as nursing homes, it is recognized that long-term care is also provided to older people in their own homes. Receiving long-term care and dying at home is a stated wish of many older people (8, 9). However, as with care in other settings, provision of quality care is a challenge. The proportion of older people who have been cared for and then die at home is low compared to hospital as a place of death. An emphasis on a home for life and a home death, supported by government policies and public opinion worldwide (10), seeks to increase the number of people who die in their own homes. There is investment in models of care that enable people to remain in their own homes, be they domestic dwellings or part of a wider sheltered/supported housing complex.

Policy initiatives aimed at giving more choice and control to older people about where they choose to live and die have implications for other locations of long-term care such as supported or extra care housing (11, 12). In these settings, tenants' needs are increasing as the age and complexities of health conditions advance for this group of people, including the growth in numbers of people with dementia. There is a limited literature in this area. However, a UK evaluation identified trends in greater end-of-life awareness and staff development in three extra care housing schemes where a training and education programme was introduced. This evaluation especially highlighted the need to establish, record, and share tenants' wishes, and also the critical importance of partnership working between professionals and services in order to achieve prior wishes and desired outcomes for tenants (11). Other research reinforces these key messages. However, Jones et al (13) also identified significant barriers to interagency working whereby confidentiality issues prevented the sharing of information, with this being a particular problem when a tenant was discharged from hospital following an in-patient stay.

Developments in palliative care in long-term care settings

Palliative care provision in long-term care settings has been the subject of research for over 15 years now (14), but there is limited rigorous evidence in the area (15). However, more recent reports and literature have consolidated and extended earlier work that sought to conceptualize and identify palliative care provision in long-term care settings (5, 16, 17). The EAPC Taskforce in Palliative Care in Long-term Care Settings (16) mapped examples of palliative care initiatives in long-term care settings across 13 countries. These interventions addressed service development, educational strategies, and/or clinical interventions. A typology was constructed from this work to classify the complex, cross-organizational and multi-level arrangements of palliative care in such settings. Relevant findings from this work are presented throughout this chapter.

In a climate of caring for older, frailer residents with complex and often multiple health conditions, long-term care settings draw on expertise and resources external to their organizations, from specialist palliative care or general care sectors, while at the same time they need to respond to relevant national and regional regulation and legislation. This complex landscape of development in palliative care indicates the extent to which it necessarily cuts across organizational, sector, and professional boundaries. Long-term care settings provide palliative care for residents in varied ways, while operating within sectors that share cultures, approaches, and dimensions to their work.

In order to understand the multi-level, cross-cutting nature of this context, a whole-systems perspective enables all dimensions of palliative care service development and implementation, as well as the diversity of provision (5), to be considered. It also permits specific focus on the role of the organization (the long-term care institution) as the mediator of change developments in palliative care. Diversity in long-term care settings is reflected in: the different features of provision (be it private, public, or not-for-profit funded); the variation of size (between larger national, smaller scale care home chains, or individually owner-managed); the health or social care sectors in which care for older people is provided; as well as the types of care provided (whether it be personal, nursing, social, or a mix).

The EAPC Taskforce on Palliative Care in Long-term Care Settings collected information on a wide range of palliative care developments and initiatives. While an approach to categorizing these was established through this work, it should be stated that there is a limited evidence base with respect to the impact and outcomes of these initiatives. It is also not possible to ascertain the on-going sustainability of existing or new practices in long-term care settings, where there can often be project-based initiatives that are underpinned by time-limited funding or working arrangements.

A typology of organizational change was used in the EAPC Taskforce to classify the interventions at: *individual, group/team, organization, regional/network,* and *national* levels. These levels capture individual palliative care initiatives as they are implemented at more local and organizational levels, while regional and national developments are also included at macro levels of policy and wider organizational implementation. The latter categories recognize how, in the area of palliative care in long-term care settings, cross-organizational initiatives and developments facilitate broader collaborations, and also serve to foster the development of a palliative care culture.

It should be noted that individual initiatives do not necessarily fall exclusively within a specific level of classification, but often bridge more than one level of organizational change. This is indicative of the complex nature of developing services where it is necessary for change and processes to occur across different levels to achieve impact at the point of delivery of care to residents and their family members. At the end of this chapter, we summarize these developments in the category levels and give further details of country specific initiative examples (see Table 3.1).

Table 3.1 Approaches to palliative care development in long-term care settings

Level of change	Where is development focused? On knowledge, behaviours, and practices of:	Initiative example
Individual	Long-term care setting staff / External staff	*Integrated care pathway and Gold Standards Framework* (21) (Scotland, UK)
		Implementation of an integrated care pathway in nursing care homes, alongside an organizational tool.
	Residents / Family	*Palliative care for older people with dementia: a guide for caregivers* (22) (Netherlands)
		Introduction of a booklet about comfort care for people with advanced dementia.
Group/team	Long-term care setting staff groups External staff groups Interdisciplinary groups	*MOBIQUAL* (France)
		Aim to enhance knowledge, skills, and practices of the caregivers. Through development of toolkits, national inter-professional education in nursing homes is promoted for a wide range of care issues including pain, palliative care, and depression. Embedded in a continuous quality improvement process across all settings for older people care. http://www.mobiqual.org/ (Accessed May 2013)
Organization	Long-term care setting staff Hospice staff Palliative care services staff Primary care staff	*Living until the end: palliative care in long-term care settings* (23) (Germany)
		Initiated top–down by a care provider. Uses a bottom–up approach with staff and residents, leading to changes in palliative care culture.
Region/networks	Regional / Provincial government bodies Networks for care providers	*Hospice and Palliative Care Plan in Tyrol* (24) (Austria)
		Aimed to collaboratively develop a regional concept for integrated palliative care and work with different key stakeholders.
National (larger system/ environment)	Long-term care setting staff Hospice staff Palliative care services staff Primary care staff	*End-of-life Care Programme* (25) (England, UK)
		Case studies, publications, and resources drawing upon practical examples of initiatives that have worked to support the development of palliative care in care homes. Incorporates Routes to Success and Six Steps to Success education programmes (Kennedy et al. 2009). <http://www.endoflifecare.nhs.uk/> (Accessed May 2014)

Levels of initiatives in palliative care provision: individual, group/team, organization

Individual (resident, family, staff) level

Types of interventions at the individual level of palliative care provision include: assessment tools and specialist clinical assessment tools; communication and information strategies; educational provision; and leadership developments. Direct assessment of resident palliative and long-term needs is addressed by initiatives that use tools to inform care or support strategies. An evaluation scale used in Belgium, for example, establishes when a resident or patient enters the terminal phase so that appropriate care can be put in place. Further tools introduced in Norway assess pain in patients with mental impairment and, in France, nutritional needs of those receiving palliative care are addressed in clinical long-term care.

Family members of people with dementia are supported through information and communication resources. A guide for carers of people with dementia requiring palliative care that originated in Canada was adapted, evaluated, and translated for Dutch, Italian, and Japanese languages. And, in a further example of supporting family members, their care needs are included in a Spanish Comprehensive Care Programme for advanced illnesses.

Care staff working in long-term care settings were the focus of a number of initiatives at this individual level. These aimed at delivering quality clinical care through educational, developmental, or clinical assessment approaches. Education and training were particularly favoured means of developing palliative care, with the majority of countries that took part in the EAPC mapping exercise able to report initiatives in this area. Some particular examples of interest existed in Ireland, Norway, and Sweden. Respectively, these involved a five- day hospice-delivered programme for residential care link nurses who, in turn, provided education within their own care facilities; a similar 'training for trainers' approach in Norway focused on long-term care staff in home care and nursing homes, where these staff receive teaching materials and presentations in order to establish a teaching programme back in their localities. Finally, a Swedish development saw over three and a half thousand nurses and care assistants involved in increasing skills through education and consultancy support from specialised palliative care teams. Four different models were evaluated, but all had an overall objective of fewer transfers to emergency care for old and terminally ill people.

Group/team level

At this level, there are examples of initiatives for inter-professional education in palliative care and 'inter-professional rounds' in health care settings. Reported initiatives are especially pertinent given the predication of effective palliative care on productive interdisciplinary working and good communication across staff groups, organizations, and sectors. Essentially, this means individual professionals or teams understanding each other, talking with each other, and being prepared and willing to meet the challenges in doing so. Over and above the specialist educational initiatives previously outlined, there are examples of interdisciplinary and inter-professional educational developments. France and Sweden offered examples of a tool for working in long-term care settings and of a collaborative project, which lead to the establishment of a specialist palliative care team. The latter emerged from a joint county council and municipal collaborative education project. In both of these initiatives, a particular feature was the use of case studies and real situation scenarios to enhance learning for a range of care staff in long-term care settings.

'Professional rounds' occur in interdisciplinary contexts whereby daily work is shared between team members enabling the formation of alternative perspectives and, in some cases, supporting joint ethical decision making. A French initiative illustrates the value of interdisciplinary collaboration and cooperation in an area of sensitive care provision for residents with long, terminal illnesses and for dying patients. A stepped decision-making guide supports all professionals working with these groups of residents and patients, in a process of deliberation and resolution, while incorporating residents' wishes and assessing capacity for withdrawing or withholding treatments in accordance with the Leonetti law in geriatric care. The practice-based guide used in this work is based on a mix of clinical situations that have undergone multi-professional team analysis, and these act as the guide to decision making and to improving preparation and skills in order to enhance patient care (18).

A similar approach has been developed in Australia, using palliative care case conferences to communicate between staff, general practitioners, family, and, where possible, the resident. The conference provides an opportunity to assist residents and family members to clarify goals of care, consider site of care options, and to share information in a proactive way. The conferences are ongoing as required (19, 20).

Organization level

Organisational level initiatives across Europe highlighted shared working between palliative care, hospice teams, and long-term care settings, and identified specialist palliative care units. As previously noted, forms of shared, joint, and interdisciplinary working are conducive to more effective palliative care and enhance a culture for the implementation of new initiatives (19, 20). Essential to supporting such work and cultures is the organizational context within which professionals are enabled to provide palliative care services. Initiatives at this typological level, then, are important in order to integrate palliative care into long-term care settings. Examples at this level were recorded in: knowledge management/transfer; specialist palliative care units in long-term care settings; and in approaches to organizational development.

In the area of knowledge management/transfer, specialist palliative care teams were seen to play a particular role in supporting long-term care settings in developing practice competences. Change developments were also enhanced by opportunities for reflection and connection between attitudes, current knowledge, and experiences within organizations. Developments highlighted in this area included one where practical tools for integrative palliative care were set out in a Dutch initiative called *This is how we do it*. This comprehensive multi-organizational care programme is used in nursing and residential homes and aims to improve the quality of care received by patients with life-threatening illnesses, from the point of receiving a diagnosis, through their illness trajectory, to the terminal phase. Underpinning the programme are national policies and guidelines, the implementation of care pathways, research, and cooperation between specialist palliative care teams and the general hospital. Specific strategies ensure the inclusion of each organization within the catchment area. These involve: the establishment of a programme steering group on which each organization is represented; specialist support for care homes with less experience in palliative care; and the installation of a 'quality care award' scheme.

Finally, at this level, organizational developments have been seen to engender important influences on palliative care culture supporting the work of staff at the point of delivery and with initiatives that ensure the inclusion of residents and their families. Whole organization strategies implemented in this way exist in a number of countries. The example from the United Kingdom is the Gold Standards Framework that seeks to promote high-quality care for residents in their last year of life through organizational and practice change. An accreditation system has seen over 2,000 care homes in the United Kingdom participating in a two-year programme that focuses on seven areas, termed the '7Cs': Communication, Coordination, Continuity, Control of symptoms, Care of the dying, Carer support, and Continued education.

Change developments in palliative care in long-term care settings

In this section, we consider what drives change and brings about the impetus to support the introduction of palliative care initiatives in health and social care systems. Key drivers for such change can be identified at local, regional, and national levels, and may be from the area of palliative care, the long-term care sector, or general health care. Thus, national palliative care programmes of development have been undertaken, for example, in England, Ireland, Spain, and Sweden. Other development has occurred under the auspices of aged and/or dementia care, which is evident in France, Norway, Sweden, and the United Kingdom.

While influences of change and development can be shown at different levels, the organizational level has particular significance here. Organizations fulfil a mediating function whereby developments can come about either in a top–down way (through broader, higher level changes, e.g. legislation) or a bottom–up fashion (through specific, locality level changes or initiatives, e.g. professional networks). In this way, we see organizations as pivotal to new developments coming about in palliative care institutions and other long-term care settings.

Extending Ferlie and Shortell's (26) organizational change typology to include regional/network and national levels permits a more nuanced framework that accounts for the complex positioning of organizations providing long-term palliative care. A picture emerges of long-term care settings as conduits of change, since they operate within a matrix of influences that shape change, developments, and initiatives. As such, they bridge different sectors and multiple organizational boundaries, are influenced by top–down or bottom–up policy drivers, and are subject to influential factors that may be exerted from within, or externally to, the organization.

Here, we present specific initiatives and strategies that have been implemented across Europe at these higher levels of development. They are in the form of legislative and regulatory frameworks that introduce standards and funding provision that are aimed at both improving the quality of care more generally and also specifically targeting palliative care provision.

Levels of change developments and initiatives in palliative care provision: regional and national

Regional/network level

Initiatives aimed at developments across inter-organizational boundaries are evident at regional levels or through networks that support cooperation or collaboration. Types of regional or network developments in palliative care include regulatory initiatives and inter-professional networks. These initiatives can be indicative of regional contextual characteristics or common experiences, for example, those that may be found in rural areas or through religious affiliation.

A mix of initiatives are evident at this level whereby some follow a more standard top–down process of implementation, while others have locality grown or 'grass roots' origins. An interesting example of the latter is a 'virtual network' in the Bavarian region of Germany. This mostly involves sharing information across a number of projects, through e-mail newsletters, in order to support integration between hospice care and palliative care in long-term care settings. Direct contact between network members is facilitated through an annual conference. Further examples of the development of networks that facilitate groups and teams to come together were evident in different countries. National umbrella organizations also promote work in this way, as seen in Scotland with the Scottish Partnership for Palliative Care and across a number of regions in the Netherlands in the form of the Netherlands Palliative Care Network for Terminally Ill Patients (NPTN). In South Western Norway, an inter-community cooperative is supported through links between long-term care settings in the main city with eight municipalities/communities in the region. The main city's local hospital and a development centre for nursing home and home care work together, through this initiative, to ensure quality palliative care delivery in the regional communities involved. A different approach, seen in an initiative in Austria, follows an action research methodology and includes nursing homes and other key providers and stakeholders in the region. The project seeks to create a regional-specific model of integrated palliative care that is relevant across the region's health care systems and that facilitates communication and knowledge generation amongst those involved in a three-year hospice and palliative care plan.

Regulatory frameworks exist at regional (or principality) level and can be strong drivers for change. These may relate to national regulation, as is the case in Germany where federal state level statute governs quality in long-term care settings, while national laws stipulate the content, range, and quality of care in long-term care settings. Similarly, in Italy, regional regulation sets accreditation standards for institutional care settings. And again, in the United Kingdom, national minimum standards are in place for the inspection of care homes within the four nations.

National level

Many countries worldwide demonstrate national level initiatives that shape and influence palliative care standards and culture. At this national level, developments are initiated through legal frameworks, national strategies, funding policies and standards, and guidelines in long-term care.

Legal and policy frameworks

While legal and policy frameworks exist in most countries, there is variation in how palliative care is addressed. Specific regulation for palliative care in relation to provision for older people is largely absent. Legislation exists, for example, in regard to pain assessment, within nursing homes and, more generally, across varied provision in long-term care settings, setting minimum standards for palliative care. However, these spheres of regulation do not directly extend to targeted provision for older people as residents in these settings. Of the thirteen countries surveyed, just two have specific regulations for palliative care in nursing homes-namely, Germany and France. Since 2005, it has been a legal requirement that palliative care is implemented in French nursing homes and, similarly, since 2007, Germany has had specialist palliative care law to cover long-term care settings.

While palliative care has very limited focus, it is possible to identify national strategic initiatives that specifically focus on long-term care settings for older people, although again there is variation in how these are interpreted and implemented. In some countries, there are multiple and related strategies that target specific services for older people, while addressing different dimensions of provision, and these combine to give strong parameters for palliative care provision. An example of this very broad approach can be seen in The Netherlands, where a specific government objective is that older people are enabled to remain at home, or in a nursing home, to receive palliative care. A range of initiatives implemented in the United Kingdom, reported at this level of the typology, are comprehensively collated and presented under the auspices of the National End-of-life Care Programme (27). Some United Kingdom initiatives come out of cross-cutting national policies (for example, the End-of-life Care Strategy), while other developments have been adapted for region-specific implementation. The Six Steps to Success Training Programme for Care Homes, in the North West of England, is an example of the latter, whereby a workshop and training programme has been developed to address the six steps as they are set out in the aforementioned National End-of-life Care Strategy (25).

Setting up specialist units within long-term care settings establishes palliative care as an integrated feature of care provision. Approaches vary; however, over a 10–15 year period, across Norway, units for palliative care in nursing homes have been developed under the auspices of the Norwegian National Palliative Care Programme. Its recommendations cover: tasks, clinical services, organization, personnel, facilities, and equipment for both nursing homes that have specialist units and those without a dedicated palliative care provision. To support developments, grants have been made available for staff training courses including post-graduate level education.

Standards and guidelines

In terms of standards and guidelines that address quality in palliative care (quality management and assurance), some countries report that national quality schemes are in place for example, the National Certificate of Quality for nursing homes in Austria, Care Quality Commission national minimum standards in England, and in Ireland, the National Quality Standards for Residential Care Settings for Older People. When considering these and the other areas reported here at national level, a complex palliative care landscape is evident and we can identify interrelated areas of provision. These might address the needs of older people and their family members, where strategies and initiatives are applicable to long-term care settings, dementia care, and specialist palliative care strategies. Internationally, national guidelines are also used. For example, in Australia, evidence-based guidelines have been written to support the delivery of palliative care in long-term care settings (28).

Palliative care funding brings further complexities where this often, again, cuts across different long-term care and health settings. Significant demands on public health care budgets and projected increasing demands of ageing populations are well rehearsed (6, 29). However, these juxtapose patient, family, public, and political calls for provision of quality palliative care in long-term care settings. Some countries are tackling this through national schemes to support the extra costs incurred of ensuring palliative care for older people in such settings. This is the case in Belgium, for example, where a daily allowance contributes towards a 'Palliative Support Team' in each long-term care setting.

Reflecting the multidimensional nature to change developments set out in this section, we conclude by returning to consider local level initiatives that give rise to broader levels of organizational change, e.g. at regional/network level. We highlight here how hospice and palliative care sectors have been key to stimulating and bringing about changes in palliative care culture and developments in palliative care in long-term care settings. At the team/group level, in this respect, there are specific initiatives to engage a single, long-term care setting, or a group of providers, with specialist palliative care services. Such influence is evident in a number of countries across Europe, including: Austria, Germany, Ireland, Italy, and the United Kingdom. A particular example is the presence of hospices located within nursing homes. These can influence palliative care provision within the wider nursing home institution through the transfer of knowledge and practices, as is the case in Italy, where 24 (14.6%) hospices are located in nursing homes. Although, also reported in this area are cultural challenges that come about through different clinical disciplines working in the area of palliative care.

The development of long-term palliative care for older people has been supported in all settings where older people reside (in their own homes, in supported or extra care housing, and in long-term care settings). Most attention has been paid to long-term care settings and, in the main, learning has come from this sector. As is the case in long-term care settings, Jones et al.'s (13) study recognized the pivotal role of managers in ensuring information reached frontline housing staff. Research (30, 31) has shown that there continues to be a lack of large-scale studies that evaluate interventions for palliative care for older people with respect to long-term care.

Challenges to future development

There are a number of challenges as regards all these developments which reflect the complex health and social care economy within which older people receive long-term care, and where organizations providing long-term care are located. Care provision for older people requiring palliative care involves multiple and inter-agency working (external to and across agency sectors). In most countries (with the exception of The Netherlands), medical care is provided in long-term care settings by external agencies. Dependence upon external organizations and practitioners adds another level of complexity to care provision, often through a lack of clarity regarding roles, funding, and ways of working. Cross disciplinary working is required which can include: specialist palliative care, geriatrics, general medicine, and primary care. This requires time and an investment in coordinated working.

The sustainability of palliative care developments and individual initiatives that provide palliative care in long-term care settings often hangs in the balance. Many initiatives are the result of short-term funding, with no ongoing commitment to continue the work once funding has finished, creating insecure and limited development opportunities.

Conclusions and future developments of palliative care in long-term care settings

This chapter provides an overview of context, domains, and approaches to palliative care in long-term care settings across and beyond Europe. Specific examples have illustrated policy and practice initiatives implemented at different levels, which aim to provide and improve palliative care in long-term care settings for older people. It has drawn on the work of the European Association for Palliative Care Taskforce on Palliative Care in Long-term Care Settings for Older People, the work of which developed a network and framework that captured expertise and experience in this sphere of provision and provided a baseline for future work within clinical practice and research domains.

While many innovative initiatives are being undertaken, they are often locally initiated and delivered, sometimes with short-term funding. While there is some evidence about these initiatives, it is limited, and further quality larger-scale studies, which rigorously evaluate and compare interventions, are required to build the foundations for high-standard care in long-term care. Cross-cultural studies will also broaden the evidence base, as different cultural contexts help identify what is common in care provision and what is unique to different health and social care systems. A continuing movement to share good practice across Europe, and internationally, will help support the development of evidence-based practice. This needs to continue to address the whole system, at all levels-individual, team, organization, and the wider health and social care economy.

Acknowledgements

We acknowledge the work of the European Association for Palliative Care Taskforce on Palliative Care in Long-term Care Settings for Older People, in particular, the Steering Group (Elisabeth Reitinger, Kevin Brazil, Katharina Heimerl, Jo Hockley, Roland Kunz, Deborah Parker, Bettina Sandgathe-Husebø) and the country informants, without whom the Taskforce could not have been completed.

References

1 European Association for Palliative Care, European Union Geriatric Medicine Society. *Better Palliative Care for Older People: Joint Manifesto*. Available at: <http://www.eapcnet.eu/Themes/Specificgroups/Olderpeople/EuropeanParliamentMeeting.aspx> (Accessed January 2014). Ref. type: online source.

2 World Health Organization. *Palliative Care for Older People: Better Practices*. Denmark: World Health Organization; 2011.

3 World Palliative Care Alliance. *Global Atlas of Palliative Care at the End of Life*. London: 2014.

4 Bradshaw SA, Playford ED, Riazi A. Living well in care homes: a systematic review of qualitative studies. *Age Ageing* 2012; **41**(4):429–40.

5 Froggatt K, Brazil K, Hockley J, Reitinger E. Improving care for older people living and dying in long-term care settings: a whole system approach. In: Gott M, Ingleton C (eds). *Living with Ageing and Dying*. New York: Oxford University Press; 2011, 213–25.

6 Organisation for Economic Co-operation and Development, European Commission. *A Good Life in Old Age? Monitoring and Improving Quality in Long-term Care*. 2013.

7 World Health Organization. *Good Health Adds Life to Years: Global Brief for World Health Day 2012*. Geneva: WHO; 2012. WHO/DCO/WHD/2012.2.

8 Gott M, Seymour J, Ballamy G, Clark D, Ahmedzai S. Older people's views about home as a place of care at the end of life. *Palliat Med* 2004; **18**(5):460–7.

9 McCarthy EP, Pencina MJ, Kelly-Hayes M, et al. Advance care planning and health care preferences of community-dwelling elders: the Framingham Heart Study. *J Gerontol Biol* 2008; **63**(9):951–9.

10 Gomes B, Cophen J, Deliens L, Higginson I. International trends in circumstances of death and dying amongst older people. In: Gott M, Ingleton C (eds). *Living with Ageing and Dying*. Oxford: Oxford University Press; 2011, 3–18.

11 Easterbrook L, Vallelly S. *Is It That Time Already? Extra Care Housing at the End of Life: A Policy-into-practice Evaluation*. Housing 21, Beaconsfield; 2008.

12 Gillick MR. *The Denial of Aging*. London: Harvard University Press; 2006.

13 Jones A, Croucher K, Rhodes D. *Evaluation of Learning Resources for End of Life Care in Extra Care Settings*. York: Centre for Housing Policy, The University of York; 2011.

14 Froggatt K. Palliative care and nursing homes: where next? *Palliat Med* 2001; **15**:42–8.

15 Hall S, Kolliakou A, Petkova H, Froggatt K, Higginson IJ. Interventions for improving palliative care for older people living in nursing care homes. *Cochrane Database of Systematic Reviews*, 2011 (3). Art. no.: CD007132; doi:10.1002/14651858.CD007132.pub2.

16 **Froggatt K, Reitinger EO.** *Palliative Care in Long-Term Care Settings for Older People: EAPC Taskforce 2010–2012*; 2013. Ref type: online source.

17 **Reitinger E, Froggatt K, Brazil K, et al.** Palliative care in long-term care settings for older people: findings from an EAPC taskforce. *Eur J Pall Care* 2013; **20**(5):251–3.

18 Societé Française d'Acompagnement et de soins Palliatifs. *Implementing a guide for decision-making to withdraw or withhold treatments in geriatric situations relative to the Leonetti law*. Available at: <http://www.sfap.org> (Accessed February 2014). Ref. type: online source.

19 **Tuckett A, Parker D, Clifton K, et al.** What general practitioners said about the palliative care case conference in residential aged care: an Australian perspective. Part 1. *Prog Pall Care*, doi:10.1179/174 3291X13Y.0000000066.

20 **Tuckett A, Parker D, Clifton K, et al.** What general practitioners said about the palliative care case conference in residential aged care: an Australian perspective. Part 2. *Prog Pall Care*, doi:10.1179/174 3291X13Y.0000000069.

21 **Hockley J, Watson J, Oxenham D, Murray SA.** The integrated implementation of two end-of-life care tools in nursing care homes in the UK: an in-depth evaluation. *Pall Med* 2010; **24**(8):828–38.

22 **van der Steen JT, M. A, Toscani F, et al.** A family booklet about comfort care in advanced dementia: three-country evaluation. *JAMDA* 2012; **13**(4):368–75.

23 **Kittelberger F, Von der Sterbebegleitung bS.** Palliativbetreuung im Pflegeheim. In: Heller A, Kittelberger F (eds). *Hospizkompetenz und Palliativ Care im Alter Eine Einführung*. Lambertus Verlag: Freiburg; 2010.

24 **Heimerl K, Wegleitner K.** Organisation and health system change through participatory research. In: Hockley J, Froggatt K, Heimerl K (eds). *Participatory Research in Palliative Care Actions and Reflections*. Oxford: Oxford University Press; 2013, 27–39.

25 **Kennedy S, Seymour JE, Almack K, Cox K.** Key stakeholders' experiences and views of the NHS End of Life Care Programme: findings from a national evaluation. *Palliat Med* 2009; **23**:183–294.

26 **Ferlie EB, Shortell SM.** Improving the quality of health care in the United Kingdom and the United States: a framework for change. *Milbank Q* 2001; **79**(2):281–315.

27 Department of Health. *End of Life Care Strategy: Promoting High Quality Care for All Adults at the End of Life*. London; 2008.

28 **Parker D.** The development and implementation of evidence-based palliative care guidelines for residential care: lessons for other countries. In: Gott M, Ingleton I (eds). *Living with Ageing and Dying: Palliative and End of Life Care for Older People*. Oxford: Oxford University Press; 2011, 226–36.

29 **Hughes-Hallett T, Craft A, Davies C.** *Funding the Right Care and Support for Everyone: Creating a Fair and Transparent Funding System; the Final Report of the Palliative Care Funding Review*. 2011.

30 **Froggatt KA, Wilson D, Justice C, et al.** End-of-life care in long-term care settings for older people: a literature review. *International Journal of Older People Nursing* 2006; **1**:45–50.

31 **Hall S, Longhurst S, Higginson I.** Challenges to conducting research with older people living in nursing homes. *BMC Geriatrics* 2009; **9**(1):38.

Chapter 4

Development of integrated and person-centred palliative care

Hubertus J.M. Vrijhoef and Liesbeth Borgermans

Introduction to development of integrated and person-centred palliative care

This chapter describes integrated and person-centred care and explores why and to what extent older people requiring palliative care may benefit from this approach. Further, future developments considered necessary to develop, evaluate, and implement integrated and person-centred palliative care are discussed. The case of the Liverpool Care Pathway for the Dying Patient is also briefly discussed. Use is made of various recently published resources derived from both 'white' and 'grey' literature about integrated and patient-centred care, palliative care, and the combination of these fields.

Definition and concept of integrated and person-centred palliative care

Integrated care is a key strategy designed to address complex and costly health needs by reducing undesired fragmentation and improving continuity and coordination of services across the entire care continuum, with the goal of improving outcomes. Despite its importance for health care systems around the world, a common definition of integrated care is still lacking. 'One size fits all' approaches to integrating health services or systems are lacking; integrated care draws on a wide range of techniques including case management and disease management. Various dimensions of integration can be distinguished, including type, breadth, degree, and process (1, 2).

Perhaps the most influential framework for care integration has been the Chronic Care Model developed by Wagner et al. (1). Recognizing the failures of health systems largely based on an acute, episodic model of care with little emphasis on patient self-management, the Chronic Care Model aims to provide a comprehensive framework for the organization of health care to improve outcomes for people with chronic conditions. Drawing on a synthesis of the evidence of effectiveness of various chronic disease management interventions, the Chronic Care Model comprises four interacting system components that are considered key to providing good chronic care: self-management support, delivery system design, decision support, and clinical information systems (3, 4). The Chronic Care Model has been applied in various countries (including Australia, Belgium, Canada, Denmark, England, Germany, the Netherlands, New Zealand, Switzerland, and the United States of America) and is also adopted by the World Health Organization (WHO) in its global strategy towards high-quality, people-centred, and integrated care (5).

The WHO's Regional Office for Europe makes use of the concept 'coordinated/integrated health services delivery (CIHSD)' and defines it as 'the management and delivery of health services such that people receive a continuum of health promotion, health protection and disease prevention services, as well as diagnosis, treatment, long-term care, rehabilitation and palliative care services through the different levels and sites of care within the health system and according to their needs' (5). Efforts towards CIHSD must take into account the services provided and the settings of care and, further, the alignment of the two according to the unique health needs of a given individual. The extent to which services along the full continuum of care are experienced in a coordinated/integrated manner can be depicted from the perspective of an individual him/herself. This perspective is defined by the concept of continuity of care as 'the degree to which a series of discrete health care events are experienced by people as coherent and interconnected over time, and consistent with their health needs and preferences' (5). The WHO talks about a people-centred approach meaning an approach where care is focused and organized around the health needs and expectations of people and communities, rather than on diseases themselves. The latter is known as the closely related patient-centred care focus (5). The WHO definition is in line with the definition of patient-centred care as provided by the Institute of Medicine, i.e. 'providing care that is respectful of and responsive to individual patient preferences, needs and values, and ensuring that patient values guide all clinical decisions' (6).

What is missing in both the WHO and Institute of Medicine definitions is an explicit emphasis on compassion. Patients, and those close to them, emphasize that paramount among their needs, preferences, and values are compassionate human interactions. For care to be truly patient-centred, a foundation of compassion is essential. Research from health care systems around the world demonstrates the fallacy of assuming that compassion is a current or prevalent feature of the care experience (7). Concurrently, a growing evidence base highlights the supreme importance of compassion driving high-quality, high-value care (8). Patient-centred communication is a critical element of patient-centred care, which the Institute of Medicine promulgates as essential to improving health care delivery. However, as with patient-centred care, no comprehensive measure of patient-centred communication exists, though there is agreement that it includes exchanging information, fostering healing relationships, recognizing and responding to emotions, managing uncertainty, making decisions, and enabling self-management (9).

The concept of integrated and person-centred palliative care

As palliative care can be provided throughout the continuum of care for patients with chronic, serious, and life-threatening diseases (10), an integrated and patient-centred approach to the provision of care seems highly relevant to this particular phase. In the last year or years of life, patients often present with multiple and complex needs and this results in their care being provided by multiple providers and in multiple settings. Patients and families in this situation require the deliberate organization of patient-centred care to optimize and integrate appropriate service delivery, both within and across care settings, and over time (11). In its publication about palliative care, the WHO's Regional Office for Europe underlines the importance of whole-system or integrated approaches to improve palliative care for older people. Moreover, it advocates that palliative care is offered from the time of diagnosis, alongside potentially curative treatment, to disease progression and the end of life (12).

In its manual of palliative care, the International Association for Hospice and Palliative Care states that palliative care incorporates the whole spectrum of care, i.e. medical, nursing, psychological, social, cultural, and spiritual. The manual mentions that a holistic approach is essential in palliative care and describes various principles of palliative care, e.g. consideration of individuality, comprehensive inter-professional care, coordinated care, and continuity of care. With regard to models of care, the manual describes in-patient beds, community services, day units, and hospital palliative care teams and points out that palliative care should be integrated into clinical care. Moreover, it suggests that palliative care should be integrated in a seamless manner with other aspects of care (13).

One recent example of combining the related concepts of integrated care and patient-centred palliative care is the European Integrated Palliative Care Study (InSup-C). The aim of this study is to find agreement on the very best ways to provide integrated palliative care, which is described as 'bringing together administrative, organizational, clinical and service aspects in order to realize continuity of care between all actors involved in the care network of patients receiving palliative care. It aims to achieve quality of life and a well-supported dying process for the patient and the family in collaboration with all care givers (paid and unpaid)' (14). There is a need for more initiatives to accelerate the adoption and application of integrated and person-centred palliative care. Moreover, palliative care may significantly contribute to the conceptualization and experimentation of integrated care, as will be outlined in the following section.

Rationale for integrated and person-centred palliative care for older people

Improving palliative care is a policy objective in many countries. Palliative care services have been developed within health care systems, resulting in both diversity and inequity of provision (15) and lack of unified standards and accepted definitions (16). Palliative care for people with cancer is relatively well developed, in terms of its conceptual framework and evidence base. However, the evidence base for those dying from other causes, such as dementia, is less well developed, although evolving (17).

In the past, palliative care was provided in the last few months of life. With advances in treatment, time of death has become less predictable. The range of life-limiting diseases has been expanded, leaving the traditional focus on specialist palliative care teams caring for people (mostly in a hospice) inadequate in volume and setting (18). Changes in living and social circumstances mean that current generations can no longer expect the informal caregiving taken for granted by their forebears, forcing people to look to formalized health care and social services. At the same time, individualistic, consumerist attitudes mean that people demand greater choice in determining and tailoring their health care, including the opportunity to be cared for and to die in their place of preference (19).

Given the increasing numbers of people with life-limiting illness and the changing profiles of the illnesses, it is neither feasible nor desirable that more traditional specialist palliative care teams provide care for everyone. Rather, these services should be reserved for patients with the most complex palliative care needs (20). In general, health care systems want to reduce inappropriate and costly hospital and emergency admissions by providing more cost-effective care in the community. However, despite the need for patient-centred palliative care, integrated care is often lacking at the end of life, resulting in increased hospitalizations, missed appointments and reduced access to care, suboptimal clinical outcomes, fragmented care, and wasted time (11).

The aforementioned raises the following two questions: what is known about the effectiveness of the elements of integrated and person-centred palliative care models and how does one build these models in daily practice? Both questions are addressed in the next section.

Evidence of integrated and person-centred palliative care for older people

Luckett et al. (21) recently published a rapid review to identify evidence-based models of palliative care. In short, they found only a few well-designed studies comparing models of palliative care with each other, or with usual care. It turned out that they had to move away from whole models to focus on service elements featured in models found to be effective. Luckett and colleagues decided to include elements of case management via integration of specialist palliative care teams with primary and community care services and to enable transitions across settings, including residential aged care. Further, the authors recommend that dynamic, less homogeneous models are increasingly required to accommodate rapidly changing population demands and health system structure and drivers. They write 'the current focus on medical and nursing service delivery should also be broadened to incorporate services addressing social and environmental determinants of health as required' (21). The focus in the literature on elements rather than models raises important questions about how these elements might interact to the betterment or detriment of care quality, outcomes, and costs (21).

In another recent systematic review by Smith et al. (22) of international evidence on the costs and cost effectiveness of palliative care interventions (in any setting), consistent patterns were found. Interventions included hospice care, hospital-based palliative care programmes, and home-based palliative care programmes. Authors write that 'the definitions of palliative care interventions vary across studies, and in a number of cases, adequate descriptions of the intervention being studied were relatively limited, making international comparisons more difficult' (22). Despite the wide variation in study type and methodological quality, it was concluded that palliative care is most frequently found to be less costly than care utilized by comparator groups, and, in most cases, the difference in cost is statistically significant (22).

In an unsystematic review by the Canadian Hospice Palliative Care Association (23), 11 innovative models of the integrated palliative approach to care from Canada, England, New Zealand, and Australia were identified. It was found that these models seem to take different approaches to providing integrated palliative care, yet all share common elements that make them successful and transferable to other locations. All are focused on increasing the capacity of different parts of the health care system; all have interdisciplinary teams and services; and all work to create 'a seamless network of primary-community-hospital-hospice services that support individuals and families as their needs change' (23). From the models, success factors were derived and grouped into four components. The first group refers to 'vision' and includes commitment to person-centred care, focus on building capacity in the community and on changing organizational culture, and senior management support. The second group, 'people', includes dedicated coordinators, inter-professional teams, a strong role and more support for family physicians, support for providers in long-term care facilities, and key roles for nurses, relationships, partnerships, and networks. The third group is about 'delivery of care' and includes integration of primary, secondary, and tertiary care, cultural sensitivity, single access points and case management, 24/7 community support and care, and advance care planning. The fourth group refers to 'supportive tools' and consists of a common framework, standards and assessment tool, flexible approaches to education, shared records and research, evaluation, and quality improvement. It was concluded that although the models may target different providers or settings, they all report having similar positive impacts on people who are dying and their families, health care providers, and the health care system (23).

From a paper by Labson et al. discussing two United States home health-based programmes for palliative care (TriCentral Palliative Care Program by Kaiser Permanente, and Advanced Illness Management by Sutter Health) that have reported improved patient satisfaction, better utilization of services, and significant cost savings, similar elements were described. In brief, the two programmes both moved the focus of care from the hospital to the home and community by integrating services (10).

Based on information from key informant discussions, grey literature, and a basic scan of research articles in the academic literature, ten steps for the development, implementation, and evaluation of integrated palliative care models were synthesized by Vancouver Island University (24). A selection of frameworks and models were compared by their commonalities and differences. This revealed four key themes: stakeholder involvement, patient-centred care, structural considerations, and communication and ongoing monitoring. From these themes, the following ten steps were derived and are considered critical in building an integrated care model:

1 'identify the form, type, and level of integration';

2 'develop a common working definition';

3 'define patient-centred care';

4 'interpret single point of entry';

5 'identify the population of focus and support structures';

6 'examine operational considerations';

7 'identify the relevant stakeholders';

8 'determine strategies for stakeholder commitment';

9 'establish communication channels';

10 'determine methods of evaluation'.

The order and categorization of these steps is not fixed but rather serves as a starting point for a discussion of the development, implementation, and integration of an integrated model for palliative care (24).

Not included in the reviews previously mentioned are the recent experiences from the Liverpool Care Pathway for the Dying Patient (LCP). The LCP was developed about a decade ago by the Royal Liverpool University Hospital and the Marie Curie Hospice in Liverpool for the care of terminally ill cancer patients (25). The LCP became embroiled in controversy as some doctors, religious leaders, and pro-life groups alleged that patients were being put on the 'pathway to death' without their consent, or that of their families, in response to financial incentives from the National Health Service (26). The Minister of State for Care Support commissioned a panel to review the use and experience of the LCP in England. In the light of this chapter, two main findings from the review are presented here.

First, the term 'care pathway' is often misunderstood. It often gets confused with terms such as protocols, standards, operating procedures, guidelines, guidance, and best practice models. Further, the LCP aims to support mutual decision making and organization of care processes for people in the dying phase. As such, the LCP is only one of several integrated end-of-life care approaches. The review panel concludes that when the LCP is used properly, patients die a peaceful and dignified death. But the review panel is also convinced that implementation of the LCP is not infrequently associated with poor care (25). Second, the review panel argues that adherence to the LCP cannot be enough: 'a system-wide approach to professional practice and institution provision, measurable and monitored, is required to bring about improvements in care for the dying' (25). The panel recommends a strategic approach or a coalition of stakeholders 'to lead the way in creating and delivering the knowledge base, the education training and skills and the long term commitment needed to make high quality care for dying patients a reality' (25). In doing so, the patient, their relatives, and their carers need to be put first, starting with defining what good-quality end-of-life services should look like and then measuring against those standards (25).

Recommendations for development of integrated and person-centred palliative care

Despite its importance for health care systems around the world, a common definition of integrated palliative care is lacking. Considering that palliative care should be offered based on the needs of the patient, the work by National Voices, a national coalition of 130 health and social care charities in England, could be taken into account. This coalition defines integrated care as 'I can plan my care with people who work together to understand me and my carer(s), allow me control, and bring together services to achieve the outcomes important to me' (27). Following from this definition, integrated care means person-centred coordinated care (27).

It would be very helpful to develop a broad consensus about a common terminology and typology regarding integrated palliative care. This lack of specificity and clarity hampers systematic understanding and successful, real-world application and challenges policy making (2). Nonetheless, an increasing number of publications report the effectiveness and implementation of integrated and person-centred palliative care, as previously described. This contributes to overcoming the difficulties experienced in resolving fragmentation in palliative care. Experimentation with integrated palliative care, including evaluation of outcomes and the involvement of stakeholders, will provide useful lessons for its further development.

Applying integrated and person-centred care to palliative care implies that issues such as the following should be addressed: how health governance should react to the challenges and what needs to be done in terms of legal requirements for integrating palliative care into existing health systems settings; how the funding of health systems can influence options to better integrate palliative care and facilitate the cooperation of health and social services; the human resource implications of integrating palliative care in terms of education and retraining of existing professionals and professions or creating new job profiles; the expected effects on the organization and the provision of services. Since palliative care services are multifaceted, they should be integrated within the health system. In this light, joint working and new models of integrated care between specialists in palliative care and specialists in care for older people are suggested (12).

It seems that experiences with palliative care may be exemplary for other populations and phases of life. Too many existing initiatives in this field are either based on diagnosis or over-emphasize the perspective of health care professionals or organizations. If well understood, palliative care is concerned with total care, i.e. 'control of pain, of other symptoms, and of psychological, social and spiritual problems. The goal of palliative care is achievement of the best quality of life for patients and their families. Palliative care is concerned both with patients and their families and with the enhancement of quality of life from an early stage in a life-threatening illness' (28).

Conclusion on development of integrated and person-centred palliative care

Palliative care services need to be further developed to meet the complex needs of mostly older people. These services should be offered in different settings, including the community, nursing homes, and hospitals, according to a systems-wide approach. The development, evaluation, and implementation of integrated and person-centred palliative care is likely to contribute to the broader agenda of integrated care for people with complex needs.

References

1 **Nolte E, McKee M.** Integration and chronic care: a review. In: Nolte E, McKee M (eds). *Caring for people with chronic conditions—a health system perspective.* Berkshire: Open University Press; 2008, 64–91.

2 **Kodner D.** All together now: a conceptual exploration of integrated care. *Healthc Q* 2009; **13**:6–15.

3 **Wagner EH, Austin BT, Von Korff M.** Improving outcomes in chronic illness. *Manag Care Q* 1996; **4**(2):12–25.

4 **Wagner EH, Austin BT, Von Korff M.** Organizing care for patients with chronic illness. *Millbank Quarterly* 1996; **74**:511–44.

5 World Health Organization Regional Office for Europe. *Strengthening people-centred health systems in the WHO European region. A framework for action towards Coordinated/Integrated Health Services Delivery (CIHSD).* Copenhagen: World Health Organization; 2013.

6 Institute of Medicine. *Crossing the Quality Chasm: A New Health System for the 21st Century.* Washington, D.C: National Academy Press: 2001.

7 **Frampto, S, Guastello S, Lepore M.** Compassion as the foundation of patient-centered care: the importance of compassion in action. *J Comp Eff Res* 2013; **2**(5):443–55.

8 **Olsson L, Jakobsson U, Swedberg K, Ekman I.** Efficacy of person-centred care as an intervention in controlled trials: a systematic review. *J Clin Nurs* 2013; **22**:456–65.

9 **McCormack L, Treiman K, Rupert D, Williams-Piehota P, Nader E, et al.** Measuring patient-centered communication in cancer care: a literature review and the development of a systematic approach. *Soc Sci Med* 2011; **72** (7):1085–95.

10 **Labson MC, Sacco MM, Weissman DE, Fache BG, Stuart B.** Innovative models of home-based palliative care. *Cleveland Clin J Medicine* 2013; **80**(E-Suppl 1):e-S30–eS35.

11 **Daveson BA, Harding R, Shipman C, et al.** The real-world problem of care coordination: a longitudinal qualitative study with patients living with advanced progressive illness and their unpaid caregivers. *PLos One* 2014; **9**(5):e95523.

12 World Health Organization Regional Office for Europe. *Palliative care for older people: better practices.* Copenhagen: World Health Organization; 2013.

13 IAHPC. *The IAHPC manual of palliative care* (3rd edn). Available at: <http://hospicecare.com/uploads/2013/9/The%20IAHPC%20Manual%20of%20Palliative%20Care%203e.pdf> (Accessed June 2014). Ref. type: online source.

14 Integrated Palliative Care InSup-C. *Definition of integrated palliative care.* Available at: <http://www.insup-c.eu> (Accessed June 2014). Ref. type: online source.

15 **Clark D, Ten Have H, Janssens R, on behalf of the Palliative Care Ethics (Pallium) Project.** Common threads? Palliative care service developments in seven European countries. *Palliat Med* 2000; **14**:479–90.

16 **Centeno C, Clark D, Lynch T, et al.** Factors and indicators on palliative care development in 52 countries of the WHO European region: results of EAPC task force. *Palliat Med* 2007; **21**:463–71.

17 **Iliffe S, Davies N, Vernooij-Dassen M, et al.** Modelling the landscape of palliative care for people with dementia: a European mixed methods study. *BMC Palliat Care* 2013; **12**(30).

18 **Watson M.** Changing emphasis in end-of-life care. *Br J Gen Hosp Med* 2010; **71**(1):6–7.

19 **Doron I.** Caring for the dying: from a 'negative' to a 'positive' legal right to die at home. *Care Manag J* 2005; **6**(1):22–8.

20 **Quill T, Abernethy AP.** Generalist plus specialist palliative care—creating a more sustainable model. *N Eng J Med* 2013; **368**(13):1173–5.

21 **Lucket T, Philips J, Agar M, Virdun C, Green A, Davidson PM.** Elements of effective palliative care models: a rapid review. *BMC Health Serv Res* 2014; **14**:136.

22 **Smith S, Brick A, O'Hara S, Normand C.** Evidence on the cost and cost-effectiveness of palliative care: a literature review. *Palliat Med* 2014; **28**(2):130–50.

23 Canadian Hospice Palliative Care Association. *Innovative models of integrated hospice palliative care, the way forward initiative: an integrated palliative approach to care*; 2013.

24 Vancouver Island University. *A selective review of applied models and promising practices for seniors' integrated care*; 2013. Available at: <http://cha.viu.ca/wp-content/uploads/2013/04/Review-of-Integrated-Care-Models-August-2013.pdf> (Accessed June 2014). Ref. type: online source.

25 **Neuberger J, Guthrie C, Aaronovitch D, et al.** *More care, less pathway. A review of the Liverpool Care Pathway*; 2013. Available at: <https://www.gov.uk/government/uploads/system/uploads/attachment_data/file/212450/Liverpool_Care_Pathway.pdf> (Accessed June 2014). Ref. type: online source.

26 **Laurance J.** 'Liverpool Care Pathway: a way of death worth fighting for?' *The Independent*; 8 January 2013. Available at: <http://www.independent.co.uk/life-style/health-and-families/health-news/liverpool-care-pathway-a-way-of-death-worth-fighting-for-8443348.html> (Accessed 24 June 2014). Ref. type: online source.

27 National Voices. A narrative for person centered coordinate care. Available at: <http://www.england.nhs.uk/wp-content/uploads/2013/05/nv-narrative-cc.pdf> (Accessed 24 June 2014). Ref. type: online source.

28 World Health Organization. *Cancer pain relief and palliative care*. Report of a WHO Expert Committee (WHO Technical Report Series, No. 804). Geneva: WHO; 1990.

Chapter 5

Policies on palliative care for older people in Africa

Richard Harding, Richard A. Powell, and Liz Gwyther

Introduction to policies on palliative care for older people in Africa

The operational definition of 'older people' for the African continent varies from that advanced by the United Nations (UN). The UN definition of 60 years is considered inappropriate in especially rural African areas, where birth dates may be indeterminate, the concept of 'retirement' does not exist, and life expectancy is lower (1). The term 'older people' in Africa encompasses more complex definitions, reflecting socio-cultural differences that entail a combination of chronological, functional, and societal factors (e.g. differing social roles, modification in work patterns, adult roles of children, and differing life expectancy).

Ageing in Africa

Within Africa, there has been an increase in longevity, achieved primarily through significant declines in mortality rates from prevention and treatment of diseases associated with premature death. By 2050, the number of persons aged at least 60 will be approximately 2.03 million (22% of the global population), with four-fifths living in developing countries (2). Compared with other continents, Africa is projected to experience an accelerated growth in this older demographic group by that time, amounting to 215 million (10% of the region's population) (2). While moderate variation existed, in 2005, in the proportion of the population aged over 60, between Northern Africa and sub-Saharan Africa (6.8% and 4.8%, respectively), by 2050, it is projected these differences will be more significant (19.6% and 8.8%, respectively), reflecting differences in the rapidity of sub-regional demographic transitions (3). While it is essential to understand that Africa has great differences between the Northern, largely Arab, countries and their sub-Saharan counterparts, this chapter largely discusses sub-Saharan Africa (which also has greater palliative care activity compared with Northern Saharan countries) (4).

More than half of the African population is aged 19 years and younger (3), and there are competing national priorities addressing economic development issues, plus a considerable infectious and non-communicable disease burden (5, 6). Therefore, ageing on this continent has had a relatively low priority among national policy makers and planners, and in public discourse (7). A number of seminal documents have been published over the last decade that highlight the needs of older persons globally, noting the omission of their needs from the mainstream development dialogue. In 2002, the Second UN World Assembly on Ageing, and the ensuing Madrid International Plan of Action on Ageing (8), stressed that population ageing is an integral developmental challenge in Africa, the latter calling for it to be included in national socio-economic development policies. These global declarations were echoed regionally by the African Union's adoption of the *Africa Health Strategy, 2007–2015* (9) which referred to the burgeoning growth of chronic noncommunicable disease linked to demographic changes. These documents were recently augmented by reports issued by the World Health Organization (WHO) (10), the World Economic Forum (11), and the United Nations Population Fund, together with HelpAge International (12), that emphasized the necessity for coherent action to ensure the well-being of an expanding older population as an integral part of societies' development.

However, while some nations, especially in Eastern and Southern Africa, have adopted policies on ageing, few are supported by dedicated budgetary provisions (12). Indeed, for the vast majority of the continent's 54 fully recognized states, there have been minimal policy and programmatic advances in caring for older people's needs since 2002. In an era when extending life expectancy rather than improving quality of life is a stated UN millennium development goal (13), one area of neglected and under-researched gerontological care provision across the continent is palliative care.

Health and social care systems in Africa

Generally, there are three different types of formal health and social care systems across the continent: the *public system,* which is based around specialist, regional, district, and home-based care providers, with services largely free to in-patients and out-patients; an *insurance-based system,* which is either founded on individual, private contributions or on an employer-related health scheme; and the *private-sector system,* for a relatively small percentage of the population with sufficient financial resources (14). The informal sector provides popular traditional medicine and healing activities, often involving diagnostic incantations, indigenous herbalism, and African spirituality. These traditions are important in end-of-life care practices (15).

Within health and social care provision, as a middle-income country, South Africa is the only country providing social welfare grants, although they are of low value and are often the only household income. The grants available are the older person's grant (for those over 60 years old), disability grant (converted to older person's grant when the grantee turns 60), war veteran's grant for veterans of the Second World War or Korean War, and Grant-in-Aid for persons receiving any of the previous three grants who are not able to care for themselves. The children's grants are also important in the context of grandparents caring for orphaned children.

However, in most African countries, health inequalities and differential service access continue to pose a considerable challenge. Impoverished households are excluded from accessing affordable quality health care services, with members often resorting to self-medication, home-based health-seeking behaviour (16), or accessing informal traditional healers. The lack of service access is also a direct result of health systems' weakness across the continent due to low governmental financial resources, with more than 20% of total health expenditure provided by external sources in nearly half of the 46 countries in the WHO African Region (17). There is overwhelming disease burden, inadequate institutional capacity, inefficient use of potential national expertise, weak coordination of health development partners, and a lack of adequate focus in government policies and legislation.

The status of palliative care in Africa

Following initiation of the first African palliative care service in Zimbabwe (18), for many years, palliative care development across the continent was minimal. Based upon the WHO's definition of palliative care (19), services now aspire to the organization's public health approach, founded upon appropriate government policies. This includes a national health policy, an essential medicines policy, and education policies, the adequate availability of medicines, the education of health professionals, and integration of palliative care, at all levels, in national health care systems (20).

In 2004–05, a global study of African hospice and palliative care services was conducted that used the following four-part typology to depict levels of service development by country: Group 1: no known hospice/palliative care activity; Group 2: capacity-building activity; Group 3: localized hospice/palliative care provision; and Group 4: countries where hospice/palliative care services were reaching a measure of integration with the mainstream health care system (21). The study reported not only that 21 of 47 African countries surveyed had no identified hospice or palliative care activity, but also that just 4 of the 47 could be classified as having services approaching some measure of integration with mainstream service providers. While those 26 countries with palliative care activity constituted approximately 136 hospice and palliative care organizations operating in 15 countries and a capacity-building presence in the other 11 (18), the majority were based in a single country—South Africa.

Five years later, and employing a modified ranking system to reflect the extent and quality of clinical coverage, follow-up research noted a number of significant advances against this baseline data (22). This most recent data has found that although 28 African countries fell into Group 1 (no known activity), nine countries progressed from no known activity/capacity building (Groups 1/2), to isolated provision (Group 3a), and four countries moved from Group 3 to Group 4a (preliminary integration into mainstream service provision). Uganda was the only African country ranked as Group 4b (advanced integration into mainstream service provision, equivalent to industrialized countries such as Australia, the United Kingdom, and the United States of America). The sub-Saharan countries in Group 4 (i.e. approaching integration) are Kenya, Malawi, South Africa, Tanzania, Uganda, and Zambia.

Despite this progress in advancing service provision in Africa (14), palliative care coverage on the continent remains inconsistent (23, 24). Where it is available, palliative care is primarily provided by non-governmental organizations with limited geographic and patient coverage, rather than integrated fully within national health systems, using a home-based care model of service provision centred around trained health professionals, community-based volunteers, and family carers (25). There is, however, a growing consensus that if palliative care is to reach all in need, service development should focus on embedding models of care within mainstream health care systems (26). An example of this is evident in Kenya, where 220 health professionals were trained to integrate palliative care into 11 major public and provincial government hospitals (27).

Policy and context on the aged, caregivers, and palliative care in Africa

As mentioned, despite a number of critical regional and global publications highlighting the needs of older persons, very few African countries (i.e. Ghana, Kenya, Mozambique, South Africa, Tanzania, Tunisia, and Uganda) have adopted national policies on ageing since the African Union's Policy Framework and Plan of Action on Ageing was instituted (12).

A global study to determine the care arrangements for people with dementia in developing countries concluded: 'Older people in developing countries are indivisible from their younger family members. The high levels of family strain identified in this study feed into the cycle of disadvantage and should thus be a concern for policymakers in the developing world' (28). Interestingly, the study found that caregivers in low- and middle-income countries reported caregiver strain (using standard outcome measures) at least as great as those in high-income countries, and caregivers from the poorest countries were most likely to be paying for expensive private medical services (28).

In South Africa, the Older Persons Act, No. 13 of 2006 and the Constitution of South Africa comprise some of the guidelines regarding the rights of older persons. The aim of the Act is to: 'deal effectively with the plight of the older persons by establishing a framework aimed at the empowerment and protection of older persons and at the promotion and maintenance of their status, right, well-being, safety and security; and to provide for matters connected therewith'. South Africa's National Action Plan for the Protection and Promotion of Human Rights of 1998 encourages the provision of adequate state funding for the care of older persons, establishing and improving the quality of care in homes and frail care centres and providing home-based care funding. These key issues are addressed by the Hospice and Palliative Care Association's publication on the legal aspects of palliative care (29).

What we know about palliative care needs of older people in Africa

While there are positive developments occurring in palliative care across Africa, they are primarily associated with addressing the impact of the HIV/AIDS pandemic and with the non-aged. The specific requirements of the African aged (e.g. potentially enduring age-related conditions, compounded by HIV/AIDS, poverty, social isolation, bereavement and loss arising from their children's premature death, and the burden of caring for their grandchildren and/or orphans and vulnerable children) are largely neglected, with few organizations targeting their needs (30), and who generally lack the specialized skills and experience necessary to deliver palliative care effectively to this group.

In order to deliver public health palliative care services in line with the WHO strategy (i.e. underpinned by drug availability, policy, and education), evidence is essential (31). Although there has been a growth in research activity and the evidence base for African palliative care in recent years (32), there has been minimal attention paid to the needs of older people. As HIV treatment access rolls out, HIV-diagnosed people live longer, and the ageing population present greater non-communicable diseases (e.g. malignancies and organ failure). Research to inform policy and practice is therefore urgently required. Moreover, people living with HIV in Africa self-report a higher number of symptoms with increasing age (33), and this presents the future challenge of how best to provide services to an ageing HIV-infected population.

Examples of good practice in Africa

The Hospice Palliative Care Association of South Africa has developed a strategy of providing on-site training and mentorship in palliative care for all staff in care homes for older people, with three key features of the training model: first is liaison with management and confirmed buy-in at this level; second is that professional staff and all lay care workers at a care home receive palliative care training; and third is that support staff (e.g. cleaning staff) are oriented to the programme and receive input on the key aspects of a palliative care approach to care. The training material for both professionals and caregivers has been specifically designed to address the palliative care needs in a care home context. A self-assessment questionnaire, completed by both professional and lay carers during the pilot phase of this training in 2012, indicated a lack of knowledge and confidence in some of the key areas of end-of-life care. This highlighted the need for training and support to enable them to provide effective pain and symptom management and to deal with the psychosocial issues facing residents and their families, particularly at the end of life.

Conclusion: future directions in Africa

Sophisticated advocacy and donor strategies have transformed the adult palliative care landscape in Africa. This is due to non-governmental organizations such as the African Palliative Care Association, the Hospice Palliative Care Association of South Africa, the Palliative Care Association of Uganda, and the Kenyan Hospice Palliative Care Association pioneering education, engaging with policy makers, and influencing legislators. Two further key and essential features of African palliative care advocates have been their strong belief in research and evidence to underpin advocacy, and their implementation of routine patient-reported measurement to demonstrate needs and outcomes (34–37). A wealth of research capacity and methodological development have been achieved, and now the evidence of an ageing population requires research to develop and evaluate effective and culturally appropriate models of palliative care for older people across the African continent.

References

1 Health Statistics and Health Information Systems, World Health Organization. *Definition of an older or elderly person: proposed working definition of an older person in Africa for the MDC project*; 2007. Available at: <www.who.int/healthinfo/survey/ageingdefnolder/en/index.html>. (Accessed January 2014). Ref. type: online source.

2 HelpAge International. *Global AgeWatch Index* 2013: *insight report*. London: HelpAge International; 2013. Available at: <www.helpage.org/download/52949da702099>. (Accessed January 2014). Ref. type: online source.

3 United Nations. *World population prospects: the 2006 revision*. New York: United Nations; 2007.

4 El Ansary M, Nejmi M, Rizkallah R, Shibani M, Namisango E, Mwangi-Powell FN, et al. Palliative care research in Northern Africa. *Eur J PallCare* 2014; **21**(2):98–100.

5 Joint United Nations Programme on HIV/AIDS. *UNAIDS report of the global AIDS epidemic*. Geneva: UNAIDS; 2012.

6 Jemal A, Bray F, Forman D, O'Brien M, Ferlay J, Center M, et al. Cancer burden in Africa and opportunities for prevention. *Cancer* 2012; **118**(18):4372–84.

7 Aboderin I, Ferreira M. *Linking ageing to development agendas in sub-Saharan Africa: challenges and approaches*. WDA-HSG Discussion Paper Series, No. 2008/1. Geneva: World Demographic Association; 2008.

8 UN Department of Economic and Social Affairs. *Madrid International Plan of Action on Ageing*. United Nations Programme on Ageing; 2002. Available at: <http://undesadspd.org/Ageing/Resources/MadridInternationalPlanofActiononAgeing.aspx> (Accessed January 2014). Ref. type: online source.

9 African Union. *African health strategy, 2007–2015*; 2007. Available at: <http://www.nepad.org/system/files/AFRICA_HEALTH_STRATEGY(health).pdf>. (Accessed January 2015). Ref. type: online source.

10 World Health Organization. *Good health adds life to years: global brief for World Health Day 2012*. Geneva: World Health Organization; 2012.

11 Bear JR, Biggs S, Bloom DE, Fried LP, Hogan P, Kalache A, et al. (eds). *Global population ageing: peril or promise*. Geneva: World Economic Forum; 2012.

12 United Nations Population Fund and HelpAge International. *Ageing in the twenty-first century: a celebration and a challenge*. New York: United Nations Population Fund; 2012.

13 United Nations. *Millennium development goals*. New York: United Nations; 2000.

14 Mwangi-Powell FN, Downing J, Ddungu H, Kiyange F, Powell RA, Baguma A. Palliative care in Africa. In: Ferrell BR, Coyle N (eds). *Textbook of palliative nursing* (3rd edn). New York: Oxford University Press; 2010, 1319–29.

15 Graham N, Gwyther L, Tiso T, Harding R. Traditional healers' views of the required processes for a 'good death' among Xhosa patients pre- and post-death. *J Pain Symptom Manage* 2013; **46**(3):386–94.

16 Council for the Development of Social Science Research in Africa. *Access and equity in African health systems*; 2005. Available at: <www.codesria.org/spip.php?article290>. (Accessed January 2014). Ref. type: online source.

17 Kirigia JM, Diarra-Nama AJ. Can countries of the WHO African Region wean themselves off donor funding for health? *Bull World Health Org* 2008; **86**(11):889–92.

18 Wright M, Clark D. *Hospice and palliative care in Africa: a review of developments and challenges.* Oxford: Oxford University Press; 2006.

19 World Health Organization. *WHO definition of palliative care*; 2002. Available at: <www.who.int/ cancer/palliative/definition/en/>. (Accessed January 2014). Ref. type: online source.

20 Sternsward J, Foley K, Ferris F. The public health strategy for palliative care. *J Pain Symptom Manage* 2007; **33**(5):486–93.

21 Clark D, Wright M, Hunt J, Lynch T. Hospice and palliative care development in Africa: a multi-method review of services and experiences. *J Pain Symptom Manage* 2007; **33**(6):698–710.

22 Lynch T, Connor S, Clark D. Mapping levels of palliative care development: a global update. *J Pain Symptom Manage* 2013; **45**(6):1094–106.

23 Powell RA, Mwangi-Powell FN, Kiyange F, Radbruch L, Harding R. Palliative care development in Africa: how we can provide enough quality care? *BMJ Support Palliat Care* 2011; **1**(2):113–4.

24 Grant L, Brown J, Leng M, Bettega N, Murray SA. Palliative care making a difference in rural Uganda, Kenya and Malawi: three rapid evaluation field studies. *BMC Palliat Care* 2011; **10**:8.

25 Mwangi-Powell FN, Powell RA, Harding R. Models of delivering palliative and end-of-life care in sub-Saharan Africa. *Curr Opin Support Palliat Care* 2013; **7**(2):223–8.

26 Mwangi-Powell F. APCA's role in the development of palliative care in Africa. *Progress in Palliative Care* 2012; **20**(4):230–3.

27 Achia G. Palliative care key in cancer management. *Science Africa* 2011, Oct 18; 5.

28 Prince M, 10/66 Dementia Research Group. Care arrangements for people with dementia in developing countries. *Int J Geriatr Psychiatry* 2004; **19**(2):170–7.

29 Hospice Palliative Care Association of South Africa. *Legal aspects of palliative care.* Pinelands, South Africa: Hospice Palliative Care Association of South Africa; 2012.

30 Lau C, Muula AS. HIV/AIDS in sub-Saharan Africa. *Croat Med J* 2004; **45**(4):402–14.

31 Harding R, Selman L, Powell RA, Namisango E, Downing J, Merriman A, et al. Research into palliative care in sub-Saharan Africa. *Lancet Oncol* 2013; **14**(4):e183–8.

32 Powell RA, Harding R, Namisango E, Katabira E, Gwyther L, Radbruch L. Palliative care research in Africa: an overview. *European Journal of Palliative Care* 2013; **20**(4):162–7.

33 Harding R, Selman L, Agupio G, Dinat N, Downing J, Gwyther L, et al. Prevalence, burden, and correlates of physical and psychological symptoms among HIV palliative care patients in sub-Saharan Africa: an international multicenter study. *J Pain Symptom Manage* 2012; **44**(1):1–9.

34 Harding R, Selman L, Agupio G, Dinat N, Downing J, Gwyther L, et al. Validation of a core outcome measure for palliative care in Africa: the APCA African Palliative Outcome Scale. *Health Qual Life Outcomes* 2010; **8**:10.

35 Logie DE, Harding R. An evaluation of a morphine public health programme for cancer and AIDS pain relief in Sub-Saharan Africa. *BMC Public Health* 2005; **5**:82.

36 Harding R, Gwyther L, Mwangi-Powell F, Powell RA, Dinat N. How can we improve palliative care patient outcomes in low- and middle-income countries? Successful outcomes research in sub-Saharan Africa. *J Pain Symptom Manage* 2010; **40**(1):23–6.

37 Lowther K, Simms V, Selman L, Sherr L, Gwyther H, Kariuki H, et al. Treatment outcomes in palliative care: the TOPCare study. A mixed methods phase III randomised controlled trial to assess the effectiveness of a nurse-led palliative care intervention for HIV positive patients on antiretroviral therapy. *BMC Infect Dis* 2012; **12**:288.

Chapter 6

Policies on palliative care for older people in Asia

Noreen Chan, Sumytra Menon, and Cynthia Ruth Goh

Introduction to policies on palliative care for older people in Asia

Asia covers a vast geographical area with more than half the world's population and huge diversity in terms of socioeconomic, cultural, and political development. Many Asian countries are experiencing sweeping demographic changes caused by falling birth rates and rising life expectancy, as shown by the accompanying population pyramids. Together with the changes in traditional family structure, exacerbated by economic migration, governments are faced with major challenges in providing care for a rapidly ageing population.

According to the *Global Atlas of Palliative Care at the End of Life* published in 2014 by the Worldwide Palliative Care Alliance and the World Health Organization (WHO), 20.4 million people were in need of palliative care at the end of life in 2011 (1). Of these, 69% were adults aged 60 and over, of whom 22% live in the WHO South-East Asian Region and 29% in the Western Pacific Region. This accounts for 51% of the global need for palliative care at the end of life.

This chapter highlights some of the challenges facing governments in the provision of palliative care at the end of life and the policies which they have come up with. A questionnaire was designed, based on the WHO public health strategy for palliative care, asking about local contextual background, the health and social care system, education and workforce issues, and governmental policies on ageing, availability of essential drugs, and existence of a national strategy for palliative care and its implementation (2). This was sent to key members and contacts of the Asia Pacific Hospice Palliative Care Network, the regional palliative care organization whose members come from many South-East Asian Region and Western Pacific Region countries (3). Detailed replies were received from six countries at different levels of development. Unfortunately, there was little information from the two most populous countries of the world, China and India.

A snapshot of six countries in Asia

Local demographic and care context

Responses to the questionnaire were received from Indonesia, Japan, Malaysia, the Philippines, Singapore, and South Korea. The most populous country was Indonesia at 237 million, and the least was Singapore with 5.4 million. According to the WHO Human Development Index, the countries range from 'Very high' to 'Medium' (Table 6.1).

All the countries are ageing rapidly. Taking Singapore as an example, it is estimated that by 2025, the proportion of residents aged 65 and above will have more than doubled, from 10% in 2012 to 21.5%, and there will be fewer economically active adults to support them. This trend is evident in the other countries ranking 'Very high' on the Human Development Index, Japan and South Korea. Japan has the oldest population with 24.5% aged 65 and above in 2012, rising to 28.9% by 2025. In contrast, countries lower on the Human Development Index, such as Malaysia, the Philippines, and Indonesia, have much younger populations—4–5.1% aged 65 and above in 2012, with a far less marked increase in 2025 to 6.8–9% aged 65 and above. (Table 6.1) Life expectancy is increasing in all countries.

Cancer was the top-ranking cause of death in Japan, South Korea, and Singapore, followed by cardiovascular disease or pneumonia. In Malaysia, the Philippines, and Indonesia, cancer ranked lower (third or fourth) as a cause of death behind cardiovascular disease.

All the six Asian countries reported that care for older people is provided mainly by family members (ranked number 1 by all countries), followed by domestic workers. Malaysia, South Korea, and Singapore reported relying on foreign as well as local domestic workers to provide care.

Only Japan, South Korea, and Singapore provided data on place of death. In all these countries, most deaths occurred in the hospital setting—Japan 76.1%; South Korea 68.5%; Singapore 60.6% (4).

The *Global Atlas of Palliative Care at the End of Life* categorizes countries into four palliative care development groups:

◆ Group 1—no known activity;

◆ Group 2—capacity-building activity;

◆ Group 3a—isolated palliative care provision (patchy in scope; funding often heavily donor-dependent; limited availability of morphine);

◆ Group 3b—generalized palliative care provision (a number of locations with local support, independent of the health care system; availability of morphine);

◆ Group 4a—preliminary integration into mainstream health service provision;

◆ Group 4b—advanced integration into mainstream health service provision.

Indonesia, the Philippines, South Korea are categorized as Group 3a (isolated provision); Malaysia as Group 4a (preliminary integration); and Japan and Singapore as Group 4b (advanced integration). For comparison, India is categorized as Group 3b (generalized palliative care provision) and China as Group 4a (preliminary integration) (1).

Table 6.1 Demographic profile of selected countries (survey respondents) in Asia

Country	Pop^n in millions (13) (2010)	Human Development Index (14)			% Pop$^n \geq 65$ yrs 2012 (15)	% Pop$^n \geq 65$ yrs 2025 (16)	% Pop$^n \geq 65$ yrs 2050 (16)	Life expectancy 2012 in yrs at birth Male/ Female (17)	Life expectancy 2012 in yrs at 60 yrs Male/ Female (17)	Global Atlas of Palliative Care Development Category (1)
		Category	Index	Rank						
Japan	127.3	Very high	0.912	10	24	28.9	36.4	80/87	23/29	4b
S. Korea	48.4	Very high	0.909	12	12	16.9	27.4	78/85	21/27	3a
Singapore	5.07	Very high	0.895	18	10	21.5	28.6	80/85	23/27	4b
Malaysia	28.2	High	0.769	64	5	9.0	15.4	72/76	18/20	4a
The Philippines	93.4	Medium	0.654	114	4	6.8	13.9	65/72	15/19	3a
Indonesia	240.6	Medium	0.629	121	5	8.4	16.4	69/73	17/19	3a
China	1359.8	Medium	0.699	101	9	13.2	22.7	74/77	18/21	4a
India	1205.6	Medium	0.554	136	5	8.3	14.8	64/68	16/18	3b

Government and policy

Of the six countries, only Japan and the Philippines did not have a national palliative or end-of-life care strategy or guidelines, but the presence or absence of such does not correlate with the level of development of palliative care. Japan is regarded as highly developed (Group 4b), with advanced integration of palliative care into mainstream service provision, while the Philippines is in Group 3a, with isolated palliative care provision and limited availability of morphine. Every country, except Japan, stated that palliative care is under the purview of a government ministry or department. Only the Philippines has a law that specifically mentions palliative care; The Palliative and End-of-life Care Bill allows a relative compassionate leave of 60 days on full pay to take care of a critically ill person.

In contrast, all countries had policies on active ageing, covering health, employment, and social service aspects. This is particularly well developed in Japan. Support services that enable older people to stay at home include in-home services (home help, bathing service, nurse visits, and night service), out-patient care, respite care, and community-based long-term care. Some municipalities have an integrated community care system that provides housing, medical care, long-term care, prevention services, and livelihood support in an integrated manner. A multi-faceted approach to aged care is also adopted by countries like Singapore, which has a Ministerial Committee on Ageing. All of the six countries, apart from Indonesia, have laws to support caregiving by families, in the form of family or childcare leave, with Korea having the most generous allowance of 90 days per family per year. Singapore passed the Maintenance of Parents Act in 1996, which allows impecunious old parents to sue their children for maintenance.

With the increasing likelihood of impaired decisional capacity towards the end of life, advance care planning is an important facet of palliative care for this group. None of the six countries has laws covering advance care planning, although Singapore has enacted two laws on advance medical directives and surrogate decision making. The Singapore Advance Medical Directive Act (1996) allows persons to state, in advance, that they do not wish to have extraordinary medical treatment should they be terminally ill, on the point of death, and unable to communicate (5). The practical application has been limited because of stringent safeguards that forbid health care institutions and doctors from asking whether patients have signed an advance medical directive, and the level of uptake by the public has been low. The Singapore Mental Capacity Act (2008) allows individuals to appoint a surrogate decision maker for health care decisions should they lose capacity to make those decisions in the future (6). However, the surrogate does not have the power to make decisions on life-sustaining treatment or treatment to prevent a serious deterioration in the patient's health. The doctor makes those decisions in the patient's best interests.

In Japan, the Cancer Control Act (2006) played a very important role in developing palliative medicine in oncology care. The Act requires facilities providing cancer treatment to supply palliative care also, and this has led to a network of hospitals treating cancer with palliative care services. Similarly, in South Korea, the Revised Cancer Control Act 2011 requires the Ministry of Public Health and Welfare to provide guidelines, medical facilities, professional and public education on palliative care, and to implement a home visiting programme for cancer patients.

Outside of the six respondent countries, certain local practices have led to laws being enacted to deal with specific situations. For example, in Taiwan, existing laws require medical institutions and practitioners to save a patient at all times, making it illegal for a doctor not to resuscitate a patient. The Taiwanese palliative care community lobbied strongly for a natural death act, and the Hospice Palliative Care Act was passed in 2000, which allows a patient's do-not-resuscitate wishes to be honoured (7).

Financial models

Countries have a variety of ways for funding general health care and palliative care. In Japan, there is universal national insurance coverage for all health care, including palliative care, and no other forms of funding are necessary. National insurance initially covered hospital in-patient palliative care services in 1990. It was extended to community home care nursing services in 1992. Though this funding was not specific to palliative care, but included aged care and disability care, hospice home care services began to flourish as a result of this funding stream. In 2002, hospital palliative care teams were reimbursed by the national insurance scheme and, in 2006, both home hospice clinics and day care hospices were reimbursed.

In all of the other five countries, funding for palliative care comes from a combination of patient contributions and charitable donations. In South Korea, Singapore, and Malaysia, there are government subsidies for certain types of palliative care services, usually those provided by government hospitals, though in Singapore, government subsidies are also available for hospice home care and in-patient hospice, after means testing. Private insurance does not cover palliative care services in any of the countries, apart from South Korea.

Service and drug availability issues

A range of palliative care services can be found in all six countries. These include hospital consultative services, in-patient palliative care beds, and hospice home care. Availability of hospice for day care was more variable, with Japan and South Korea reporting nil. Estimates of coverage of patients who need palliative care range from around 30% in Singapore to single-digit figures, even in Japan and South Korea.

Commonly used opioids, in oral immediate release, slow release, and injectable forms, are available in all six countries through the palliative care services. But barriers to access are reported in several countries. Even in Japan, there is partial unavailability in community pharmacies due to licensing and stock issues. In Indonesia and the Philippines, where palliative care provision is patchy (Global Atlas Group 3a), barriers include complicated and restrictive bureaucratic rules around prescribing, and a lack of supply in areas beyond regional hospitals. Malaysia, Indonesia, and the Philippines report 'opiophobia' and lack of knowledge in health care workers leading to inappropriate or underprescribing.

Educational and workforce issues

Five of the six countries (the exception being Indonesia) report that there is a palliative care component in most undergraduate medical curricula. However, only Japan, Singapore, and the Philippines have palliative care in undergraduate nursing training.

Palliative medicine was recognized as a speciality or sub-speciality in the Philippines in 2002, in Malaysia in 2005, in Singapore in 2006, and in Japan in 2011. It is not a recognized speciality in Indonesia or South Korea. In contrast, South Korea has specialist nursing qualifications up to advanced practice level for hospice palliative nursing and geriatric nursing. Most of the other countries, apart from Japan, do not have specialist palliative nursing qualifications.

Role of non-governmental organizations

Non-governmental organizations (NGOs) often played a strong role in the starting of palliative care services in all of these countries. As integration into the mainstream health care system progresses, the role of non-governmental organizations changes from service provision to advocacy, raising public awareness, education of health care professionals and the public, fund raising, and attracting volunteers.

Japan seems to be the only country which does not report current involvement of charities or other non-governmental organizations in palliative care service provision, because of their universal national insurance coverage. Palliative care started at the Presbyterian Yodogawa Christian Hospital in 1973. Services grew rapidly after national health insurance funding became available for hospital palliative care services in 1990. Now, Japan has several associations for medical and nursing professionals, some with an emphasis on research, and a national umbrella body, Hospice Palliative Care Japan. The Japan Foundation for Hospice Palliative Care provides charitable funds for research and professional and public education.

In South Korea, a hospice was opened in 1964 by Catholic nuns belonging to the Little Company of Mary and later championed by the Catholic Kangnam St Mary's Hospital. There are groups such as the Korean Catholic Hospice Association and the Korean Hospice Association. The national association is the Korean Society for Hospice Palliative Care.

In Singapore, community palliative care services comprising home care and in-patient hospice beds are run by eight Christian, Buddhist, and secular charities. All government hospitals have consultative palliative care services. The Singapore Hospice Council is the umbrella body representing both hospital and community hospice services. Professionals are represented by the Chapter of Palliative Medicine Physicians of the College of Physicians Singapore and the Singapore Palliative Nurses Chapter of the Singapore Nursing Association.

In Malaysia, hospice home care services are run by charities such as Hospis Malaysia. The Malaysian Hospice Council is the umbrella body that represents local charities providing hospice care. Malaysia has a dual system of small palliative care units at government hospitals which run alongside hospice home care services provided by the charitable sector.

Many charities have provided hospice care, largely in the form of home care, in the Philippines. Some government hospitals have palliative care services, which may be in-patient or out-patient and may include home care services. There are two national advocacy groups: the National Hospice and Palliative Care Council (now re-named Hospice Philippines), whose primary goal is raising awareness and promoting networking of service providers, and the Philippine Society of Hospice and Palliative Medicine, which provides training for physicians and promotes research.

In Indonesia, palliative care services started at the government-run Dr. Soetomo Hospital in Surabaya in the 1990s. Currently, there are services in major centres like the Dharmais National Cancer Centre. The umbrella body is the Palliative Care Society of Indonesia. Charities, such as Rachel House, work in niche areas like HIV children, and have strengths in advocacy.

The involvement of NGOs seems to be closely linked to the local context. Where palliative care is less well developed, NGOs can play a role by increasing awareness, advocating for change, contributing to service development or provision (either directly or indirectly), promoting capacity building, and even in quality assurance. But unless NGOs are able to work with one another and with government, it may be difficult to bring about widespread and sustainable change (8).

Palliative care for older people in China and India

There is little information on palliative care policy developments in Asia's two largest countries, India and China. It has been an enormous challenge to get an overall picture of palliative care development in those two countries. While there are undoubtedly centres of excellence, vast numbers of people have no access to palliative care services.

India now has two palliative care-related World Health Organization Collaborating Centres at Kozhikode (Calicut) and Thiruvananthapuram (Trivandrum) in the southern state of Kerala, where over 80% of India's palliative care services are situated. There have been three major policy breakthroughs of late. In 2010, the Medical Council of India approved palliative medicine as a speciality and announced a Doctor of Medicine course in palliative medicine. The Doctor of Medicine is the standard postgraduate medical qualification in India (9). In November 2012, the Government of India announced a National Programme in Palliative Care, including an action plan to integrate palliative care into medical practice (10). In February 2014, following 19 years of advocacy, the Indian Parliament amended the infamous Narcotic Drugs and Psychotropic Substances Act of India. This amendment declares access to pain relief as one of the objectives of the Act and makes provision for a countrywide, uniform, simple licensing procedure, removing bureaucratic barriers while retaining essential control via a system run by a single governmental agency (11).

China has at least three umbrella bodies representing palliative care. Much of the work in the 1990s was in making opioids available, linked to efforts to advocate cancer pain relief. It is unclear how much of palliative care service provision is led from oncology units or by the pain management community. The charitable Li Ka Shing Foundation, whose headquarters are in Swatow, Fujian province, runs over 30 hospice home care services all over China. Little is known about government policies affecting palliative care, although end-of-life care is a recognized speciality in China.

Conclusion on policies on palliative care for older people in Asia

The rapidly ageing societies of Asia provide huge challenges to governments in terms of health care provision, funding, and caregiving. Palliative care forms just part of the package that needs to be addressed. Most governments are now aware of the need to ramp up palliative care services in their countries and to formulate policies to achieve this. However, many hospice palliative care services are still focused on cancer and do not extend to chronic disease management or elder care programmes. The recent passing of the World Health Assembly resolution, 'Strengthening of palliative care as a component of comprehensive care throughout the life course', on 24 May 2014, reiterates the importance all countries should give to the development of quality palliative care services (12).

Acknowledgements

The authors thank Dr. Chan Kin-Sang, Dr. Karin E. Garcia, Dr. Ednin Hamzah, Dr. Hyun-Jung Jho, Professor Hyun-Sook Kim, Dr. Richard Lim, Professor M.R. Rajagopal, Dr. Maria Astheria Witjaksono, and Dr. Akemi Yamagishi for their help with the country survey, and Ms. Luo Zhifei for research assistance.

References

1 Worldwide Palliative Care Alliance, World Health Organization. *Global Atlas of Palliative Care at the End of Life*; 2014. Available at: <http://www.who.int/nmh/Global_Atlas_of_Palliative_Care.pdf?ua=1> (Accessed May 2014). Ref. type: online source.

2 **Stjernsward J, Foley KM, Ferris FD.** The public health strategy for palliative care. *J Pain Sympt Manag* May 2007; **33**(5):486–93.

3 Asia Pacific Hospice Palliative Care Network. Available at: <http://aphn.org/category/home/> (Accessed May 2014). Ref. type: online source.

4 Immigration and Checkpoints Authority of Singapore. Report on Registration of Births and Deaths 2013. Available at: <http://www.ica.gov.sg/data/resources/docs/Media%20Releases/SDB/Annual%20RBD%20Report_2013.pdf> (Accessed January 2015). Ref. type: online source.

5 Attorney General's Chambers, Singapore. Advance Medical Directive Act. Available at: <http://statutes.agc.gov.sg/aol/search/display/view.w3p;page=0;query=DocId%3Ac3137d32-215d-4bd1-a935-fc4770fc5850%20%20Status%3Ainforce%20Depth%3A0;rec=0> (Accessed May 2014). Ref. type: online source.

6 Attorney General's Chambers, Singapore. Mental Capacity Act. Available at: <http://statutes.agc.gov.sg/aol/search/display/view.w3p;query=DocId%3A7f933c47-8a34-47d1-8d0a-0a457d6fa1c2%20%20Status%3Ainforce%20Depth%3A0;rec=0;whole=yes> (Accessed May 2014). Ref. type: online source.

7 **Chen R.** The spirit of humanism in terminal care: Taiwan experience. *The Open Area Studies Journal* 2009; **2**:7–11.

8 Shaw R. The development of palliative medicine in Asia. In: Bruera E, Higginson I, Ripamonti C, von Gunten CF (eds). *Textbook of Palliative Medicine*. Boca Raton: CRC Press; 2006, 58–63.

9 Khosla D, Patel FD, Sharma SC. Palliative care in India: current progress and future needs. *Indian J Palliat Care* 2012; **18**(3):149–54.

10 Directorate General of Health Services: Ministry of Health and Family Welfare. *Proposal of Palliative Care Strategies for India*; 2012. Available at: <http://palliumindia.org/cms/wp-content/uploads/2014/01/National-Palliative-Care-Strategy-Nov_2012.pdf> (Accessed May 2014). Ref. type: online source.

11 Ministry of Law and Justice, India. The Narcotic Drugs and Psychotropic Substances (Amendment) Act 2014. Available at: <http://www.prsindia.org/uploads/media//Recent%20Acts/Narcotic%20Drugs%20and%20Psychotropic%20(Amendment)%20Act,%202014.pdf> (Accessed May 2014). Ref. type: online source.

12 World Health Organization. *Strengthening of Palliative Care as a Component of Integrated Treatment Throughout the Life Course*; 2014. Available at: <http://apps.who.int/gb/ebwha/pdf_files/WHA67/A67_31-en.pdf> (Accessed May 2014). Ref. type: online source.

13 United Nations, Department of Economic and Social Affairs. *World Population Prospects: The 2012 Revision*. Available at: <http://esa.un.org/unpd/wpp/Excel-Data/population.htm> (Accessed May 2014). Ref. type: online data.

14 United Nations Development Programme. *Human Development Report* 2013. *The Rise of the South: Human Progress in a Diverse World*. United Nations Development Programme; 2013. Available at: <http://hdr.undp.org/sites/default/files/reports/14/hdr2013_en_complete.pdf> (Accessed May 2014). Ref. type: online source.

15 The World Bank. *Population Ages 65 and Above (% of Total)*. Available at: <http://data.worldbank.org/indicator/SP.POP.65UP.TO.ZS> (Accessed May 2014). Ref. type: online data.

16 Population Division, DESA, United Nations. *World Population Ageing: 1950–2050: Countries or Areas*. Available at: <http://www.un.org/esa/population/publications/worldageing19502050/countriesorareas.htm> (Accessed May 2014). Ref. type: online data.

17 World Health Organization. *Life Expectancy at Birth*. Annual World Health Statistics Reports 2012. Available at: <http://gamapserver.who.int/gho/interactive_charts/mbd/life_expectancy/atlas.html> (Accessed May 2014). Ref. type: online data.

Chapter 7

Policies on palliative care for older people in Australia

David Currow and Jane Phillips

Introduction to policies on palliative care for older people in Australia

Similar to other developed nations, Australia's population is ageing, with the median age at death currently 80.9 years and rising (1, 2). Life expectancy has increased by more than three decades over the last century. The percentage of people over the age of 65 in 1970 was 8.3%, rising to 14% in 2011 (3). Disability-adjusted life expectancy is second only to Japan (4). National policies in Australia continue to evolve to reflect these demographic changes.

The Australian health care system

Australia is a federation of states and territories ('jurisdictions'), with health care respon-sibilities shared between the federal and jurisdictional governments (5). The Federal Government funds universal health insurance ('Medicare') for all permanent residents, covering individual medical consultations in the community, including general practice, private hospital admissions, and access to subsidized pharmaceuticals. 'Medicare' is paid for by a surcharge on income tax. The Jurisdictions are responsible for funding public hos-pital in-patient care. Increasingly, people are facing co-payments for out-patient specialist or general practice consultations and many Australians have national insurance to fund private health care.

The Australian health care system is built around primary care, triaging access to spe-cialist care. General practitioners can directly access almost all diagnostic investigations. People are free to choose their own general practitioner without having to register. Many general practices now employ practice nurses, who often have a focus on care of older peo-ple. On average, 90% of the population visit a general practitioner at least once each year and 9% of these encounters include a practice nurse.

Australian aged care programmes are highly regulated and run largely by government-subsidized private (for-profit and not-for-profit) providers. Aged care is subsidized by the Federal Government but most operators would insist that, as a minimum, 85% of the pen-sion goes towards providing that person's care. There is additional funding for the provi-sion of intensive nursing or complex pain management. In a market-driven system, the quality of care varies widely.

Entry into aged care requires assessment by a Federal Government funded aged care assessment team who recommend the level of care to be offered. The three levels of care are:

i) community-based programmes where resources support aged people 'in place';

ii) lower-level care in hostel-like residential accommodation; and

iii) higher-level care provided by residential aged care facilities (nursing homes).

The registered nursing input into residential aged care facilities has gradually declined. Most care is now provided by unregulated care assistants, supervised by a small number of registered nurses. Medical cover is provided by general practitioners, a small number of whom exclusively work in residential aged care facilities (6).

If a person who would otherwise be eligible for care in a residential aged care facility is in an acute care hospital, and clinical assessment suggests that the acute needs have been adequately addressed, they are deemed to have long-term care needs and are charged the daily co-payment for residential aged care facility care. Very few people are admitted directly to residential aged care facilities, with most admissions occurring after an acute hospital admission. It is not clear that this is the most effective use of resources.

The Australian social care system for older people

Australia has a publically-funded means-tested pension. The age at which people can first draw the age pension recently increased from 65 to 67 years. The age pension, at below half the median wage, and is just above the poverty line when rental assistance is included (7).

For the last two decades, Australia has had a compulsory superannuation system, aiming to provide adequate income for retirement. The compulsory superannuation levy now sits at 12% of income. Although there have been some taxation incentives to do this, the actual quantum of money that can be saved is very modest.

People caring ('carers') for people who have chronic or complex illnesses are currently able to draw on two financial resources: a non-means-tested *carer's allowance* which helps with co-payments for pharmaceutical therapies, allied health, and community nursing; and a *carer payment* which is more substantial and means-tested. The *carer payment* approximates with the age pension.

National policy and standards in Australia

'National Palliative Care Strategy'

Australia has had a 'National Palliative Care Strategy' since 2000 (8), endorsed by all jurisdictions. Updated in 2010, key priorities include:

i) support for patients, families, and carers in the community;

ii) community access to symptom control medications;

iii) workforce education, training, and support; and

iv) research and quality improvement.

The National Strategy also seeks to increase coverage of palliative care services—geographically and in its reach to all groups within the community including, but not limited to, older people. (One in three people referred to specialist services are under the age of 65.) A derivative document from the national peak body helps to operationalize this document (9).

Derived from the National Strategy are funded programmes to improve capacity and coverage of palliative care services including:

◆ the Palliative Care Clinical Studies Collaborative—the world's largest palliative care phase III clinical trials group, improving evidence for prescribing at the end of life (10);

◆ CareSearch (www.caresearch.com.au)—an evidence resource that includes real-time interrogation of the National Libraries of Medicine (PubMed) (11);

◆ adopting the Wisconsin-developed *Respecting Patients' Choices*, for advance care planning (12, 13).

Palliative care standards, quality, and outcomes

'National Standards Assessment Program'

In 2007, work was undertaken to introduce a national self-assessment programme in palliative care against 13 key initiatives (14). The 'National Standards Assessment Program' supports services, to improve the quality of care they provide, through existing quality improvement and accreditation cycles (15). The majority of services have completed at least one cycle to date.

'Palliative Care Outcomes Collaborative'

Since its commencement in 2006, this quality improvement programme benchmarks patient outcomes between services (16). Currently, more than 80% of all patients referred to specialist palliative care have point-of-care symptom data collected (17). Data demonstrate improved outcomes systematically and evidence that services have redesigned to improve care processes. Benchmarking happens between services in national and jurisdictional meetings. This has allowed the sharing of key success factors as well as reflecting on the shared challenges in providing the best possible care.

'Aged Care Standards' and accreditation

The Australian 'Aged Care Standards' are underpinned by legislation, enforcing the Federal Government's expectation of aged care providers. Failure to comply with the continuous monitoring and accreditation results in immediate withdrawal of accreditation and funding (18). While it is expected that the comfort and dignity of terminally ill residents is maintained, each facility has to demonstrate how this is achieved. The lack of measurable outcomes contributes to variability of uptake and impact of the programme. For instance, while many residential aged care facilities now require patients to have advance care plans, there has been lower uptake of a systematized approach to palliative care.

National initiatives in Australia

'Living Longer—Living Better'

Healthy ageing underpins national policy, while understanding that the majority of people will need increasing levels of care at some stage. The 2012 federally-funded 'Living Longer—Living Better' aged care reforms included developing a palliative aged care advisory service to build capacity amongst providers (19). This initiative is in the early stages of development and aims to better support families and aged and primary care providers address residents' unmet palliative care needs.

Evidence-based palliative approach guidelines

'Therapeutic Guidelines'

Australia has published *Therapeutic Guidelines* (20), now in its third edition. Reflecting the best available evidence (or consensus when evidence is not available), these prescribing guidelines help to align therapies nationally.

Needs-based assessment tool

A needs-based assessment tool (21–25) facilitates rapid assessment of a patient for any health professional seeing someone with life-limiting illness and assesses the carers' and health professionals' ability and willingness to provide the care required. A randomized trial showed significantly fewer informational needs when the tool was used.

Australian 'Cancer Pain Guidelines' and opiate calculator

Most recently, national 'Cancer Pain Guidelines' have been launched, incorporating acute, chronic, and cancer pain (26). Given the complexity of opiate conversions and the risks associated with conversion errors, an online opiate calculator has been developed, with an in-built age-related prompt. With the prevalence of pain in older people, these resources can assist clinicians to better manage pain.

Aged and community care

Australia is the first country internationally to introduce evidence-based guidelines for the delivery of palliative aged care (27). These were endorsed by the National Health and Medical Research Council and drew on the best available evidence (much of which was not derived from randomized control trials). These guidelines have been introduced into all Australian residential aged care facilities and been adapted for use in the community (28).

Primary care—'Medicare' benefits

General practitioners have been supported with financial incentives, through the national insurance scheme (Medicare), to provide more complex care. This includes reimbursement for an annual comprehensive health assessment for people over 75 years or living in residential aged care facilities (29), the ability to undertake case conferencing with at least two other health professionals, and, most recently, the introduction of reimbursed *home medication reviews*.

Dying in place

Reflecting *ageing in place*, there is increasing emphasis on helping people to die in their place of choice. Community nursing and allied health services are widely available, for a small co-payment, together with a nationwide network of palliative care service providers who support generalist providers, ideally in the place of the person's choice. These initiatives have not seen significant change in the place of care at the time of death to date.

The role of non-government organizations in Australia

Palliative Care Australia

For more than 20 years, Australia's national peak advocacy body for palliative care has been Palliative Care Australia. Key accomplishments that relate to palliative care and aged care include the national census of palliative service provision in 1998, which informed planning for the next decade; the documents around service planning that came out early this century; and, more recently, its role as the facilitator of the national self-assessment programme. The organization has a strong relationship with government, other peak bodies, and its state and territory counterparts.

Council of the Ageing

Council of the Ageing is a national peak body seeking to represent older Australians. It collaborates with aged care organizations to improve the well-being of older people. It is partnered with Palliative Care Australia to promote community discussions about end-of-life care. Their advocacy is around broad political issues, with some focus on the infirm.

Alzheimer's Australia

Alzheimer's Australia is the peak body providing support and advocacy for the 280,000 Australians living with dementia, their families, and caregivers.

Future development required in Australia

Although Australia has foundations in place to support older people nearing the end of life, there is the continuing challenge of how to best engage the community to ensure care is provided in the right place, at the right time, by the right health and social professionals. The referral base in Australia has not reflected that of the United States where far higher rates of older people are referred to palliative care services (30). More research needs to be done to understand the optimal care for those with multi-morbidities, fragility, and advancing age.

The emphasis on ageing in place needs to more actively identify people who do want to be cared for at home in the terminal stages of their life-limiting illness, in order to ensure the system is geared to deliver this.

Conclusion on policies on palliative care for older people in Australia

In summary, Australia has strong national policies for delivering palliative care in aged care, including advance care planning. The quality of care is assured through accreditation and refined through clinical benchmarking. The particular issues of palliation in older people are still an area that needs further research, both in Australia and around the world. Specific to Australia are its health and social systems which seek to ensure support for older people and the infirm in either being cared for at home or in making a smooth transition to supported living environments.

References

1 Australian Bureau of Statistics (ABS). *Deaths, Australia. 2008*. Canberra, Australia: ABS; 2009.

2 Australian Bureau of Statistics (ABS). *Deaths, Australia 2010*. Canberra, Australia: ABS; 2011. Contract No. 3302.0.

3 Australia Bureau of Statistics (ABS). *Australian Historical Population Statistics*. Canberra, Australia: ABS; 2008. Contract No. 3105.0.65.001.

4 Mathers CD, Sadana R, Salomon JA, Murray CJL, Lopez AL. *Estimates of DALE (Disability Adjusted Life Expectancy) for 191 Countries: Methods and Results*. Geneva, Switzerland: World Health Organizaion; 2000. Working Paper 16.

5 Gordon R, Eagar K, Currow D, Green J. Current funding and financing issues in the Australian hospice and palliative care sector. *J Pain Symptom Manage* 2009; **38**(1):68.

6 Royal Australian College of General Practitioners. *A Best Practice Guide for Collaborative Care Between General Practitioners and Residential Aged Care Facilities*. East Melbourne, Victoria, Australia: The Royal Australian College of General Practitioners; 2013.

7 Clare R. *The Age Pension, Superannuation and Australian Retirement Incomes*. Association of Superannuation Funds of Australia; 2008.

8 Care CDoHaA (ed). *National Palliative Care Strategy—A National Framework for Palliative Care Service Development*. Canberra, Australia: Publications Production Unit (Public Affairs, Parliamentary and Access Branch); 2000.

Commonwealth Department of Health and Aged Care. National Palliative Care Strategy: A National Framework for Palliative Care Service Development. Canberra. 2000. Available at: <http://elibrary.zdrave.net/document/Australia/natstrat.pdf>.

9 Currow DC, Nightingale EM. 'A planning guide': developing a consensus document for palliative care service provision. *Medical J Australia* 2003; **179**(6 Suppl):S23–5.

10 Currow DC, Shelby-James TM, Agar M, Plummer J, Rowett D, Glare P, et al. Planning phase III multi-site clinical trials in palliative care: the role of consecutive cohort audits to identify potential participant populations. *Support Care Cancer* 2010; **18**(12):1571–9.

11 Tieman J, Sladek R, Currow D. Changes in the quantity and level of evidence of palliative and hospice care literature: the last century. *J Clin Oncol* 2008; **26**(35):5679–83.

12 Detering KM, Hancock AD, Reade MC, Silvester W. The impact of advance care planning on end of life care in elderly patients: randomised controlled trial. *BMJ Clinical Research Ed* 2010; **340**:c1345.

13 Silvester W, Detering K. Advance care planning and end-of-life care. *Medical J Australia* 2011; **195**(8):435–6.

14 Palliative Care Australia. *National Standards Assessment Program Canberra, Australian Capital Territory*; 2013. Available at: <http://www.palliativecare.org.au/Policy/TheNationalStandards.aspx> (Accessed December 2014).

15 Palliative Care Australia. *National Standards Assessment Program Canberra, Palliative Care Australia*; 2012. Available at: <http://www.palliativecare.org.au/Policy/TheNationalStandards.aspx> (Accessed December 2014).

16 Eagar K, Watters P, Currow DC, Aoun SM, Yates P. The Australian Palliative Care Outcomes Collaboration (PCOC)—measuring the quality and outcomes of palliative care on a routine basis. *Aust Health Rev* 2010; **34**(2):186–92.

17 Currow DC, Eagar K, Aoun S, Fildes D, Yates P, Kristjanson LJ. Is it feasible and desirable to collect voluntarily quality and outcome data nationally in palliative oncology care? *J Clin Oncol* 2008; **26**(23):3853–9.

18 Australian Government, Australian Aged Care Quality Agency. *Aged Care Standards and Accreditation Agency Limited—Accreditation Standards*; 1997. Available at: <http://www.aacqa.gov.au/for-providers> (Accessed December 2014).

19 Australian Government, Department of Health *Living Longer, Living Better*. Canberra, Australia: 2012. Available at: <http://webarchive.nla.gov.au/gov/20140802080607/http://www.health.gov.au/internet/main/publishing.nsf/Content/palliativecare-pubs-compac-guidelines.htm> (Accessed December 2014).

20 Palliative Care Expert Group. *Therapeutic Guidelines: Palliative Care, Version 3*. Melbourne, Australia: Therapeutic Guidelines Limited; 2010. Available from: <http://www.tg.org.au/?sectionid=47> (Accessed December 2014).

21 Waller A, Girgis A, Currow D, Lecathelinais C. Development of the palliative care needs assessment tool (PC-NAT) for use by multi-disciplinary health professionals. *Palliat Med* 2008; **22**(8):956–64.

22 Waller A, Girgis A, Johnson C, Lecathelinais C, Sibbritt D, Forstner D, et al. Improving outcomes for people with progressive cancer: interrupted time series trial of a needs assessment intervention. *J Pain Symptom Manage* 2012; **43**(3):569–81.

23 Waller A, Girgis A, Johnson C, Lecathelinais C, Sibbritt D, Seldon M, et al. Implications of a needs assessment intervention for people with progressive cancer: impact on clinical assessment, response and service utilisation. *Psycho-Oncology* 2012; **21**(5):550–7.

24 Waller A, Girgis A, Johnson C, Mitchell G, Yates P, Kristjanson L, et al. Facilitating needs based cancer care for people with a chronic disease: evaluation of an intervention using a multi-centre interrupted time series design. *BMC Palliat Care* 2010; **9**:2.

25 Waller A, Girgis A, Lecathelinais C, Scott W, Foot L, Sibbritt D, et al. Validity, reliability and clinical feasibility of a Needs Assessment Tool for people with progressive cancer. *Psycho-Oncology* 2010; **19**(7):726–33.

26 Australian Adult Cancer Pain Management Guideline Working Party. *Cancer Pain Management in Adults. Evidence Based Clinical Practice Guidelines Adapted For Use in Australia Sydney*. Australia: Cancer Council Australia. Available at: <http://wiki.cancer.org.au/australia/Guidelines:Cancer_pain_management> (Accessed December 2014).

27 Australian Government: Department of Health and Ageing. *Guidelines for a Palliative Approach in Residential Aged Care—Enhanced Version*. Canberra, Australia: Department of Health and Ageing; 2004. Available at: <http://www.health.gov.au/internet/main/publishing.nsf/Content/palliativecare-pubs-workf-guide.htm> (Accessed December 2014).

28 Australian Government: National Health and Medical Research Council. *Guidelines for a Palliative Approach for Aged Care in the Community Setting. Best Practice Guidelines for the Australian Context*. Canberra, Australia: Department of Health and Ageing; 2011. Available at: <http://www.clinicalguidelines.gov.au/browse.php?treePath=&pageType=2&fldglrID=1914> (Accessed March 2014).

29 Australian Government: Department of Human Services. *Medical Benefits Schedule* 2014. Available at: <http://www.medicareaustralia.gov.au/provider> (Accessed December 2014).

30 Morrison RS, Meier DE. Palliative care. *NEJM* 2004; **350**(25):2582–90.

Chapter 8

Policies on palliative care for older people in Europe

Carlos Centeno, José Miguel Carrasco, Kathrin Woitha, and Eduardo Garralda

Introduction to policies on palliative care for older people in Europe

The ageing of the European population demands management and socio-health services that correspond to their needs, including an increase in long-term care, social inclusion, safety and well-being.

The national socio-health systems are based on two large patterns. The first pattern centres on solidarity and the redistributive principle of wealth, and it permits universal access to all services which are financed by a tax system in which part of the resources are progressively obtained from income, complemented by value-added tax and taxes applied to different products (e.g. Denmark and Spain). The second pattern is financed by obligatory National Service contributions paid by companies and workers, and the resources are principally directed toward the workers and their beneficiaries; the general taxes finance disadvantaged sectors and areas that have no coverage (e.g. Germany and France). In some countries, the borderline between public and private insurance is hazy, with existing compensation mechanisms directed at promoting universal coverage (1).

Although many countries have designed strategies for coordinating socio-health services, Europe lacks a common strategy and there are important social, cultural, economic, and access inequalities regarding socio-health resources.

This chapter describes the situation regarding palliative care for the older people in Europe using examples from three different countries (Germany, Spain, and Hungary), as well as the role of European institutions and non-governmental organizations.

Geo-health background of Europe

In 2010, the WHO estimated the European Union at approximately 900 million people. The European population over 65 years of age was 15% in 2010 and is expected to be 25% in 2050.

The last few decades have been characterized by large, rapid demographic changes, with important decreases in birth and death rates, with progressively ageing populations, and a pyramid of rhomboid-shaped population (Figure 8.1). Thanks to the control of

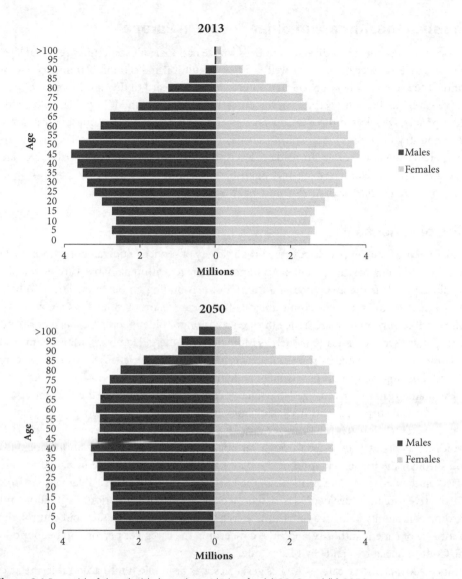

Figure 8.1 Pyramid of thomboid-shaped population for (a) 2013 and (b) 2050

Reproduced from EUROSTAT, *Population Structure and Ageing*, Figures 4 and 5, 2014. Original published: <http://epp.eurostat.ec.europa.eu/statistics_explained/index.php/Population_structure_and_ageing#>.

transmission diseases, the delay of the appearance of chronic diseases, and the reduction of premature mortality, the life expectancy now surpasses 76 years of age in both sexes. This is due to the improvement of life styles and conditions. At the same time, the risk of developing neurodegenerative diseases and cancer has increased, resulting in great social dependency (2, 3).

The socio-health care of older people in Europe

Europe is compounded by diverse countries whose national and sometimes regional laws are quite diverse. Such diversity, as well as different cultural and economic influences, have contributed to relatively large country differences with regard to the development of palliative care. To allow an overview of the differences in development of palliative care for older people, we selected three European countries as particular cases: one Central European country (Germany), one South European country (Spain), and one Eastern European one (Hungary). For an up-to-date description of the development of palliative care across Europe we refer to the recently published *Global Atlas of Palliative Care at the End of Life* (4) and the *European EAPC Atlas on Palliative Care* (2013) (5).

Case one: Germany

Palliative care for older people covers a broad variety of services, equivalent to those solely dedicated to palliative care patients. An important aspect within palliative care provisions for older people is the assurance of a domestic surrounding and care facilities. To help carry out said provisions, the community palliative care teams or volunteers are very significant. Recently, an increase in health care provision for older people has been observed in in-patient services. Locations such as Munich, Heidelberg, Hamburg, Mannheim, and Darmstadt can be named as showcases, joining the areas of geriatrics and palliative care and establishing the specific provision of palliative geriatrics.

The main organizations engaged in palliative care for older people are the German Association for Palliative Medicine, in close collaboration with the German Hospice and Palliative Care Association. Representing geriatrics is a task of the German Society for Geriatrics. Professional vitality is reflected through various recent and significant position papers (2) and through the implementation of the national plan for older people in palliative care based on the Budapest Commitments of the European Association for Palliative Care (6).

Palliative care for older people is also protected by current legislation. Regulations regarding community palliative care teams, in- and out-patient hospices, opioid control, the certificate of patient authority, and rules concerning the caregiver person can be found in the Code of Social Law and Civil Law Code.

Since 2009, palliative care, as well as geriatrics, has been taken into account in the academic education of students. Based on a large degree of self-commitment, such as in Hamburg, student teaching is organized as bedside teaching in small groups, presentations, and seminars.

Up to now, the existence of a Chair of Geriatrics and a Chair of Palliative Medicine at the University Hospital of Cologne has been a unique structure among German university hospitals, offering a variety of medical, educational, and scientific cooperation. In addition to the academic training, the Federal Hospice Association and the Robert-Bosch-Stiftung are engaged in supporting further coaching of workforces for older people and of volunteers (7, 8).

Financial reimbursement is provided through health insurance. Services included are out-patient services (e.g. community palliative care teams or general out-patient palliative care consultation) and in-patient services (e.g. palliative care units or hospices). In the special case of hospices, 10% of the costs have to be borne by the institutions themselves, mainly through donations. In addition, human resources, such as coordinators for the out-patient service, are rewarded. The most outstanding projects are selected and funded by the federal states (9). Furthermore, financial issues via the health insurance remain expensive and the pay off the complex palliative care treatment remains deficient in the pricing system for hospital services in German hospitals (Diagnosis-Related-Groups System).

However, barriers in these two young disciplines, palliative care and geriatrics, still exist. Frequently, the type of hospitalization given to the patient is incorrect due to a lack of knowledge regarding both health sectors; patients that need to be in a palliative care setting are in geriatric one, and vice versa. The referral of older people with multi-morbidities or dementia, from care homes to palliative care units, can be accomplished without any problem, whereas the transition of patients from nursing homes to an in-patient hospice is sometimes problematic. Furthermore, a future challenge will be the health provision of dementia patients at home or in long-term settings, e.g. ensured by the general out-patient palliative care consultation. Therefore, practitioners in the field need to join forces to ensure holistic competences. The adjustment of the source of financing (care funding versus health insurance) can be complicated.

The range of organizational structures for the provision of palliative care for older people is divergent; for example, they can differ between enclosed wards or integrative concepts. In addition, the focus of long-term care facilities concentrates on rehabilitative and activating aspects, instead of hospice or palliative care responsibilities. The level of care in these institutions is considered to be poor and more hospice and palliative care is needed.

Case two: Spain

Just as in other countries of southern Europe, a social model of marked family solidarity is what dominates most in Spain, with 30% of older people living with a family member (descendent). Of the older people who live alone, the majority (94%) live in their own homes, with a smaller or larger degree of socio-family support. After losing one's spouse, the option to remain living in one's own residence is gaining preference with older people in Spain (20–30% of older people live alone). The primary health care centres have social workers who assess and coordinate social assistance (10).

A small part (5%) of the older population lives in public nursing homes (partially or totally financed by the governmental system) or in private nursing homes. The residences financed by the government have limited access; assignments are made using a pre-established scoring system. Access to these nursing homes is slow and complicated.

The number of private nursing homes has multiplied during the past 15 years due to the interest shown from foreign investment and companies working under franchises, which can jeopardize the quality of service given to the older people.

The model of assistance to older people is dichotomous, either strictly health or strictly social; this is a problem in today's society because no integral response is being offered to address the needs and assisted care demands of older people. However, especially in the region of Catalonia, more and more nursing homes have evolved from simple catering/hotel types into specialized care centres, having equipment and technology quite similar to that available in the national health network.

Health assistance for older people by a decentralized governmental system is the responsibility of each autonomous community, and they all differ from each other to a certain degree. In the north-east area of Catalonia, the care system is more advanced and follows the model of the programme 'life for older people' that began in the 1990s: interdisciplinary teams act as inter-consultants in acute hospitals and if a longer hospitalization period is required, they transfer the patients to socio-health hospitals where there are specialized units and also palliative care units. In Andalusia and the Basque Country, geriatrics is not offered in the menu of services, possibly due to the interests of other specializations. The remaining Spanish regions have developed in a variety of ways, characterized by coordination of insufficient resources, although structurally, they have developed support hospitals for 'chronic patients' or for 'medium- to long-term stays with resources dedicated to older patients' (11).

Palliative care is usually part of the clinical activity and training of all geriatricians. A total of 10% of their activity is dedicated to caring for advanced stage or terminal patients in their homes or in an acute unit. In Catalonia, palliative care units ('hospice units') are very much integrated into the geriatric units and handle 80–90% of cancer palliative care patients and 10–20% of non-cancer palliative care patients. There are approximately 400 different palliative care units in Spain, and it is estimated that their development is intermediate with respect to other countries, and similar to the levels of France, Germany, and Italy. In Spanish palliative care services, the average age of the patients is frequently over 60 years of age. In general, they care for cancer patients, and this was the main reason these units were developed. However, more and more patients with other profiles are being accepted and regional plans in Extremadura, Madrid, and Andalusia have been developed to reflect this.

On a national level, no national plan or strategy for caring for older people has been developed. In the last few years, and in order to adjust health costs, more emphasis has been placed on providing assistance to chronic and pluripathological patients, including older patients, who would be the prototype group for any national health policy on providing palliative care to older people.

Social assistance to dependent persons was regulated in 2007 by the National Law of Dependency, which provides for aid to the sick and their families, including financial aid. However, such aid is irregular and slow because applications have to be made to the autonomous communities.

The specialty of geriatrics has existed since 1978, around the time when the first special-ties emerged. It is supported by a professional society that produces a journal and holds congresses, the latest being in 2014, marking the 56th edition of the journal. The Euro-pean Congress of the European Geriatric Medicine Society has been hosted three times in Spain. Training in this specialty follows the residency system in hospitals that are specifi-cally accredited for it. The first accredited centre was the Hospital de la Cruz Roja (Red Cross Hospital) of Madrid. Geriatrics is included at the undergraduate level of education, but often only as an elective course within medicine. The professors currently in charge of this course are usually not specialists in geriatrics.

Case three: Hungary

Hungary adopts a purchaser/provider split model, with output-based payment methods (12), in which care for the older people does not exist as a separate legal subject of care and is subsequently covered by 'general' palliative and social care.

The provision and organization of palliative care services in Hungary have improved over the last two decades. Overall progress has been made in home-based services as they have become more widely available across the country (69 teams). Nevertheless, there has been none or very limited development in the rest of the resources (13). The coordination and promotion of this activity have relied on the commitment of the Hungarian Hospice Palliative Association since 1995.

Recognition of palliative care is reflected and theoretically guaranteed in the general legislation. Since 1995, a national palliative care training programme has been accredited by the Ministry of Health and immediately afterwards, in 1997, hospice palliative care was recognized by the New Health Care Act (Article 99). Palliative care was included in the national cancer control programme in 2006 and a number of minimum palliative care standards (2004, 2012) and professional guidelines (2000, 2002) have been developed and constantly updated (guidelines last updated as a Ministerial Decree in 2010).

However, despite this well-developed legal mandate, government support, and finan-cing (features that are perceived as strengths when examining the system of Hungarian hospices), a lack of a comprehensive conceptualized health policy has also been identified. This is due to the fragmented governmental measures that are a result of continuous pol-itical changes. Palliative care or hospice treatment was provided and funded for only 7862 patients by 76 hospice care providers in 2013 (14).

With regard, in particular, to geriatrics, this area of medicine was approved as a spe-cialty in 2000 (15). Existing as a department at Semmelweis University (Budapest) and as a sub-department in Debrecen, it is taught to nurses, social workers, physiotherapists, and social caregivers at the undergraduate level, but little to medical students. However, the vitality of the discipline is well represented by the Preventive Geriatrics and Gerontol-ogy Association and the Hungarian Association of Gerontology and Geriatrics (which has held around 25 conferences and produces a journal entitled 'Hungarian Gerontology').

Social services in Hungary are organized separately from health services. This is deemed as a problem in itself, as no integrated models for older people currently exist. These services are provided mostly by nurses lacking training in palliative care, in independent nursing homes, long-term care facilities, hospice homes, gerontology wards, etc. Social assistance is still reported as a weakness and a threat in relation to its scope and quality of care, although all the development goals are stated in the national strategy concerning senior citizens (21). Services are provided according to the dependency level in long-term care and might be given at home or in old people homes, depending on the hours of care needed. Therefore, the services do not reflect the potential multidisciplinarity and complexity of this form of care. A good practice example occurs, however, in Pécs hospice, where social services are well integrated (14).

Local governments offer social assistance to older people at home in the forms of social caregivers and diverse, but generally low, financial support. These governments are in charge of residences and nursing homes, where residents must pay up to 80% of the costs, with long waiting lists before admission. Social caregivers provide care for two to three hours a day and the patient pays little if the caregiver is employed by the local government. Day care centres are mostly available at no cost but there are also private residences and nursing homes.

The greatest challenge that Hungary needs to face is the integration of palliative care in the health system, potentiating and simultaneously coordinating health services and social services.

Role of European institutions in palliative care for older people

In recognition of the importance of palliative care for European citizens, the Council of Europe implemented the nine-section Supplementary Recommendation 24, Rec (2003) 24 in 2003 (22) to emphasize the responsibility of developing a coherent, integrated national policy-making framework for palliative care. As a follow-up report to the Rec (2003) 24, the European Union (EU) Parliament commissioned a technical report in 2008 (23), which formulated, among other recommendations, policy options to advance palliative care in the EU, including national plans on palliative care and possible areas of legislation (16).

The WHO Regional Office for Europe published the booklet 'Better palliative care for older people' in 2004 in order to present evidence for health policy and decision makers in a clear and understandable form (17). The booklet presents the needs of older people, the different trajectories of illnesses they suffer, evidence of underassessment of pain and other symptoms, their need to be involved in decision making, evidence for effective palliative care solutions, and issues for the future. After this report, in 2011, WHO Europe also published 'Palliative care for older people: better practices' (18). This publication builds on the previous one by giving specific examples of promising or better practices in palliative care for older people, along with evidence of their effectiveness when available. This project was the work of a European Association for Palliative Care Task Force and the guide is developed for countries in the WHO European Region.

Role of European non-governmental organizations in palliative care for older people

Over the past few years, the European Association for Palliative Care (EAPC) has promoted several task forces related to palliative care for older people. One of these was 'Palliative Care in Long-term Care Settings for Older People'. The task force identified the development of palliative care in long-term care settings across Europe. Although now completed, this work is part of a broader process of international collaboration, and it is anticipated that expertise and experience will continue to develop and be exchanged in the new task force 'Mapping Palliative Care Systems in Long-term Care Facilities in Europe'. This task force is being established under the auspices of the recently European Union funded FP7 project, 'PACE (Comparing the effectiveness of palliative care for elderly people in long term care facilities in Europe)', and aims to perform comparative research concerning the effectiveness of palliative care in long-term care facilities.

Another EAPC effort was the 'White paper on palliative care in dementia—recommendations from the EAPC' published in 2013 (19). This contains a set of recommendations, with explanatory text, based on evidence and extensive references from the literature.

Although not specifically focusing on older people, but supported by the European Association for Palliative Care, an up-to-date description of the development of palliative care across Europe was published in 2013 (5). From this Atlas, it becomes clear that further developments are needed to ensure palliative care coverage for older people, especially for those who are living and cared for in nursing and residential care homes.

The first ever dialogue between palliative medicine and geriatrics, on an EU level, took place at the European Parliament in Brussels on 25 September 2012 with the cooperation of the European Association for Palliative Care and the European Union Geriatric Medicine Society. A joint manifesto, 'Palliative care for older people in the European Union', was unveiled (20). This sought to assist policy makers and national organizations in improving palliative care for older people in Europe.

The future of palliative care for older people in Europe

In the next few decades, Europe will face a serious public health problem due to the increase in the prevalence of chronic and degenerative diseases, with a greater demand for palliative services. Common strategies for ensuring coordination between the health services and social services involved in the provision of palliative care should be defined, and, at the same time, the social inequalities should be reduced so as to guarantee equality in the access to this type of care.

Acknowledgements

The authors wish to express their gratitude for the special contributions made regarding the country cases—Spain: Javier Gómez-Pavón; Hungary: Katalin Hegedüs and Ágnes Csikós; Germany: Lukas Radbruch, Johannes Vogel, Birgit Jaspers, Norbert Krumm, and Gabriele Röhrig-Herzog.

References

1 Subdirección General de Información Sanitaria e Innovación. *Los Sistemas Sanitarios en los Países de la UE: Características e Indicadores de Salud, 2013*. Madrid: Ministerio de Sanidad, Servicios Sociales e Igualdad; 2014.

2 World Health Organization. *The European Health Report 2012: Charting the Way to Well-being*. Copenhagen: WHO Regional Office for Europe; 2013.

3 EUROSTAT. *Population Structure and Ageing*; 2014. Available at: <http://epp.eurostat.ec.europa.eu/statistics_explained/index.php/Population_structure_and_ageing#>. (Accessed June 2014). Ref. type: online data.

4 World Palliative Care Alliance. *Global Atlas of Palliative Care at the End of Life*. London: 2014.

5 Centeno C, Lynch T, Donea O, Rocafort J, Clark D. *EAPC Atlas of Palliative Care in Europe 2013—Full Edition*. Milan: EAPC Press; 2013.

6 Radbruch L, Bausewein C, Simon ST, et al. Europäische Empfehlungen zur Palliativversorgung und Hospizarbeit und ihre Umsetzung in Deutschland. *Zeitschrift für Palliativmedizin* 2011; **12**:175–83.

7 Klapper B, Kojer M, Schwänke U. Palliative Praxis–Ein Curriculum zur Begleitung alter Menschen am Ende des Lebens. In: Heller A, Heimerl K, Husebø S (eds). *Wenn Nichts Mehr Zu Machen Ist, Ist Noch Viel Zu Tun Wie Alte Menschen Würdig Sterben Können*. Freiburg: Lambertus Verlag; 2007, 445–56.

8 Kompetenzzentrum Pflegeunterstützung Berlin, Arbeitskreis-Arbeit mit Ehrenamtlichen in Niedrigschwelligen Betreuungsangeboten. *Mustercurriculum für die Arbeit mit Ehrenamtlichen der Anerkannten Niedrigschwelligen Betreuungsangebote für Menschen mit Demenz in Berlin*. Berlin: Kompetenzzentrum Pflegeunterstützung Berlin; 2012 [February 2012; 12.6.2014]. Available at: <http://www.pflegeunterstuetzung-berlin.de/uploads/media/Mustercurriculum_NsBA_Arbeit_mit_Ehrenamtlichen_Demenz_01.pdf> (Accessed June 2014). Ref. type: online source.

9 Union Hilfswerk—Kompetenzzentrum Palliative Geriatrie. *Hospiz auf dem Weg in die Altenpflege*. Berlin: © 2009 UNIONHILFSWERK. Available at: <http://www.palliative-geriatrie.de> (Accessed June 2014). Ref. type: online source.

10 Comunidad de Madrid. *Plan Estratégico de Geriatría de la Comunidad de Madrid 2011–2015*. Madrid: Edita Salud Madrid; 2010

11 Gómez Pavón J. Asistencial al final de la vida. In: López Soto A, Formiga Pérez F, Ruiz Hidalgo D, Duaso Magaña E (eds). *Clínicas en Geriatría Hospitalaria*. Barcelona: Elservier; 2006, 171–90.

12 Gaál P, Szigeti S, Csere M, Gaskins M, Panteli D. Hungary: health system review. *Health Systems in Transition* 2011; **13**(5):1–266.

13 Centeno C. et al. *EAPC Atlas of Palliative Care in Europe 2013—Full Edition*. Milano: EAPC (European Association for Palliative Care); 2013, 385.

14 Hegedus K. The SWOT analysis of Hungarian hospice palliative care. *Advances in Palliative Medicine* 2010, **9**(4):111–16.

15 Gyula B. The state and models of specialisation in geriatrics in Europe and Hungary. *Orv Hetil* 2005 Apr 10; **146**(15):707–10.

16 Davies E, Higginson I (eds). *Better Palliative Care for Older People*. Copenhagen: World Health Organization, Regional Office for Europe; 2004.

17 Martin-Moreno J, Harris M, Gorgojo L, et al. *Palliative Care in the European Union*. Brussels: European Parliament Economic and Scientific Policy Department; 2008.

18 Hall S, Petkova H, Tsourous A, Costantini M, Higginson I. *Palliative Care for Older People: Better Practices*. Copenhagen: World Health Organization Regional Office for Europe; 2011.

19 Van der Steen J, Radbruch L, Hertogh CMPM, et al. White paper defining optimal palliative care in older people with dementia: a Delphi study and recommendations from the European Association for Palliative Care. *Pall Med* 2013; **28**(3):197–209.

20 Fondazione Maruzza Lefebvre D'Ovidio Onlus. 'Palliative Care for Older People in the European Union'. Available at: <http://www.maruzza.org/en/key-projects/pc-for-older-people/> (Accessed June 2014). Ref. type: online source.

21 Hungarian Parliament (2009), National Strategy concerning the Elderly, Decision No 81/2009 (X.6.) of the Parliament, accessed from <http://www.parlament.hu/irom38/10500/10500.pdf>.

22 Council of Europe,Recommendation Rec(2003)24 of the Committee of Ministers to member states on the organisation of palliative care and explanatory memorandum. Available at: <http://www.coe. int/T/E/Social_Cohesion/Health/Recommendations/Rec(2003)24.asp>.

23 Martín-Moreno JM, Harris M, Gorgojo L, Clark D, Normand C, Centeno C. European Report- 2008. Palliative Care in the European Union. Avaiable at <http://www.pavi.dk/Libraries/EAPC_white_ paper/Pall_Care_Eur_Parliament.sflb.ashx>.

Chapter 9

Policies on palliative care for older people in North America

Katherine Ornstein and Diane Meier

Introduction to policies on palliative care for older people in North America

In the United States, palliative care is defined as specialized medical care focused on providing relief from the symptoms, pain, stress, and treatments of a serious illness—whatever the diagnosis. The goal is to provide the best possible quality of life for the patient and the family (1). Palliative care is provided by an interdisciplinary team that works with patients, families, and other health care professionals to provide an added layer of support. It is appropriate at any age, for any diagnosis, at any stage in a serious illness, and provided together with curative and life-prolonging treatments.

Palliative care (predominately located in hospitals in the United States) and hospice (limited to the last six months of life for patients who choose to forego disease treatment) programmes improve physical and psychosocial symptoms, family caregiver well-being, bereavement outcomes, and patient, family, and physician satisfaction (2, 3). The benefits of integrating a palliative care approach into the care of people with serious illnesses now extends far beyond cancer. Evidence increasingly suggests that as a result of better quality of care, palliative care is cost saving (4, 5). Studies have even demonstrated that palliative care may be associated with a significant prolongation of life for some patient populations (6).

This chapter will explore policies on palliative care for older people in North America. We will provide a comprehensive discussion of American-based palliative care policy and will also include a discussion of the state of palliative care in Canada and Mexico.

Use of palliative care in the United States

The American health care system has both private insurers and a public scheme. The Medicaid programme serves poor families and the disabled. The Medicare programme covers those aged 65 and over and some disabled younger persons. Veterans are covered under a separate programme. Health care reforms enacted through the 2010 Affordable Care Act are being phased in through to 2020 and aim to decrease the number of Americans without health insurance, improve health care outcomes and delivery, and lower costs.

Palliative care in the United States is provided both within and outside hospice programmes. Hospice palliative care is appropriate when curative treatments are no longer beneficial, when the burdens of these treatments exceed their benefits, or when patients are entering the last weeks to months of life. Hospice services are delivered in a model established by statute in Medicare, and followed by most other insurers. Eligibility for hospice services requires that two physicians certify that the patient will die within six months 'if the disease runs its normal course' and that the patient agrees to forego regular insurance coverage for life-prolonging and curative treatments.

While the Medicare hospice benefit has existed since 1982, non-hospice palliative care developed within academic medical centres in the early 1990s in the United States and is offered simultaneously with life-prolonging and curative therapies for persons living with serious, complex, and life-threatening illness. While most non-hospice palliative care is currently hospital-based, community-based programmes are increasing.

The prognosis-based distinction between palliative care (eligibility based on need, with no prognostic restriction) and hospice (eligibility based on a prognosis of living less than six months) is unique to the United States, whereas in other countries the terms 'palliative care' and 'hospice' are largely synonymous. In fact, it was the need for palliative care for those patients not meeting the hospice eligibility requirement that led to the recent rapid growth in palliative care in the United States.

In the last decade, there have been huge advances in American palliative care. In 2002, the American Board of Nursing Specialties established a certification in hospice and palliative nursing. In 2006, the National Quality Forum published a National Framework and Preferred Practices for Palliative and Hospice Care Quality that established consensus quality guidelines for standardized palliative care (7). In 2011, a certification programme for hospitals was created by the Joint Commission. Additionally, in 2008, palliative medicine was recognized as a formal sub-speciality by ten parent boards of the American Board of Medical Specialties. Currently, over two-thirds of American hospitals and more than 80% of large American hospitals (those with more than 300 beds) have palliative care teams, and over 6000 physicians are board certified in palliative medicine by the American Board of Medical Specialties (8, 9). Hospice use is also increasing overall (10) with 46% of deaths occurring under the care of one of over 5000 hospices (11). Within the veterans' health care system, the Veterans' Health Care Eligibility Reform Act of 1996 standardized the provision of hospice and palliative care to eligible veterans (12).

Barriers to access to palliative care in the United States

The development of palliative care services has been largely influenced by the American fee-for-service reimbursement system. Current reimbursement mechanisms fail to provide support for the interdisciplinary palliative care team beyond physician reimbursement. Therefore, palliative care teams have largely developed within hospitals where the demonstration of the enhanced quality provided by these teams, in combination with the significant cost savings to hospitals, has provided a strong business case to support their development. Unlike the ambulatory care settings, hospitals receive a lump sum diagnosis-related group payment for an episode of patient care. Thus, interventions like palliative care, that reduce overall patient care costs for hospitals, improve profit margins.

Patients living in the community who are not hospice eligible have had few palliative care options available to them and very little palliative care is provided by generalists. There remains huge regional variation in palliative care. The overall prevalence of hospital palliative care is highest in the densely populated North-east (74%), whereas the South has the lowest prevalence (42% in 2011) (1). Additionally, access to care is itself impacted by physician awareness and practice patterns, as referral to palliative care at most hospitals requires a request for consultation by an attending physician.

Barriers to more widespread use of hospice services in the United States include the inability to accurately prognosticate non-cancer diagnoses, the requirement to relinquish expensive but often beneficial treatments (e.g. radiation therapy, palliative chemotherapy) because such treatments are either forbidden under the hospice benefit or prohibitively expensive given hospice per diem reimbursements, and the link in the minds of clinicians and patients of hospice care with the end of life. As a result, many patients who could bene-fit from hospice care are not eligible or do not receive it under the current programme (13).

Palliative care for patients with dementia is an area of growing importance. A minority of decedents with dementia are referred to a hospice before death (11) and burdensome interventions (e.g. feeding tube placement) are common, despite comfort being a primary goal of care (14). Lack of hospice use may be explained by rigid Medicare prognostic cri-teria, the requirement for facilities to bring in an outside team, and failure to recognize dementia as a terminal illness (15). Although there will be three million Americans in nursing homes in 2030, and these residents (both with and without dementia) want pallia-tive care, palliative care in nursing homes is currently not widely available (16, 17).

Promoting access to and quality of palliative care in the United States

Incentives for delivery of palliative care services for hospitals, nursing homes, and all providers receiving Medicare or Medicaid payment can improve access to care (see Table 9.1). This includes both increased payments to hospitals providing quality pallia-tive care services to patients in high-need categories and financial penalties for failure to provide these services. A key component of the Affordable Care Act for palliative care, in order to increase efficiency and cost savings, is the restructuring of Medicare reim-bursement from 'fee-for-service' to 'bundled payments' in which a single payment is paid to a hospital or physician group for a defined episode of care, rather than individual payments to individual service providers. The Affordable Care Act provides incentives to deliver palliative care outside of hospitals. Despite the potential for palliative and hos-pice care to enhance the ability of new delivery and payment models to improve quality and reduce cost, there is currently no mandate for their inclusion and no certainty about their integration.

Table 9.1 Policies to promote access to and quality of palliative care in the United States*

Category	Initiatives
Health professional training and certification	◆ Invest in palliative care workforce through loan repayment programmes and career development awards. ◆ Increase current cap on graduate medical education slots nationwide. ◆ Ensure adequate numbers of palliative care teaching faculties in the nation's nursing, social work, chaplaincy, and medical schools. ◆ Mandate demonstration of core palliative care competences at both undergraduate and postgraduate medical and nursing education levels as a condition of accreditation. ◆ Require palliative care training for all levels of staff in nursing homes.
Financial licensing and regulatory incentives for care delivery	◆ Increase payments to hospitals and nursing homes providing quality palliative care and hospice services to patients in high-need categories. ◆ Require access to quality non-hospice and hospice palliative care services for eligible beneficiaries in all *Affordable Care Act* proposed models of payment reform (including bundled payments, accountable care organizations, and the patient-centred medical home). ◆ Direct deemed regulatory bodies to develop either a voluntary certificate programme or accreditation requirements for quality palliative care programmes. ◆ Require palliative care services meeting quality guidelines as a condition of accreditation and payment as a regulatory requirement for health care organizations receiving Medicare and Medicaid financing. ◆ Reduce financial incentives to hospitalize nursing home residents and require access to hospice.
Strengthening evidence base through research	◆ Designate government funding to conduct research on prevention and relief of pain and other symptoms and to improve communication, decision support, and care transitions in advanced illness. ◆ Designate funding for career development awards in palliative and hospice care in all appropriate government research funding agencies. ◆ Direct government research funding agencies to develop research centres of excellence in palliative and hospice care. ◆ Direct comparative effectiveness research funding to evaluate palliative care and hospice delivery models, alternative approaches to pain and symptom management, and effective means of communication, decision support, and transitional care coordination for seriously ill patients and their families. ◆ Direct the Secretary of Health and Human Services to conduct demonstrations and pilot projects testing hospital-, nursing home-, and community-based palliative care and hospice programmes for patients with multiple chronic conditions, functional decline, and/or serious illnesses.

* For more expansive list, see Meier 2011 (13).

Furthermore, an inadequate workforce with expertise in palliative care is one of the greatest barriers to access (18). The current capacity of fellowship programmes is insufficient to fill the physician shortage. As outlined in Table 9.1, changes in graduate medical education funding and structures are needed to foster the capacity to train sufficient numbers of physicians and other staff.

Finally, it is imperative that we strengthen our evidence base through research that will guide and measure quality of care. While research funding towards palliative care has increased recently (19), it remains a small percentage of overall funding. A number of initiatives have been undertaken to stimulate and support new palliative care research, e.g. new funding initiatives in palliative care research from the National Institute for Nursing Research, the National Institute of Aging, and the American Cancer Society, and the development of the National Palliative Care Research Centre.

Use of palliative care in Canada

Canada has a universal, publicly funded health care system. Private insurance can be purchased to cover any gaps in the coverage. The federal government sets national standards and provides financial support, but each of the provincial and territorial governments are responsible for administering services.

Palliative care began in Canada with the creation of hospital palliative care units in the 1970s. An institute for research and education in palliative care was created at the University of Ottawa in 1983. The Canadian Hospice Palliative Care Association was developed as a national organization in 1991 (20). In 2000, the Senate of Canada created The Quality End-of-Life Care Coalition of Canada in order to develop a national Canadian strategy for end-of-life care. In 2001, a Minister with Special Responsibility for Palliative Care was appointed and the Secretariat on Palliative and End-of-Life Care at Health Canada was created (21). The Canadian Federal Health Accord of 2003 provided the provinces with federal funding to improve end-of-life care service delivery, home care, and compassionate care benefit for caregivers (22). Canada currently has over 200 palliative care physicians who work either full-time or part-time. All 17 medical schools in Canada provide education in palliative care, and education programmes for nurses, social workers, pharmacists, and pastoral care providers include training in end-of-life care. The national Compassionate Care Benefit gives family caregivers six weeks of paid leave to care for a loved one.

Despite these initiatives, significant disparities across Canada still remain with respect to access and quality of care and out-of-pocket costs to the patient (23). Only a small number of provinces have designated palliative care as a core service under their provincial health plans, leaving funding vulnerable to budget reductions (21). While Canada's physicians are salaried and are not subject to the same 'fee for service' payment incentives as American physicians, a restructuring of the system of care provision is still required, including strengthening the role of palliative care within specialty versus primary care practice.

Palliative care research has remained a priority in Canada over the last decade. The Canadian Institutes for Health Research (Institute of Cancer Research) identified palliative and end-of-life care as one of six original strategic research priorities in 2002. The Canadian Institute for Health Research has a longstanding and growing independent multidisciplinary palliative care study section.

The 'Way Forward Initiative' project, led by the Quality End-of-Life Care Coalition of Canada, is currently working to develop a national framework for the integration of palliative care. The initiative includes specific goals for long-term care residents, acute care, home care, primary care, and federal provincial and territorial governments (24). The Coalition's current priorities, through to 2020, are as follows: (i) ensure all Canadians have access to high-quality end-of-life care; (ii) provide more support for family caregivers; (iii) improve the quality and consistency of palliative care in Canada; and (iv) increase public awareness to expand advance care planning discussion (23) (see Table 9.2).

Table 9.2 Comparison of care structure, usage, quality, and barriers across the United States, Canada, and Mexico

	United States	**Canada**	**Mexico**
Current population	316,000,000 (25)	35,000,000 (26)	112,000,000 (27)
% population 65 years and over	13.7% (25)	14.8% (28)	6.2% (27)
Health care payment system	Public—private system	National health care system	Fractionalized public system with coverage available for uninsured and private sector
Key elements of palliative care	Hospice; in-patient palliative care programmes; community-based palliative care developing	Hospice; in-patient palliative care programmes; community- based palliative care developing	Limited availability of in-patient and community-based palliative care and hospice teams
Physician training/ education	Board certification and palliative care medical sub-specialty; increased medical school training	Board certification and palliative care medical sub-specialty; training across all medical schools	250 palliative care practicing physicians; board certification
Availability/access	Regional variation	Regional variation	Increasing; highly limited in rural areas
Key policy initiatives	◆ Require palliative care services for *Affordable Care Act* models of care. ◆ Increase provider training and palliative care workforce. ◆ Increase research.	◆ Increase support for caregivers. ◆ Increase research. ◆ Increase public awareness.	◆ Build national policy on palliative care. ◆ Increase public education and awareness. ◆ Increase opioid access.

Use of palliative care in Mexico

Mexico's 112 million inhabitants receive their health care from a fractionalized health system composed of a variety of public programmes. Private insurance is mostly used by wealthy residents. A social security administered system covers those who are employed, unless they have private employer-sponsored insurance, while the Seguro Popular programme, created in 2003 (29), was set up to help cover the remaining uninsured population.

Despite major health care reforms in Mexico over the past ten years and recent advances in palliative care legislation, palliative care in Mexico remains limited. In a global comparison of palliative care services (26), Mexico is characterized by 'the development of palliative care activism that is patchy in scope and not well-supported.' The history of palliative care in Mexico is fairly recent. In 1990, an out-patient programme was initiated at the National Institute of Cancer in Mexico City. In 1992, the first palliative care unit was opened in Guadalajara. The first hospice was created in Mexico in 2002 in Guadalajara.

National health policy on palliative care is developing, with new regulations currently underway. The Federal Palliative Care Act was enacted in 2009 and, in 2011, the Ministry of Health included palliative care in insurance coverage. Also in 2011, the Mexican Association of Palliative Care was formed, followed by the Mexican College of Palliative Care in 2012 (30). In 2013, regulation on palliative care was enacted. The Mexican 'Standard of Palliative Care Practice' has been drafted, although not finalized, and calls for the provision of palliative care in the in-patient, out-patient, and home setting.

Board certification is now available to physicians through the Mexican Society of Anesthesiology, and palliative care is in the process of becoming a medical specialty. As of 2012 (30), there are 250 doctors who provide palliative care, 7 hospices, 47 home care teams, 16 community care teams, and 34 in-hospital palliative care units.

It is widely recognized that staff resources and current services in Mexico are simply not sufficient to cover the palliative care needs of the population, despite increased efforts to increase physician and nurse training. In general, health care supply is low. Care for complex or serious medical conditions is heavily regionalized in Mexico and availability of services is especially limited outside of Mexico City, Guadalajara, and Monterrey. There has been an effort to offer training to providers in rural areas where there are few care options. Access and availability of opioids in Mexico is very limited. While there remains little knowledge on the family and provider level regarding basic palliative care (31), government educational campaigns are under way.

Conclusion on policies on palliative care for older people in North America

Table 9.2 compares palliative care structure, usage, quality, and barriers across the United States, Canada, and Mexico. Palliative care policy is at a nascent stage in Mexico, with major strides being made recently, and far more developed in the United States and Canada. Although Canada has a system of national health care, regional disparities remain regarding access to and quality of care. The United States is undergoing major health care reform that may improve access to palliative care due to the increased focus on quality as opposed to volume of care.

Overall, there has been tremendous growth in palliative care across all of North America in the past two decades. Palliative care is moving beyond the cancer setting and is better understood as appropriate for all patients with serious illness, based on patient and family need, and independent of prognosis. Expanded training opportunities, public awareness, and changing regulatory and quality incentives (such as those within the American Affordable Care Act) will expand access to palliative care in coming years. Policy changes throughout North America have, and will remain, integral to the expansion of palliative care services.

References

1 Center to Advance Palliative Care. *Growth of palliative care in US hospitals 2013 snapshot.* Center to Advance Palliative Care; 2013. Available at: <http://www.capc.org/capc-growth-analysis-snapshot-2013.pdf> (Accessed May 2014). Ref. type: online source.

2 **Wright AA, Zhang B, Ray A, Mack JW, Trice E, Balboni T, et al.** Associations between end-of-life discussions, patient mental health, medical care near death, and caregiver bereavement adjustment. *JAMA* 2002; **300**(14):1665–73.

3 **Teno JM, Clarridge BR, Casey V, Welch LC, Welte T, Shield R, et al.** Family perspectives on end-of-life care at the last place of care. *JAMA* 2004; **291**(1):88–93.

4 **Morrison RS, Dietrich J, Ladwig S, Quill T, Sacco J, Tangeman J, et al.** Palliative care consultation teams cut hospital costs for Medicaid beneficiaries. *Health Aff (Millwood)* 2011; **30**(3):454–63.

5 **Kelley AS, Deb P, Du Q, Aldridge Carlson MD, Morrison RS.** Hospice enrollment saves money for Medicare and improves care quality across a number of different lengths-of-stay. *Health Aff (Millwood)* 2013; **32**(3):552–61.

6 **Temel JS, Greer JA, Muzikansky A, Gallagher ER, Admane S, Jackson VA, et al.** Early palliative care for patients with metastatic non-small-cell lung cancer. *NEJM* 2010; **363**(8):733–42.

7 National Quality Forum. *A national framework and preferred practices for palliative and hospice care quality.* Washington, D.C.: National Quality Forum; 2006. Available at: <http://www.qualityforum.org/Publications/2006/12/A_National_Framework_and_Preferred_Practices_for_Palliative_and_Hospice_Care_Quality.aspx> (Accessed May 2014). Ref. type: online source.

8 Center to Advance Palliative Care. 'Palliative care programs continue rapid growth in US hospitals: becoming standard practice throughout the country'. [Press release, 5 April 2010]. New York: Center to Advance Palliative Care; 2010. Available from: <http://www.capc.org/news-and-events/releases/04-05-10> (Accessed May 2014). Ref. type: online source.

9 **Morrison RS.** Models of palliative care delivery in the United States. *Curr Opin Support Palliat Care* 2013; **7**(2):201–6.

10 **Teno JM, Gozalo PL, Bynum JP, Leland NE, Miller SC, Morden NE, et al.** Change in end-of-life care for Medicare beneficiaries: site of death, place of care, and health care transitions in 2000, 2005, and 2009. *JAMA* 2013; **309**(5):470–7.

11 National Hospice and Palliative Care Organization. 2011 *edition: National Hospice and Palliative Care Organization facts and figures; hospice care in America.* National Hospice and Palliative Care Organization; 2012. Available at: <http://www.nhpco.org/sites/default/files/public/Statistics_Research/2011_Facts_Figures.pdf> (Accessed May 2014). Ref. type: online source.

12 **Aldridge MD, Meier DE.** It is possible: quality measurement during serious illness. *JAMA* 2013; **173**(22):2080–81.

13 **Meier DE.** Increased access to palliative care and hospice services: opportunities to improve value in health care. *Milbank Q* 2011; **89**(3):343–80.

14 **Mitchell SL, Teno JM, Kiely DK, Shaffer ML, Jones RN, Prigerson HG, et al.** The clinical course of advanced dementia. *NEJM* 2009; **361**(16):1529–38.

15 **Unroe KT, Meier DE.** Quality of hospice care for individuals with dementia. *J Am Geriatr Soc* 2013; **61**(7):1212–4.

16 **Meier DE, Lim B, Carlson MD.** Raising the standard: palliative care in nursing homes. *Health Aff (Millwood)* 2010; **29**(1):136–40.

17 **Carlson MD, Lim B, Meier DE.** Strategies and innovative models for delivering palliative care in nursing homes. *JAMDA* 2011; **12**(2):91–8.

18 **Lupu D, American Academy of Hospice and Palliative Medicine Workforce Task Force.** Estimate of current hospice and palliative medicine physician workforce shortage. *J Pain Symptom Manage* 2010; **40**(6):899–911.

19 **Gelfman LP, Du Q, Morrison RS.** An update: NIH research funding for palliative medicine 2006 to 2010. *J Palliat Med* 2013; **16**(2):125–9.

20 Canadian Hospice Palliative Care Association. *History*. Ottawa: Canadian Hospice Palliative Care Association; 2014. Available at: <http://www.chpca.net/about-us/history.aspx> (Accessed May 2014). Ref. type: online source.

21 Canadian Hospice Palliative Care Association. *Fact sheet: hospice palliative care in Canada*. Ottawa: Canadian Hospice Palliative Care Association; 2013. Available at: <http://www.chpca.net/media/319587/fact_sheet_hpc_in_canada_fall_2013_final.pdf> (Accessed May 2014). Ref. type: online source.

22 **Dudgeon D, Vaitonis V, Seow H, King S, Angus H, Sawka C.** Ontario, Canada: using networks to integrate palliative care province-wide. *J Pain Symptom Manage* 2007; **33**(5):640–4.

23 Quality End-of-Life Care Coalition of Canada. *Blueprint for action 2010 to 2020*. Quality End-of-Life Care Coalition of Canada; 2010. Available at: <http://www.qelccc.ca/media/3743/blueprint_for_action_2010_to_2020_april_2010.pdf> (Accessed May 2014). Ref. type: online source.

24 The Way Forward. *The Way Forward National Framework*. Ontario: Canadian Hospice Palliative Care Association; 2013. Available at: <http://www.hpcintegration.ca/> (Accessed May 2014). Ref. Type: Online Source.

25 United States Census Bureau. *USA QuickFacts from the US Census Bureau*. Washington, D.C.: The United States Census Bureau; 2014. Available at: <http://quickfacts.census.gov/qfd/states/00000.html/> (Accessed March 2014). Ref. type: online source.

26 Statistics Canada. *Population by year, by province and territory*. The Government of Canada; 2014. Available at: <http://www.statcan.gc.ca/tables-tableaux/sum-som/l01/cst01/demo02a-eng.htm> (Accessed November 2013). Ref. type: online data.

27 **Knaul FM, Gonzalez-Pier E, Gomez-Dantes O, Garcia-Junco D, Arreola-Ornelas H, Barraza-Llorens M, et al.** The quest for universal health coverage: achieving social protection for all in Mexico. *Lancet* 2012; **380**(9849):1259–79.

28 Statistics Canada. *The Canadian population in 2011: age and sex*. The Government of Canada; 2014. Available from: <http://www12.statcan.ca/census-recensement/2011/as-sa/98-311-x/98-311-x2011001-eng.cfm#a6> (Accessed January 2014). Ref. type: online source.

29 **Lynch T, Connor S, Clark D.** Mapping levels of palliative care development: a global update. *J Pain Symptom Manage* 2013; **45**(6):1094–106.

30 **Pastrana T, De Lima L, Wenk R, Eisenchlas J, Monti C, Rocafort J, et al.** *Atlas care palliative Latin ALCP—Mexico*. Houston: International Association for Hospice and Palliative Care Press; 2012.

31 **Okhuysen-Cawley R, Garduno Espinosa A, Paez Aguirre S, Paniagua Nakashima Y, Cardenas-Turanzas M, Reyes Lucas MC, et al.** Pediatric palliative care in Mexico. In: Knapp C et al. (eds). *Pediatric palliative care: global perspectives*. New York: Springer; 2012, 345–58.

Chapter 10

Policies on palliative care for older people in Latin America and the Caribbean

Liliana De Lima, Lilian Hidalgo, Rocío Morante, and Jose Parodi

Introduction to policies on palliative care for older people in Latin America and the Caribbean

Latin America and the Caribbean is an area characterized by its greatly heterogeneous nature. Countries differ greatly in size, Brazil being the largest with over eight million km^2 and almost 200 million inhabitants (or 34% of the regional population) compared with countries like El Salvador which is the smallest (over 21,000 km^2) and Uruguay with only around three million people. Thirteen countries in Latin American and the Caribbean fall into the middle- to high-income levels, while six fall within the low- to middle-income levels. The percentage of people living on less than USD 1.25 per day (adjusted to exchange rate or "purchasing power parity") varies from 0% (Uruguay) to 23.3% (Honduras). the exchange rate adjusts so that an identical good in two different countries has the same price when expressed in the same currency

Non-communicable diseases are currently the main cause of mortality worldwide. An estimated 36 million deaths, or 63% of the 57 million deaths that occurred globally in 2008, were due to non-communicable diseases, comprising mainly cardiovascular diseases (48%), cancers (21%), chronic respiratory diseases (12%), and diabetes (3.5%) (1). According to World Health Organization (WHO) projections, the total number of annual non-communicable diseases deaths will increase to 55 million by 2030 (2). Currently, non-communicable diseases are also the main cause of death and disability in Latin America and the Caribbean. In 2002, they were responsible for 44% of deaths of men and women less than 70 years old and were the main cause of death in one out of two in the total population. Non-communicable diseases contributed to almost 50% of the lost disability adjusted life years in the region.

Data from the Pan American Health Organization—the WHO Regional office for the Americas—show that there is an increasing trend in the number of older people living in the region (3). The report states that:

+ there are approximately 106 million people in the Americas who are over 60 years of age and, in 2050, the number will reach 310 million, of which 190 million will live in Latin America and the Caribbean;

◆ based on demographic tendencies, in 2050, one out of five people will be over 60 years old in Latin America and the Caribbean;

◆ life expectancy is expected to rise in Latin America and the Caribbean to 80 years by the mid 2000s.

This epidemiological and demographic transition, which is replacing infectious diseases with non-communicable diseases as the most common causes of morbidity and mortality, is resulting in a large older population with particular health care needs (4). In addition, this transformation poses challenges in developing countries, including those in Latin America and the Caribbean. For some years, traditional communicable diseases will continue to occur simultaneously with non-communicable diseases, resulting in more disability and terminality (5). This has created a 'double burden of disease' on the health systems of these countries (6), a scenario that social/health services and the community must be prepared to face.

This chapter provides an overview of the health care systems in Latin America and the Caribbean, including current policies, guidelines, and quality indicators, as well as the current status of palliative care and the role of the civil society, and concludes with recommendations on future steps to provide palliative care for older people.

Palliative Care in health care systems in Latin America and the Caribbean

Health expenditure as a percentage of the GDP in the Latin American and Caribbean countries ranges between 10.9% (Costa Rica) and 4.8% (Bolivia). The number of doctors per 10,000 inhabitants ranges from 67.3 (Cuba) to 1.5 (Colombia). These differences indicate some of the challenges that countries face when implementing health care policies, especially when there are regional cross-country initiatives.

Gradually, health systems in the region are dealing with an increasing number of users with physical therapy and palliative care needs. In spite of this, provision is poor. According to data in the *Atlas of Palliative Care in Latin America* published recently by the Latin American Association for Palliative Care, many countries are unable and unprepared to meet the growing demand and it is estimated that only between 5% and 10% of patients who need palliative care services access them, that over 90% of services are located in large urban centres, and more than 50% of patients cannot afford the services or medication (7). Eighty percent of the countries do not recognize palliative care as a discipline and do not include it in public and private health systems. There are 922 palliative care services in total (1.63 services/units/teams per million). Most do not have palliative care or geriatric consultants. Forty six percent of the palliative care services are in two countries (Chile and Argentina), covering 10% of the regional population. The most frequent type of service is at the first level of health care, while the remaining services are at the third level i.e. highly specialized centres in large cities (see Table 10.1).

Table 10.1 Palliative care policies and programmes in Latin America (7)

Country	National PC law	National PC programme/ plan	Audit, monitoring, evaluation	Cancer national programme (includes PC)		HIV/AIDS national programme (includes PC)		Primary assistance national programme (includes PC)		Development resources	Research resources	Opioids: collaboration between prescribers and regulators
Argentina	No*	No	No	Yes	(Yes)	Yes	(Yes)	Yes	(No)	No	Yes†	4.0
Bolivia	No	No	No	No	—	Yes	(No)	Yes	(No)	No	No	1.0
Brazil	No	Yes +	No	Yes	(Yes)	Yes	(Yes)	Yes	(Yes)	No	No	3.5
Chile	Yes	Yes +	Yes	Yes	(Yes)	Yes	(Yes)	Yes	(Yes)	Yes	No	4.0
Colombia	Yes +	No	No	Yes	(Yes)	Yes	(No)	Yes	(No)	No	Yes	3.5
Costa Rica	No	No	Yes	Yes	(Yes)	Yes	(Yes)	Yes	(Yes)	Yes	No	5.0
Cuba	No	Yes +	Yes	Yes	(Yes)	Yes	(Yes)	Yes	(Yes)	Yes	Yes	4.0
Dominican Republic	No	No	No	Yes	(No)	Yes	(No)	Yes	(No)	No	No	3.0
Ecuador	No	No	No	Yes	(Yes)	Yes	(No)	Yes	(No)	No	No	3.0
El Salvador	No	No	No	Yes	(No)	Yes	(No)	Yes	(No)	No	No	2.0
Guatemala	No	No	No	No	—	Yes	(No)	Yes	(No)	No	No	2.0
Honduras	No	No	No	Yes	(No)	Yes	(No)	Yes	(No)	No	No	1.3
Mexico	Yes	Yes	No	Yes	(Yes)	Yes	(Yes)	Yes	(No)	No	Yes	3.0
Nicaragua	No	No	No	Yes	(Yes)	Yes	(No)	Yes	(No)	No	No	1.5

Continued

Table 10.1 (continued) Palliative care policies and programmes in Latin America (7)

Country	National PC law	National PC programme/ plan	Audit, monitoring/ evaluation	Cancer national programme (includes PC)		HIV/AIDS national programme (includes PC)		Primary assistance national programme (includes PC)		Development resources	Research resources	Opioids: collaboration between prescribers and regulators
Panama	Yes	Yes	Yes	Yes	(Yes)	Yes	(No)	Yes	(Yes)	Yes	No	3.5
Paraguay	No	No	No	No	—	Yes	(No)	Yes	(No)	No	No	1.5
Peru	No	Yes +	No	Yes	(Yes)	Yes	(No)	Yes	(Yes)	Yes	No	3.0
Uruguay	No	No	No	Yes	(Yes)	Yes	(Yes)	Yes	(Yes)	No	No	3.7
Venezuela	No*	Yes +	Yes	Yes	(Yes)	Yes	(No)	Yes	(Yes)	No	No	3.0

PC = palliative care

* Existence of federal, state, or municipal laws

+ Related to cancer control programmes

† National Cancer Institute resources

Pain relief is one of the basic components of palliative care and availability and access to opioid analgesics is essential. According to data, pain is frequent in older people and it is estimated that between 40% and 80% of older people with non-cancer pain and 40% with cancer pain do not receive any analgesic treatment (8). Morphine is recognized as essential in the WHO essential medicines list (9) and the preamble to the *Single Convention on Narcotic Drugs* (10) establishes that these medications are indispensable for the relief of pain and suffering, and gives instructions to the member states to take the necessary provisions to assure their availability. However, Latin American and Caribbean countries account for less than 2% of the global consumption of morphine (11), mostly due to stringent laws and regulations which interfere with appropriate prescription and dispensing, and lack of knowledge and skills on how to assess and treat pain appropriately with opioids (12).

Guidelines, standards, and quality indicators in Latin America and the Caribbean

The Latin American Association for Palliative Care's *Atlas* shows that ten countries have at least one published palliative care guideline or standard, and five countries have a service directory. Only Brazil publishes a palliative care journal, which is currently being indexed (7). No specific policies, standards, or quality indicators have been developed for palliative care for older people in the region.

Policy initiatives in Latin America and the Caribbean

For the past three years, the Organization of American States has been working on developing a proposal for a regional resolution for the protection of the rights of older people. This proposal is under development and being coordinated by a working group of Organization of American States representatives from Argentina, Bolivia, Chile, the Dominican Republic, and Uruguay (13).

In a recent development, which has global implications, the WHO included a list of essential medicines in pain and palliative care in the WHO *Model List of Essential Medicines*. The eighteenth edition of the *Model List* includes morphine, oxycodone, and hydromorphone (in all its available formulations) for the management of pain (9).

Role of non-governmental organizations in Latin America and the Caribbean

Civil society, including the Latin American Association for Palliative Care, plays a significant role in the improvement of the quality of the lives of older people and especially in helping to improve access to palliative care. The mission of the Latin American Association for Palliative Care is to promote the development of palliative care in Latin America and the Caribbean through communication between and integration of all groups interested in improving the quality of life of patients with advanced lifethreatening diseases and their families. This and other non-governmental organizations can contribute in many ways, including:

Legislation and norms

 ◆ providing advice to governments and law makers when drafting health programmes and regulations to ensure that the palliative care needs of older people are considered and included;

 ◆ assisting in the process of reviewing national laws and regulations to identify undue restrictions which impede legitimate access to controlled medications and finding ways to eliminate them;

 ◆ facilitating the dialogue between civil society and government representatives.

Appropriate medical and scientific use

 ◆ developing treatment guidelines on the medical and scientific use of controlled medications for the older population;

 ◆ educating and training health care providers in the rational use of controlled medicines and how to prevent diversion under the Conventions.

Monitoring

 ◆ monitoring and providing information on the number of palliative care services, number of providers, and consumption of controlled medications;

 ◆ monitoring and providing information on national policies that may interfere with or impede access to palliative care for older people.

Networking

 ◆ developing international and regional networks of support with organizations and individuals interested in palliative care for older people.

Generating awareness and informing

 ◆ providing information to the general public;

 ◆ developing and implementing advocacy campaigns to generate and increase awareness among the general public about the need to ensure safe and effective access to controlled medications.

Future development required in Latin America and the Caribbean

Policy

The importance of palliative care as an essential component of care is being recognized by health providers, government representatives, and legislators and, more recently, by the WHO Executive Committee, by the adoption of a proposal presented to the World Health Assembly on May 2014 (14).

Primary health assistance is a strategy which has been proved effective to maximize resources in health systems around the world (15) and improve equality of access, and which may be adapted to different socio-economic levels and other political, social, and cultural contexts as well as in palliative care implementation (16).

The following strategies can guide the implementation of a health policy framework for older people, including those with palliative care needs:

1 Development of policies, regulations, laws, rules, programmes, and budgets for palliative care that are compatible with human rights instruments in the UN and the Organization of American States.

2 Development of legal frameworks for palliative care and enforcement of mechanisms for older people in long-term care services. This involves assigning the mechanisms, budget, and adequate staff for supervision of intersectional activities.

3 Encouragement of cooperation among countries in the design of strategies, exchange of capacities, and resources for the building and development of political frameworks related to palliative care.

4 Adoption of the necessary steps to ensure safe access to palliative care and pain treatment medicines, as recommended by the WHO (9).

Education

There are only four countries in the region in which palliative care has official accreditation as a specialty and/or medical sub-specialty (7). Health care professionals need to have the skills, knowledge, and competences to respond to the palliative care needs of older people. Issues related to education regulation, professional accreditation, quality control, certification process, staffing needs, competences and skills, and the strengthening of staff performance are essential to ensure access to palliative care (5). In this regard, the strategy is to provide palliative care training to:

1 health care professionals, managers, and administrators in undergraduate, postgraduate, and continuing education programmes;

2 caregivers such as family members, community promoters, local councils, social services, and churches.

Services

Strategies to achieve the implementation of palliative care services for older people are:

1 establishing primary health assistance quality services for older people with palliative care needs, ensuring access to medicines (including opioids) and adopting implementation tools (17);

2 strengthening prevention and management of life-threatening illnesses and conditions by:

   ◆ including the palliative care needs of older people in the design of programmes and services for the treatment of non-communicable diseases;

- designing, adapting, and using instruments based on evidence in the palliative care treatment of non-communicable diseases and life-threatening conditions (18);
- adapting and using protocols for periodic evaluation of patients at risk of becoming terminally ill or with a terminal disease.

Auditing and monitoring in Latin America and the Caribbean

For many years, the palliative care community has advocated systematic monitoring at national and global levels. Several palliative care organizations have developed reports on the status of palliative care development (19, 20) including, more recently, the Latin American Association for Palliative Care's *Atlas* (7). Member states have no obligation to monitor and report palliative care progress, and the available reports have had limited impact on the provision of care. Recently, the Latin American Association for Palliative Care developed, in collaboration with the Pan American Health Organization and other non-governmental organizations, ten indicators for monitoring and evaluating palliative care in the region: one for public health, three for education, three for structure, and three for medications (21).

For appropriate auditing and monitoring, it is recommended that countries should:

1 implement the Latin American Association for Palliative Care indicators at national level and engage with governments and non-governmental organizations to help collect and report information;

2 strengthen the health system authorities' skills in evaluating and monitoring palliative care;

3 promote the development and spread of the scientific evidence necessary to adapt health interventions to national realities.

Conclusion on policies on palliative care for older people in Latin America and the Caribbean

Access to palliative care services and to pain treatment is limited in Latin America and the Caribbean as a result of lack of political will, insufficient education and information, and excessive regulation of the use of opioid medications. Those mainly affected are the most vulnerable, including marginalized populations, disabled people, children, and older people. Many national health programmes and strategies for life-threatening conditions such as cancer and HIV do not have provisions to ensure access to palliative care and to pain treatment for older people, and the majority do not include provisions to ensure palliative care at all. It is critical that governments in Latin America and the Caribbean, and the rest of the world, take the necessary steps to ensure that palliative care is integrated into health care programmes for all, but especially older people and other vulnerable populations.

References

1 **Alwan A.** Monitoring and surveillance of chronic non-communicable diseases: progress and capacity in high-burden countries. *The Lancet* 2010; **376**(9755):1861–8.

2 World Health Organization. *World Health Statistics 2012*. Geneva: World Health Organization; 2013.

3 Pan American Health Organization. *Health in the Americas*. Washington DC: Pan American Health Organization; 2012.

4 World Health Organization. *The World Health Report 2002: Reducing the Risks, Promoting Healthy Life*. Geneva: World Health Organization; 2002.

5 Ministerio de Salud. *Foro Nacional sobre Enseñanza de Geriatría y Gerontología en el Perú*; 2005. Available at: <http://www.medicina.usmp.edu.pe/investigacion/pdf/CAYJ45AZ..pdf>. Ref. type: online source.

6 **Palloni A, Guido P, Peláez M.** Demographic and health conditions of ageing in Latin America and the Caribbean. *Int J Epidemiol* 2002; **31**(4):762–71.

7 **Pastrana T, De Lima L, Wenk R, Eisenchlas J, Monti C, Rocafort J, et al.** *Atlas of Palliative Care in Latin America*. Houston: International Association for Hospice and Palliative Care Press; 2012.

8 **Bonilla P, Morón C, Quintero F.** Uso de opioides en el adulto mayor. In: Bonilla P, De Lima L, Díaz P, León MX, González M (eds). *Uso de Opioides en Tratamiento del Dolor: Manual Para Latinoamérica*. Houston: International Association for Hospice and Palliative Care Press; 2011.

9 World Health Organization. *Model List of Essential Medicines*. Geneva: World Health Organization; 2013.

10 United Nations. *Single Convention on Narcotic Drugs*. New York: United Nations; 1961.

11 International Narcotics Control Board. *Availability of Internationally Controlled Drugs: Ensuring Adequate Access for Medical and Scientific Purposes*. E/INCB/2010/1/Supp.1. New York: United Nations; 2010.

12 World Health Organization. *Ensuring Balance in National Policies on Controlled Substances*. Geneva: World Health Organization; 2011.

13 Organización de los Estados Americanos. *Proyecto de resolución Proyecto de Convención Interamericana sobre la Protección de los Derechos Humanos de las Personas Mayores* (Presentado por el Grupo de Trabajo y copatrocinado por Argentina, Bolivia, Chile, República Dominicana y Uruguay). Washington DC: OEA; 2013.

14 World Health Organization. *Strengthening of Palliative Care as a Component of Integrated Treatment Within the Continuum of Care*. Geneva: World Health Organization; 2014.

15 **Kickbusch I, Buse K.** Global influences and global responses: international health at the turn of the twenty-first century. In: Merson MH, Black RE, Mills AJ (eds). *International Public Health: Disease, Programs, Systems, and Policies*. Gaithersburg (MD): Aspen Publications; 2001.

16 Committee on the Future Health Care Workforce for Older Americans. *Retooling for an Aging America: Building the Health Care Workforce*. Washington D.C.: The National Academies Press; 2008.

17 **Stjernsward J, Foley K, Ferris F.** The public health strategy for palliative care. *J Pain Symptom Manage* 2007; **33**(5):486–93.

18 **van der Steen JT, Radbruch L, Hertogh CMPM, de Boer ME, Hughes JC, Larkin P, et al.** White paper defining optimal palliative care in older people with dementia: a Delphi study and recommendations from the European Association for Palliative Care. *Palliat Med* 2013; **28**(3):197–209.

19 World Palliative Care Alliance. *Mapping Levels of Palliative Care Development: A Global Update*. London: World Palliative Care Alliance; 2011.

20 **Centeno C, Clark D, Lynch T, Rocafort J, Praill D, De Lima L, et al.** Facts and indicators on palliative care development in 52 countries of the WHO European region: results of an EAPC task force. *Palliat Med* 2007; **21**(6):463–71.

21 **De Lima, L.** How can we monitor palliative care? Suggestions from the Latin American Association for Palliative Care. *Int J Palliat Nurs* 2013; **19**(4):160–1.

Part III

Socio-cultural and clinical context of dying in old age

Chapter 11

Dying in place in old age: public health challenges

Joachim Cohen and Merryn Gott

The place of death for older people as a public health issue

Place is a central concern within palliative care. The hegemonic medical-revivalist death discourse that is so central to palliative care philosophy defines a good death in terms of control, autonomy, dignity, awareness, and heroism (1, 2), and being able to die 'at home' (which may for some people may be a care home) is believed to benefit all those nodal points of a good death. Home dying is argued to promote control over quality of life, increase psychological comfort, and enable people to prepare for death together with their loved ones (3–5). Being a central and, theoretically, easily manipulable outcome, the place of death has therefore long been an important focal point of the palliative care movement and a lot of end-of-life research has focused on factors or strategies that can facilitate a home death (6). However, despite sustained attention for more than four decades, in most countries, the majority of people continue to die in hospitals and the proportion of home deaths is not increasing, and is even decreasing, in most developed countries (7).

In recent years, attention has shifted to an examination of the economic implications of place of end-of-life care. This shift is reflective of the focus within wider health policy in most countries to concentrate care in the community, endorse the desire of people to stay at home as long as possible, and, in particular, promote ageing in place as a strategy to reduce costs associated with institutional care (8). Within palliative care, there has been a particular focus upon unpicking the complex totality of factors which drive hospitalizations at the end of life, in an attempt to identify strategies to prevent hospitalizations which are viewed as not clinically justified or as 'potentially avoidable' (9–12). Indeed, there is a strong economic motive for paying increased interest to minimizing and avoiding hospital use at the end of life as such hospitalizations contribute significantly to total health care expenditure (13–15). Older people are the major users of hospitals at the end of life and are thought to be particularly at risk of potentially avoidable admissions (10) (although the role of ageism in determining attitudes to who is an 'appropriate' hospital user must also be acknowledged (16)). However, while it is important to draw attention to potential economic motivations underlying decision making about place of end-of-life care for older people, it is equally important to acknowledge there is evidence that an admission to hospital for older people can be associated with lower-quality end-of-life care, particularly in terms of psychological, spiritual, and existential care (17–20).

It is therefore apparent that the place of dying and death for older people is an important public health issue for two key reasons. Firstly, place of dying influences the health of older people and their family caregivers (with health defined in line with the WHO definition as a state of complete physical, mental, and social well-being and not merely the absence of disease or infirmity). Secondly, where people die has significant implications for the distribution and efficient use of available resources. The principal challenges for public health policy in relation to the place of death of older people are therefore twofold: firstly, there is the challenge of effectively planning and organizing available resources and care across different settings of end-of-life care, and secondly, there is the challenge of conceiving and pursuing strategies that promote an optimal health situation for people who are dying and, hence, support older people's aspirations regarding where they spend their final days.

In response to these challenges, this chapter provides robust statistical descriptions regarding the patterns of place of death for older people across various countries and continents using population-level death certificate data. The application of such a population-level and cross-national perspective provides important information to address these two public health challenges: it provides an empirical indication for policy as to where end-of-life care resources, support, and strategies should be targeted and, additionally, has the important added value of providing benchmarks for comparison. Furthermore, understanding of cross-national differences can help to identify general health care and specific end-of-life care policies that could influence where people are dying within a country. However, we will also make a case for the need of some kind of 'deconstruction' of these statistics and the truths they convey. Previous authors have tended to present this information as taken for granted evidence which is best interpreted within the context of contemporary constructions of a 'good death' (21). However, we wish to extend the scope of this discussion by helping to develop an understanding of the context within which these statistics need to be interpreted and understood. As such, we will consider some of the socio-cultural and organizational factors that underpin the patterns of place of death observed, as well as challenge some normative assumptions around the meanings of place, and the nature of choice of place, at the end of life. The chapter will conclude by discussing some of the public health challenges regarding the place of death.

Place of death statistics for people aged over 80 years

For the following statistical description of place of death, we draw on data collected as part of the International Place of Death (IPoD) Study. This study collected death certificate data from 13 countries for a full population of deaths for 2008. More information about the project design and the data can be found elsewhere (22). Individual death certificate data were integrated into a common database for analysis. In addition to place of death, the database contains a number of clinical, socio-demographic, and residential characteristics of the deceased. For the purposes of this chapter, only deaths for people aged over 80 years were retained (see Table 11.1).

Table 11.1 Place of death of people aged above 80 in 13 countries

Country	Abbrev.	Total no. of deaths of aged 80 or more	% within all deaths	Place of death (% within deaths of aged 80 or more)			
				Home	Care home	Hospital[a]	Other[b]
Italy	IT	328,270	56.8	44.0	8.9	42.9	4.2
Spain (Andalusia)	ES	30,538	53.2	40.1	11.2	48.2	0.5
England	ENG	253,744	53.3	14.2	27.2	55.2	3.5
France	FR	287,445	53.1	26.6	17.5	52.8	3.0
Wales	WAL	16,782	52.3	13.6	19.9	63.7	2.9
Belgium	BE	52,695	51.8	17.3	36.7	45.3	0.6
The Netherlands	NL	67,970	50.3	17.6	52.8	25.6	4.0
Canada	CA	88,879	48.8	9.3	29.3	56.8	4.6
New Zealand	NZ	14,282	48.7	13.2	47.9	31.6	7.3
United States	US	1,078,024	44.4	20.8	35.6	36.2	7.4
Czech Republic	CZ	41,535	40.8	19.2	24.8	55.0	0.9
Korea	KR	67,522	27.3	31.3	2.9	65.0	0.8
Mexico	MX	139,042	26.3	62.8	—*	34.0	3.2

[a] Category 'hospital' may include palliative care units in hospital in those countries where available.

[b] Category 'other' includes free-standing hospices in those countries where available.

* Not presented as a category on the death certificate in Mexico (due to the fact that there are almost no residential care homes for older people in Mexico).

Analyses revealed large cross-national differences in place of death. For example, the percentage of people dying at home ranged from 9.3% (Canada) to more than 40% (Italy and Spain) and up to 63% (Mexico). High percentages of deaths in care homes or nursing homes were found in the United States (36%), Belgium (37%), New Zealand (48%), and the Netherlands (53%), but a relatively low proportion dying in this setting were found in Spain (11%), Italy (9%), and Korea (3%). While only about a quarter of those aged 80 or above died in hospital in the Netherlands, and about a third in New Zealand, Mexico, and the United States, the proportion doing so amounted to more than 50% in France, Canada, England, and the Czech Republic, and more than 60% in Wales and Korea.

A multivariate binary logistic regression analysis with age as an independent variable and additionally controlling for sex, marital status, and underlying cause of death allowed us to evaluate how the chances of dying in a certain care setting changes as the age of older people increases (not in table). In all countries, the chances of dying in a care home, for those aged 80 or above, increased with age, and the chances of dying in a hospital decreased with age. Interestingly, however, opposing patterns were found regarding the chances of dying at home with increasing age: in most countries, the chances of such decreased with more advanced older age, but in France, Italy, Spain, the Czech Republic, Mexico, and Korea, the chances increased with more advanced older age.

The marked between-country differences in the chances for older people of dying in a nursing home were, to a small extent, explained by differences in the socio-demographic (sex, age, and marital status) and clinical characteristics (causes of death), and, to a somewhat larger extent, by the availability of nursing home beds within the different health care regions within a country. However, a large part of the variation between countries remained unexplained and, thus, needs to be attributed to other factors (Figure 11.1).

The three models shown in Figure 11.1 are binary logistic regression analyses with care home/nursing home versus all other places of death as the outcome variable. Model 1 has country as the independent variable; model 2 adds sex, age, and cause of death (36 categories) as confounders; and model 3 additionally controls for the number of available hospital beds and nursing home/care home beds per capita in the health care region. Comparing the three models allows an evaluation of whether certain variables explain part of the variation between countries. As odds ratios are closer to each other and closer to 1 by adding potentially explaining variables to the model, a part of the variation is explained. For many countries, this is particularly the case in model 3, indicating that the variables entered in this model explain part of the variation (more than the ones entered in model 2). However, the variation remains large and, hence, the conclusion that a large part of the variation between countries remained unexplained and, thus, needs to be attributed to other factors.

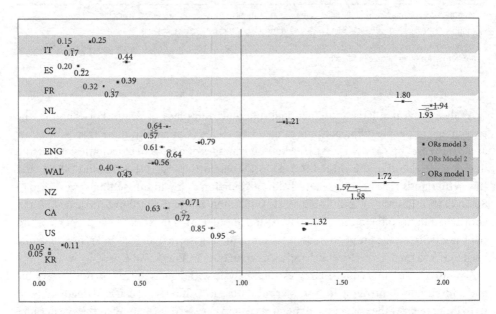

Figure 11.1 Variation between countries in the chances of older people dying in a nursing home, based on 3 logistic regression models. Belgium was used as the reference category

Mexico is not included in the analysis as there was no category of nursing home or care home on the death certificate data.

Challenges of interpretation for public health policy

Our data about the place of death provide robust indications of how different societies are managing one aspect of end-of-life care for their older population. The analyses, revealing very large cross-national differences in where older people die, provide some indications as to how different health policies, including end-of-life care policies, may result in very different places of dying. For example, some countries seem to have strategies that result in lower numbers of older people dying in a hospital. The proportion doing so is relatively low in the Netherlands, New Zealand, and the United States of America. In these countries, this is not countered by a large proportion dying at home (that proportion is rather relatively low) but by a high percentage dying in nursing homes. There are two plausible explanations as to why this pattern is observed: firstly, these countries have a high availability of beds in institutional long-term care settings (23); and/or secondly, they have developed care models in these settings that accommodate high-quality end-of-life care that addresses the specific end-of-life challenges of older people. Both these arguments could be applied to the Netherlands, which has recognized 'elderly care' (formerly called 'nursing home medicine') as a medical specialty and has developed a long-term care model in which there is a permanent presence within the nursing home of a trained 'elderly care' physician. The provision of palliative care in nursing homes is a basic competence of that physician (23, 24). The particular palliative care challenges of illnesses such as dementia are especially addressed, there is a culture of end-of-life care planning and decision making (preventing a lot of end-of-life hospitalizations), and, overall, there is evidence that the quality of end-of-life care provided is high (23, 25).

Conversely, in New Zealand, whilst there is little research evidence regarding the nature of care provided within care homes, models of end-of-life care within the aged residential care sector are not well developed. Rather, high usage of the aged residential care sector for end-of-life care appears to be driven largely by models of care adopted within acute hospitals and the high numbers of aged residential care beds. Indeed, there is evidence that acute hospitals are discharging older people who are in their last days and weeks of life to this setting to die. In a recent study, we found that 10% of people who were discharged into private hospital care (caring for those requiring 24-hour nursing/medical care) from an acute hospital, died within two weeks of their admission, 16% died within one month of their admission, and 36% within six months (26). We concluded that long-term care private hospitals are being used as 'de facto' hospices, but without the support and resources provided to mainstream hospices, or indeed, any a priori health policy directive. In this case, therefore, bed availability in itself appears to be a principal determinant of place of death for older people and additional resources are urgently needed by the aged residential care sector to meet this high level of demand for end-of-life care.

Similarly, the high percentages of older people dying in hospital in countries such as France, Canada, and Korea, can be understood in relation to historical health care organizational choices. In these countries, aspects of long-term care provision are organized in the hospital rather than in separate care homes or nursing homes, leading to a high percentage of hospital deaths. Although it is likely that dying in a long-term care ward within the hospital will be characterized by less acute and perhaps interventionist care, as compared with acute care wards, it can be questioned whether the organization of long-term care within the hospital setting is the most optimal organizational choice in terms of end-of-life care for older people.

Meaning and the need for deconstruction

As much as the presented statistics provide useful public health insights into end-of-life care provision for older people, they also beg for some kind of 'deconstruction'. After all, an overarching issue for this type of large-scale quantitative research is that it can suggest statistical patterns and patterns of association, but it does not allow us to say anything conclusive about social processes that are produced or maintained by those patterns (4) or about their meaning in terms of experiences of dying individuals. There seem to be, along with a number of socio-demographic patterns, cross-cultural patterns in place of death. However, it is difficult to move the conclusions about these patterns beyond ad hoc explanations that are focused on patient choice, funding models, or health care organization. The large country differences may be due to economic differences (for example, differences in the budget) or due to a number of end-of-life care organizational differences. However, even if we would be able to operationalize all those economic or organizational factors and test our hypotheses about them, it still remains unclear whether these political/economic factors are the cause of the changes or difference or whether they are part of broader social processes, such as varieties in processes of health care restructuring, or of wider cultural patterns. While there may be a drive among quantitative public health researchers to operationalize all potential explanatory factors and, thereby, statistically test all hypotheses, the point is that this may not be possible or even desirable. Statistical representations are not self-evident truths and must be countered with work on how we know certain truths to be true, and their meaningfulness in a social context (4).

It is quite common within the biomedical paradigm to translate findings into straightforward public health policy recommendations. A typical (ad hoc and purposely straightforward) interpretation regarding the large cross-national differences in place of death of older people, and its association with the availability of hospital and care home/nursing home beds, is that it reflects different choices of health care systems. The data seem to suggest that different countries have made different organizational choices regarding end-of-life care: some chose to focus on long-term care within specialized and skilled nursing home facilities; others chose to focus on hospitals as places for long-term and end-of-life care; and yet others have relied strongly on primary care and informal care to provide end-of-life care (23, 27). It seems likely that these different choices result in different patterns of health services' use at the end of life.

It has to be acknowledged, however, that these choices are also the result of historical contingencies and that the statistical patterns are, in themselves, probably more a result of these contingencies and the wider processes that have shaped societies than the result of conscious and rational health care system choices. The point is that the findings and their explanations are also embedded within a more complex whole of, for instance, cultural values regarding informal caregiving and the place of older people within the community. This context needs to be adequately understood first before sensible health care policies can be implemented.

Similarly, the striking differences in the proportion of older people dying at home tend to be interpreted within the wider socio-cultural context rather than as the result of rational health care organizational choices. The high proportion of home deaths in Mexico may indeed reflect a lack of alternatives to hospitals (e.g. care homes) and difficulties of accessing the hospital, but in some of the early industrialized European countries such as Italy, Spain, and (to a lesser extent) France, the relatively large proportion of older people dying at home probably also reflects culturally embedded ideas of the role family carers and the wider community should adopt in taking care of older people within the community rather than in institutional settings. These cultural ideals will, of course, influence what end-of-life care organizational strategies countries pursue in different ways. An example of how this is translated into practice was described earlier, in terms of the extent to which increasing (older) age results in a higher chance of home death in some countries but a lower chance of such in others.

An additional issue related to these findings and the tentative conclusions we may want to draw from them regarding differences in terms of quality of end-of-life care concerns the meaning of our outcome variable. What is the meaning of 'home' and what makes it so distinct from a hospital? Some of the assumptions underlying the research can indeed be questioned: for example, is the hospital, as a setting for end-of-life care, really disturbing normal social relations and is home a valid operationalization of control, dignity, or comfort (4)? The next section addresses these issues in more detail.

Meanings of 'place at the end of life' for older people

It is important to preface any discussion about older people with an acknowledgement that ageing does not confer commonality in attitudes or experience. Indeed, how ageing is both understood and experienced will differ markedly, influenced by factors such as socio-economic status, gender, and ethnicity. Cohort differences also exist—the current baby boomer generation, for example, are approaching ageing in a very different way to the generation that went before (28). It is obviously not possible in the space available to do justice to this diversity, but this is the context within which the following must be read and interpreted.

Moreover, we would also concur with key ageing theorists such as Gullette (29) and Gilleard and Higgs (30) that how individuals experience ageing is largely the result of prevailing culture. From a young age, we are socialized into thinking about ageing in terms of decline and loss (29), and ageism is prevalent in the vast majority of societies. It is this framework within which views and opinions are formed by older people and responses to 'the problem of ageing' are framed at a societal level. As we argue in the section 'Choices relating to place of death', this matters when we are thinking about the preferred place of end-of-life care and death for older people and, in particular, the concept of 'choice'. We will explore these ideas through discussions of meanings afforded to 'home' within an end-of-life context.

Meanings of 'home' for older people

As we have already argued, home dying is central to the revivalist 'good death' and accepted almost universally by researchers, practitioners, and policy makers as the ideal to which we should all aspire. While some of us may be wary of the motivating factors behind the drive to promote end-of-life care at home on the part of policy makers, there is no doubt that this discourse has gained primacy at an academic level, with home dying typically promoted in a very uncritical manner and its meaning taken for granted. In response to this trend, a recent exposition of the meanings of 'home' within an end-of-life context argued that this romanticized idealization of home can only really be fully understood in juxtaposition to contemporary concerns about over-medicalized dying. Indeed:

> The very essence of home as a concept within a palliative care context could be argued to be partly constructed in response to this threat: if hospital deaths bring to mind excessive intervention and lack of control, home comes to represent the opposite—choice and comfort. (31)

In line with new thinking by geographers working in related areas (32), this way of framing 'home' views it not as a static physical location, but rather a 'spatial imaginary: a set of intersecting and variable ideas and feelings, which are related to context, and which construct places, extend across spaces and scales, and connect places' (32). For researchers used to working within a bio-medical paradigm, this may at first glance seem nonsensical and, at second glance, not have anything to do with the practical realities of the delivery of end-of-life care. However, as we will go on to argue, it offers a new perspective on this issue that brings with it a host of very practical possibilities for reframing how we think about 'place' within the context of death and dying.

Thinking more critically about what we mean by 'home' is helpful in interpreting survey data of preferences for place of care. Many palliative care research papers cite such data to support their argument that most people want to die at home. However, these claims ignore the nuances of preference that have been identified in previous research: for example, widowed people (33) and those who live alone (34) have been found in some (but not all) previous research to be less likely to express a preference for a home death. When we turn to look specifically at older people, there is (again inconsistent) evidence that older people may be more likely to prefer non-home dying than younger people (35, 36). Despite the fact that evidence is equivocal, policy directives in many countries seem to overwhelmingly support home dying.

Nevertheless, academics from other disciplines are beginning to acknowledge that quantitative approaches by themselves are not sufficient to understand the complexities of how 'home', as a concept, is understood (32). Indeed, it is only when qualitative researchers start unpicking these preferences, as well as exploring the lived realities of home dying, that it becomes apparent that, in choosing the response category 'home', participants may not be solely, or even predominantly, expressing preferences for physical location. For example, research has highlighted the ways in which 'home' can become institutionalized when care is delivered there (37–39), as well as the converse—institutions such as hospitals can become 'homely' when the space becomes familiar and 'family-like' relationships are established with staff (9). Similarly, a recent study exploring 'the beliefs, attitudes and expectations expressed by older South Asians living in East London about dying at home' concluded that the physical place of death was perceived to be less important to participants than the opportunity for certain cultural and religious practices to be conducted at the time of death (40).

The contradictory meanings of home are exemplified well by discussions about residential or nursing care 'homes'. The Department of Health for England, for examples, asserts the following: 'The End-of-life Care Strategy states that, wherever possible, people should be able to spend their last days in the place of their choosing. Most people say that they would prefer to get this support in their own home. For people who move to live in a care home, that becomes their home.' (41) However, older residents of 'care homes' are themselves more equivocal. For example, an interesting study by Lewinson and colleagues (42) which used photo voice techniques with older residents of an 'assisted living' facility in the United States, identified that 'home' to them incorporated three elements: the physical, the psychological, and the social. The aspect of the facility that rendered it least 'home-like' for most participants was the lack of planned activities to foster a home-like community within the facility. A very practical recommendation from the study was, therefore, to increase the range and frequency of activities for residents. This is an example of how the meaning of place can be manipulated, even when the place itself remains the same.

Choices relating to place of death

The End-of-life Care Strategy for England includes the word 'choice' 45 times (43), providing a good indication of the importance afforded to choice and autonomy within palliative care policy and delivery internationally (44, 45). Place of death is one of the key 'choices' that is focused upon perhaps, as we have already argued, because it is seemingly straightforward and easy to measure. However, the extent to which choice is either desirable or practical within an end-of-life context, in particular for older people, has been questioned. Agledahl et al. (46), for example, highlight the gap between conceptual understandings of 'informed choice' and the everyday realities of medical practice, arguing that: 'The options patients do confront are somewhat arbitrarily constructed within the narrow framework of both what is deemed medically appropriate and how the health care system is organised practically' (46). Drought and Koenig (47) apply this argument to end-of-life care, identifying that choice within this context is 'predicated on three unacknowledged assumptions': firstly, that the time of death can be accurately predicted and that information shared with, and understood by, the patient; secondly, that there are actually choices to be made given 'the availability of resources or the constraints of physiology'; and finally, and they argue most problematically, that we are all able to accept, and engage with, our dying in a logical, rational manner. They finish by arguing that we need to move beyond 'meaningless recitation of non-existent choices—such as dying at home if one is elderly and alone' (47).

The ability to engage in decision making, and have these decisions enacted, is influenced by key social and demographic factors. Within palliative care, we rarely acknowledge that power is distributed unevenly within society, meaning that some groups are more able to exercise choice than others. This is perhaps one reason why in many countries, hospice and specialist palliative care services, a scarce resource, are predominantly accessed by white, middle-class people. Moreover, a recent study identified that older people would prefer to die in a hospice, but are much less likely to do so than younger people (36), adding weight to the argument that ageism is a determinant of specialist palliative care usage (48). Similarly, in New Zealand, racism has been invoked as a reason why **Māori** and Pacific people are less likely to die in hospices than New Zealand Europeans, although congruence in cultural ideals around good dying must also be a consideration (49). Culturally related constraints around choice have also been identified in New Zealand for Asian patients: hospital clinicians report that many Asian patients prefer interventionist care up until the point of death as 'good dying' within their cultural context involves demonstrating that all possible treatment was given (9). However, this view not only clashes with dominant cultural understandings of the 'good death' but also has significant resource implications which will again limit choice at an individual level.

Critical gerontologists Higgs and Gilleard (50) take the debate around choice and ageing a step further. Whilst they identify choice as a central feature of ageing for those in the 'third age', as exemplified by the current baby boomer generation who are redefining what it means to be 'old', they argue that a 'fourth age' exists beyond this, which they define, by contrast, as a time when individual agency is rarely exercised and there is 'no reason to trust that previous agentic choices will ever be honoured or acted upon' (50). Whilst this may be an oversimplification of the lived realities of the oldest old to make an important theoretical point, there is no doubt that both cohort and social contextual factors constrain choices in later life, including those relating to place of living and place of death. Lavoie et al (51), for example, identify that the ability to exercise autonomy around care decisions such as place of care and death is shaped by the availability and willingness of informal carers, a resource which may not be available to many older people (51). Moreover, as Seymour et al. (52) concluded from research conducted with older people living in the North of England, decision making is typically relational rather than individualistic as the palliative care paradigm typically assumes. Older people, in thinking about where they want to die, make decisions in the best interests of the collective (i.e. their family) rather than the individual (i.e. themselves).

Conclusions on the public health challenges of place of dying in old age

The place of dying and death for older people is an important public health issue as it influences both the health and well-being of older people and their families and the distribution and efficient use of available resources for end-of-life care. Robust population-level statistics about patterns in place of death of older people (such as the ones presented in our chapter) provide indispensable empirical indications to inform public health policy makers in deciding where end-of-life care resources, support, and improvement strategies should be targeted. Adding a cross-national comparison to this also provides an opportunity to examine policy and health care organizational factors influencing patterns of place of death and to identify strategies that may change such patterns (e.g. reduce the number of hospital deaths) if desired.

However, other types of research evidence (e.g. qualitative work), critical thinking, and an engagement with social theory are equally indispensable in order to understand the context within which statistical patterns should be interpreted, as well as their meaningfulness within this context, and in order to inform the resulting public health policy. We have highlighted some of the issues that particularly need critical consideration in order to move towards sensible public health suggestions regarding place of end-of-life care: firstly, whether statistical patterns can straightforwardly be interpreted within a 'good death' paradigm (as is usually the case); secondly, whether categories of place are fixed physical locations; and thirdly, to what extent choice is a factor that ideally and realistically underpins all decisions about place of care, especially for older people.

References

1 Seale C, van der Geest S. Good and bad death: introduction. *Soc Sci Med* 2004; **58**(5):883–5.

2 Steinhauser KE, Clipp EC, McNeilly M, Christakis NA, McIntyre LM, Tulsky JA. In search of a good death: observations of patients, families, and providers. *Ann Intern Med* 2000; **132**(10):825–32.

3 Bowling A. The hospitalization of death: should more people die at home? *J Med Ethics* 1983; **9**(3):158–61.

4 Brown M, Colton T. Dying epistemologies: an analysis of home death and its critique. *Environ Plann A* 2001; **33**(5):799–821.

5 Cohen J, Wilson DM, Thurston A, MacLeod R, Deliens L. Access to palliative care services in hospital: a matter of being in the right hospital. Hospital charts study in a Canadian city. *Palliat Med* 2012; **26**(1):89–94.

6 Tang S. Place of death and end-of-life care. In: Cohen J, Deliens L (eds). *A Public Health Perspective on End of Life Care*. Oxford: Oxford University Press; 2012, 21–34.

7 Houttekier D, Cohen J, Surkyn J, Deliens L. Study of recent and future trends in place of death in Belgium using death certificate data: a shift from hospitals to care homes. *BMC Public Health* 2011; **11**.

8 Kaspers PJ, Pasman HR, Onwuteaka-Philipsen BD, Deeg DJ. Changes over a decade in end-of-life care and transfers during the last 3 months of life: a repeated survey among proxies of deceased older people. *Palliat Med* 2013; **27**(6):544–52.

9 Gott M, Frey R, Robinson J, et al. The nature of, and reasons for, 'inappropriate' hospitalisations among patients with palliative care needs: a qualitative exploration of the views of generalist palliative care providers. *Palliat Med* 2013; **27**(8):747–56.

10 Gott M, Gardiner C, Ingleton C, et al. What is the extent of potentially avoidable admissions amongst hospital inpatients with palliative care needs? *BMC Palliat Care* 2013; **12**:9.

11 Reyniers T, Houttekier D, Cohen J, Pasman HR, Deliens L. The acute hospital setting as a place of death and final care: a qualitative study on perspectives of family physicians, nurses and family carers. *Health Place* 2014; **27C**:77–83.

12 Reyniers T, Houttekier D, Cohen J, Pasman HR, Deliens L. What justifies a hospital admission at the end of life? A focus group study on perspectives of family physicians and nurses. *Palliat Med* 2014; **28**(7):941–8.

13 Gardiner C, Ward S, Gott M, Ingleton C. Economic impact of hospitalisations among patients in the last year of life: an observational study. *Palliat Med* 2014; **28**(5):422–9.

14 Fassbender K, Fainsinger RL, Carson M, Finegan BA. Cost trajectories at the end of life: the Canadian experience. *J Pain Symptom Manage* 2009; **38**(1):75–80.

15 Fassbender K, Sutherland L. Economic and health-related consequences of individuals caring for terminally ill cancer patients in Canada. In: Cohen J, Deliens L (eds). *A Public Health Perspective on End of Life Care*. Oxford: Oxford University Press; 2012, 60–69.

16 Tadd W, Hillman A, Calnan M, Calnan S, Read S, Bayer A. From right place—wrong person, to right place—right person: dignified care for older people. *J Health Serv Res Policy* 2012; **17**(Suppl 2):30–36.

17 Yao CA, Hu WY, Lai YF, Cheng SY, Chen CY, Chiu TY. Does dying at home influence the good death of terminal cancer patients? *J Pain Symptom Manage* 2007; **34**(5):497–504.

18 Escobar Pinzón LC, Weber M, Claus M, et al. Factors influencing place of death in Germany. *J Pain Symptom Manage* 2011; **41**(5):893–903.

19 Curtis JR, Patrick DL, Engelberg RA, Norris K, Asp C, Byock I. A measure of the quality of dying and death: initial validation using after-death interviews with family members. *J Pain Symptom Manage* 2002; **24**(1):17–31.

20 Higginson IJ, Sarmento VP, Calanzani N, Benalia H, Gomes B. Dying at home—is it better: a narrative appraisal of the state of the science. *Palliat Med* 2013; **27**(10):918–24.

21 Van Brussel L, Carpentier N (eds). *The Social Construction of Death. Interdisciplinary Perspectives*. Basingstike, New York: Palgrave Macmillan; 2014.

22 Cohen J, Bilsen J, Miccinesi G, et al. Using death certificate data to study place of death in 9 European countries: opportunities and weaknesses. *BMC Public Health* 2007; **7**(1):283 .

23 van der Steen J, Helton M, Sloane P, Ribbe M. Palliative care in institutional settings. In: Cohen J, Deliens L (eds). *A Public Health Perspective on End of Life Care*. Oxford: Oxford University Press; 2012, 122–34.

24 Koopmans RT, Lavrijsen JC, Hoek JF, Went PB, Schols JM. Dutch elderly care physician: a new generation of nursing home physician specialists. *J Am Geriatr Soc* 2010; **58**(9):1807–9.

25 van Uden N, Van den Block L, van der Steen JT, et al. Quality of dying of nursing home residents with dementia as judged by relatives. *Int Psychogeriatr* 2013; **25**(10):1697–707.

26 Connolly MJ, Broad JB, Boyd M, Kerse N, Gott M. Residential aged care: the de facto hospice for New Zealand's older people. *Australas J Ageing* 2013; **33**(2):114–20.

27 Kringos D, Boerma W, Bourgueil Y, et al. The strength of primary care in Europe: an international comparative study. *Br J Gen Pract* 2013; **63**(616):e742–50.

28 Gilleard CJ, Higgs P. Third age versus fourth age studies. *Gerontologist* 2012; **52**:559.

29 Gullette M. *Aged by Culture*. Chicago: University of Chicago Press; 2004.

30 Gilleard C, Higgs P. *Cultures of Ageing: Self, Citizen and the Body*. Harlow: Prentice Hall; 2000.

31 Gott M, Moeke-Maxwell T, Williams L. The paradoxes of 'home' within a palliative and end-of-life care context. In: Roche M, Mansvelt J, Prince R, Gallagher A (eds). *Engaging Geographies: Landscapes, Lifecourses and Mobilities*. Newcastle-upon-Tyne: Cambridge Scholars Publishing; 2014 (in press).

32 Blunt A, Dowling R. *Home*. London: Routledge; 2006.

33 Wilson DM, Cohen J, Deliens L, Hewitt JA, Houttekier D. The preferred place of last days: results of a representative population-based public survey. *J Palliat Med* 2013; **16**(5):502–8.

34 Aoun SM, Skett K. A longitudinal study of end-of-life preferences of terminally-ill people who live alone. *Health Soc Care Community* 2013; **21**(5):530–5.

35 Iecovich E, Carmel S, Bachner YG. Where they want to die: correlates of elderly persons' preferences for death site. *Soc Work Public Health* 2009; **24**(6):527–42.

36 Gomes B, Higginson IJ, Calanzani N, et al. Preferences for place of death if faced with advanced cancer: a population survey in England, Flanders, Germany, Italy, the Netherlands, Portugal and Spain. *Annals of Oncology* 2012; **23**(8):2006–15.

37 Gott M, Seymour J, Bellamy G, Clark D, Ahmedzai S. Older people's views about home as a place of care at the end of life. *Palliat Med* 2004; **18**(5):460–7.

38 Brown M. Hospice and the spatial paradoxes of terminal care. *Environ Plann A* 2003; **35**(5):833–51.

39 Twigg J. The spatial ordering of care: public and private in bathing support at home. *Sociol Health Ill* 1999; **21**(4):381–400.

40 Venkatasalu MR, Seymour JE, Arthur A. Dying at home: a qualitative study of the perspectives of older South Asians living in the United Kingdom. *Palliat Med* 2014; **28**(3):264–72.

41 Department of Health. *End of Life Care Strategy: Fourth Annual Repor.* National Health System; 2012. Available at: <https://www.gov.uk/government/uploads/system/uploads/attachment_data/file/136486/End-of-Life-Care-Strategy-Fourth-Annual-report-web-version-v2.pdf>.

42 Lewinson T, Robinson-Dooley V, Grant KW. Exploring 'home' through residents' lenses: assisted living facility residents identify homelike characteristics using photovoice. *J Gerontol Soc Work* 2012; **55**(8):745–56.

43 Department of Health. *End of Life Care Strategy. Promoting High Quality Care for All Adults at the End of Life.* National Health System; 2008. Available at: <https://www.gov.uk/government/publications/end-of-life-care-strategy-promoting-high-quality-care-for-adults-at-the-end-of-their-life>.

44 Lau R, O'Connor M. Behind the rhetoric: is palliative care equitably available for all? *Contemp Nurse* 2012; **43**(1):56–63.

45 Brogaard T, Neergaard MA, Sokolowski I, Olesen F, Jensen AB. Congruence between preferred and actual place of care and death among Danish cancer patients. *Palliat Med* 2013, **27**(2):155–64.

46 Agledahl KM, Førde R, Wifstad A. Choice is not the issue: the misrepresentation of health care in bioethical discourse. *J Med Ethics* 2011; **37**(4):212–5.

47 Drought TS, Koenig BA. 'Choice' in end-of-life decision making: researching fact or fiction? *Gerontologist* 2002; **42** SpecNo 3:114–28.

48 Gardiner C, Cobb M, Gott M, Ingleton C. Barriers to providing palliative care for older people in acute hospitals. *Age Ageing* 2011; **40**(2):233–8.

49 Frey R, Gott M, Raphael D, et al. 'Where do I go from here'? A cultural perspective on challenges to the use of hospice services. *Health Soc Care Community* 2013; **21**(5):519–29.

50 Higgs P, Gilleard C. Departing the margins—social class and later life in a second modernity. *Journal of Sociology* 2006; **42**(3):219–41.

51 Lavoie JG, Forget EL, Dahl M, Martens PJ, O'Neil JD. Is it worthwhile to invest in home care? *Healthc Policy* 2011; **6**(4):35–48.

52 Seymour J, Gott M, Bellamy G, Ahmedzai SH, Clark D. Planning for the end of life: the views of older people about advance care statements. *Soc Sci Med* 2004; **59**(1):57–68.

Chapter 12

Symptoms and trajectories experienced by older people approaching and at the end of life: implications for care

Liesbeth Van Vliet, Bárbara Antunes, and Irene J Higginson

Introduction

Older people form a heterogeneous group (1). They differ according to personal, demographic, cultural, clinical, and other characteristics and should, thus, be considered as individuals. That being said, they do often suffer from physical, psychosocial, and spiritual symptoms and have one or more diseases influencing their end-of-life trajectory. These multifaceted issues highlight the demand for appropriate palliative care. However, this is not always achieved. There is an urgent need for better assessment of older people's individual palliative care needs and for action on them. In this chapter, we first discuss circumstances in which older people die, their main symptoms, comorbidities, and end-of-life trajectories, taking into account individual variability. Secondly, we address main barriers to accessing and using palliative care services for this population. Finally, we describe the importance of measurement to achieve high-quality palliative care for older people from the individual and public health perspectives, including considerations for the future of measurement. Our aim is to contribute to the setting of priorities for both clinical care and public health policy aimed at improving palliative care for older people.

Circumstances in which older people approach the end of life

Symptoms and unmet needs in older people

Not only do older people approaching the end of life experience multiple symptoms but some of these problems seem to be more common than in younger age groups (2). With increasing age, people increasingly experience problems in several physical domains (e.g. mobility) and non-physical domains (e.g. mental disorders) (1). In the physical domain, pain, urinary incontinence, constipation, and anorexia are often reported (3, 4). In the psychological domain, depression is prevalent at the end of life, with estimates of 15% (5), and that prevalence possibly increases with increasing age (4). Often occurring along-side psychological issues, older patients can also be prone to experiencing social problems (see (6) for an overview) such as receiving less informal caregiver support than younger patients (4). They can have low contact with friends and, to a lesser extent, family (7). Lastly, when spiritual issues such as 'unfinished business', 'involvement and control', and 'a positive outlook' are not responded to (e.g. by empathic, compassionate care), existential distress, including feelings of fear and hopelessness, can develop (8).

Although not all older people experience these and other symptoms, when they do, the symptoms are not always controlled. One example is pain, which seems to be both under-reported by older patients and undertreated (9). In one study among older hospitalized patients, pain was an important symptom affecting 67%. However, it was only treated in half of cases and 74% reported that therapy had little or no effect (10). The importance of relieving pain is highlighted by a qualitative study showing that only when pain is con-trolled is there room for psychosocial needs to emerge in older patients (11). Also, depres-sion seems poorly recognized and treated, as illustrated in an older sample of people with Parkinson's disease; a third met the criteria for depressive disorder, which was only treated in a third of these, while half of those taking an antidepressant still met the criteria for de-pressive disorder (12). Lastly, a study on spiritual distress found that among patients with advanced cancer (although mean age was 56.8 years), the spiritual needs of 72% were met by the medical system only in a limited way (13).

Furthermore, symptoms in this population should be interpreted alongside increasing disabilities. Davies and Higginson have pointed out that (i) the cumulative psychological impact of minor problems is greater in older people while (ii) problems of illness must be seen against a background of possible physical/mental impairment and social and eco-nomic hardship. Moreover, (iii) older people are often affected by multiple diseases and conditions and (iv) the cumulative effect of having multiple conditions might be bigger than the individual effects (9). So, despite heterogeneity, many older patients face high symptom needs that are not always controlled, and might also experience a greater burden of symptoms due to their increased vulnerability in all life domains.

Symptoms and needs with different diseases among older people

While older people approaching death are likely to suffer from multiple progressive and disabling diseases rather than a single disease (14), the level of multi-morbidity also in-creases with age. It has been estimated that more than 80% of people aged over 85 ex-perience several chronic conditions (15). Palliative care for patients with co-morbidities includes treating the primary disease while managing chronic co-morbidities and geriat-ric symptoms (16). In Europe, the most fatal diseases among people aged over 65 include cancer, heart diseases, and cerebrovascular diseases (including vascular dementia) (17).

Many studies focus on the needs of older cancer patients. Women often die from breast and colorectal cancer, and men from lung, colorectal, and prostate cancer (17). According to a meta-analysis, fatigue is the most prevalent physical symptom in older cancer patients, affecting an estimated 78%, followed by excretory problems (76%), urinary incontinence

(71%), asthenia (67%), and pain (66%) (18). Older patients experience more functional disability throughout the year before death than do younger patients (19). In the psychological domain, anxiety and depression are often mentioned as problems (18, 20), affecting an estimated 50% of patients (18). The question of whether older cancer patients are at greater risk of developing psychological distress than younger patients yields some seemingly conflicting answers (6). There is some evidence that older cancer patients have a lower need for psychosocial support than younger patients—perhaps due to a cohort effect or because younger patients are at a different stage regarding work, children, and relationships (21). However, other life events and losses pose particular challenges for the psychological functioning of older people (22). Indeed, social challenges such as isolation, living alone, and having reducing social support pose a threat to psychosocial and spiritual well-being (6).

Looking at heart disease, a different picture emerges. In England, cardiovascular diseases are the main cause of death, especially in older age groups. The prevalence of coronary heart disease is 28.6% for males and 19.3% for females aged over 75 (23). Patients with heart disease experience several physical symptoms such as pain (41–77%), fatigue (69–82%) and breathlessness (60–88%) (20). Psychosocial problems are also often reported including anger, frustration, anxiety, and depression, with carers also experiencing anxiety (24). Exacerbations, including hospital admissions, constrict the patient's social world and can produce acute anxiety. Physical disability and social isolation generate low mood. Overall, spiritual well-being decreases over time, with some fluctuations reported throughout the trajectory (25).

Lastly, an exponential increase in dementia is foreseen for the future, affecting an estimated 44 million people worldwide in 2013, rising to an estimated 136 million by 2050 (26). Most people diagnosed with dementia are older people. Their prognosis is variable and depends on factors such as age, with decreasing life expectancies for increasing age (27). During the disease trajectory, symptoms progress over time in different domains. Most notably, functional decline can be expected in memory, reasoning, communication skills, and the ability to carry out daily activities. Other symptoms include depression and aggression (28). These pose challenges to communication and to the chances of a patient's wishes at the end of life being respected. They also add to the burden on caregivers who are especially at risk when patients experience behavioural problems (29). The wish for, and the problems in enjoying meaningful activities and relationships (30) are characteristic of the spiritual needs of community-dwelling dementia patients.

Distinct trajectories—time for a new perspective

Different diseases have been linked, theoretically, to different end-of-life trajectories (31, 32). The first proposed trajectory, which has been linked to cancer, is one of steady progression and a short, clearly identifiable terminal phase. Patients can have a reasonably good level of functioning, followed by a rapid deterioration and a relatively short terminal phase. A second trajectory, illustrated by heart disease and other organ failures, is one of a more gradual decline with intermittent serious episodes. Any exacerbation may lead to death, although most people will survive and continue functioning on a somewhat lower level after each episode. The prognosis remains uncertain, and many people still die relatively unexpectedly. The last trajectory is one of frailty and prolonged dwindling, as often seen in dementia. Patients start at a relatively low baseline of functioning and gradually deteriorate over time.

There is some empirical data to support these conceptual models, although coming from cohort and retrospective studies. In one study, persons aged 65 and older were interviewed annually about their physical functioning. The participants who provided interview data in their last year of life were evenly distributed in 12 cohorts, depending on the time in months between interview and death. Results showed that cancer patients functioned relatively well early in their last year of life but functioning declined sharply in the last months of life. People dying from organ failure showed more variation in functional ability; and the frailty group were the most disabled throughout the year (33). The sharp decrease in functioning for cancer patients nearing the end of life, in comparison with other patient groups, has also been reported by a retrospective study including next of kin reports (34).

However, recent longitudinal data has challenged the existence of distinct end-of-life trajectories. In one large study of older people, disability levels were assessed monthly. Five distinct end-of-life trajectories were found in the last year of life, ranging through no disability, catastrophic disability, accelerated disability, progressive disability, to persistently severe disability. Only for dementia patients was a dominant trajectory of persistently severe disability apparent over time. The other diseases, including cancer and organ failure, were not characterized by a specific trajectory (35) (Figure 12.1). This is in line with findings from Higginson et al. (36) that in cancer patients approaching death, multidimensional

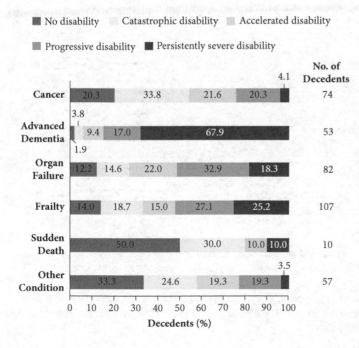

Figure 12.1 Distribution of disability trajectories in the last year of life, according to condition leading to death. The values within the bars are the percentages of decedents with the disability trajectories.

From *The New England Journal of Medicine*, Thomas M. Gill, Evelyne A. Gahbauer, Ling Han, et al., Trajectories of Disability in the Last Year of Life, 362 (13), pp. 1173-1180, DOI: 10.1056/NEJMoa0909087 Copyright © 2010, Massachusetts Medical Society. Reprinted with permission from Massachusetts Medical Society.

symptoms could both improve and worsen over time. Another study (37) reported that, over a six-month period, both a cancer cohort (using a backward trajectory) and a chronic obstructive pulmonary disease cohort (using a forward trajectory), on a group level, experienced increased breathlessness. However, at individual patient level, variable trajectories were observed and a fluctuating pattern was most present (Figure 12.2). It should be noted,

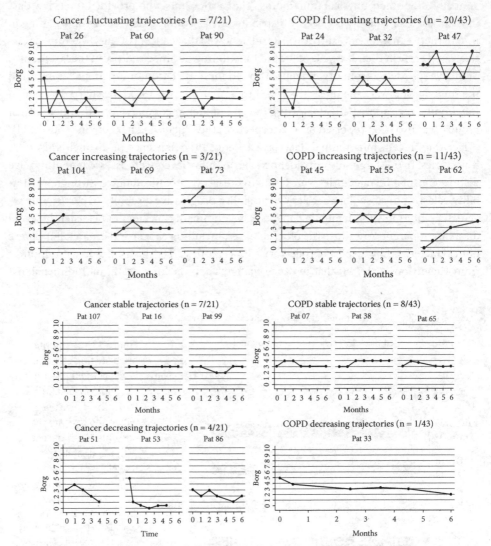

Figure 12.2 Patterns of fluctuating and increasing and stable and decreasing breathlessness trajectories in cancer and chronic obstructive pulmonary disease patients. Breathlessness measured on the Modified Borg Scale.

Reproduced from Claudia Bausewein, Sara Booth, Marjolein Gysels, Robert Kühnbach, Birgit Haberland, and Irene J Higginso, *Palliatve Medicine*, 24 (8), pp. 777–786, doi:10.1177/0269216310378785, copyright © 2010 by SAGE Publications. Reprinted by permission of SAGE.

however, that not all persons died in the study period. Finally, a longitudinal study in a small sample of heart failure patients approaching death also failed to find a clear pattern of a physical limitation trajectory 24 to 3 months prior to death (38).

So, although theoretically appealing, the concept of distinct end-of-life trajectories may need to be reconsidered. Longitudinal data at individual level shows more variation in end-of-life trajectories for discrete diseases then initially assumed. This finding does not seem to be limited to the aforementioned disease groups. For example, symptom trajectories also seem to fluctuate in Parkinson's disease (39). Moreover, even if diseases follow certain patterns (as in the study of Bausewein et al. (37), this does not mean that all individuals with that illness will follow the pattern.

When trying to explain some of the variations in end-of-life trajectories, it is useful to take co-morbidities into account. It has been suggested that when people have multi-morbidities, the most rapidly progressing trajectory dominates (32). However, this could be an oversimplification, especially for older people, as the effects of diseases can interact, and cumulate symptom burden, leading to more variable trajectories. Interestingly, these variations do not seem to imply that different older people experience very different symptoms at the end of life; on the contrary, symptoms such as pain, fatigue, and breathlessness are prevalent in many diseases, including cancer and heart failure (20). So, taking into account individual variability, commonalities at the end of life might be more noticeable than differences between different diseases.

Barriers to accessing and using palliative care

While older patients form a heterogeneous group and should, thus, be seen as individuals, they are also prone to experiencing multiple diseases and symptoms that may interact and accumulate against a background of increased vulnerability. On a population level, diseases may be characterized less by their distinct end-of-life trajectories and more by common prevalent ymptoms. Taking these findings into account, it might appear obvious that older people would access palliative care to a great extent. However, although the mean or median age of people receiving palliative care has indeed been estimated to be around the upper 60s to low 70s, the likelihood of being referred to palliative care is higher for younger patients (40).

It is not clear why older people access palliative care less, but several factors might contribute to this situation. On a patient and carer level, Walshe et al. (40) have postulated several reasons although discerned many as well. We will look at three of these possible reasons. Firstly, it has been suggested that older people have less complex symptoms or needs. However, in line with Walshe et al. (40), we have described how older people do seem to experience high needs and a high symptom burden. Secondly, older people might have different attitudes towards palliative care from younger people, affecting their use. This factor might however not be very influential (40). One study found no differences in beliefs about hospice care in the United Kingdom between younger and older adults, with 90% of both groups believing that hospices care for all age groups (41). Additionally, there is some evidence that older people are more knowledgeable about palliative care than younger people (42). A third, more convincing factor influencing the enrolment into palliative care services may be the presence or absence of younger carers; there is some evidence that older people who live with a carer have better access to palliative care, especially when that carer is of a younger age (40).

From a disease-level perspective, there might be more influential factors hindering access to palliative care for older people. The high prevalence of older people suffering from diseases other than cancer could be an important factor. Taking Europe as an example, relatively more people under 65 die from cancer than do older people (43). Even today, non-cancer patients access palliative care in the United Kingdom at disproportionately low rates compared with other patient groups (44). The (proposed) differences in end-of-life trajectories are considered to be one of the biggest barriers to palliative care provision for non-cancer patients (45). As only cancer has been believed to have a predictable prognosis, referral from other illnesses has been hindered. A related barrier seems to be that some practitioners have questioned the expertise and, thus, added value of palliative care physicians for specific non-cancer disease groups (46).

However, evidence is starting to emerge of the effectiveness of palliative care interventions in diseases other than cancer and of the added value of its early introduction. One study in multiple sclerosis showed that involvement of the palliative care team, compared with standard care, improved key symptoms for patients (e.g. pain, nausea, vomiting) (47). Another study showed the benefits of early palliative care for advanced heart failure and chronic obstructive pulmonary disease patients (48). The effects of early palliative care have been demonstrated in other studies as well, most notably, the Temel et al. (49) study focusing on lung cancer patients: early palliative care integrated with standard oncological care, compared with standard oncological care alone, improved quality of life and decreased the use of aggressive treatments while increasing survival time. As a consequence, early palliative care is currently being recommended to cancer patients by the American Society of Oncology (50). At the same time, there is data which suggests a trend in the United Kingdom towards access to palliative care by non-cancer patients (44). Moreover, there is increasing agreement in the clinical field that palliative care should not be based on prognosis but on the patient's needs. This shift might be especially promising for older people who vary in their needs and morbidities but commonly miss out on palliative care despite their high symptom burden.

Measurement of palliative care needs

Better measurement of palliative care needs is required

To achieve tailored palliative care interventions based on need rather than prognosis, an individual approach appears to be the way forward. In this, an individual's needs are considered and matched to resources and interventions provided. Such an approach would be especially useful in palliative care provision for older people as they form a heterogeneous group and are unlikely to benefit from generic palliative care provision. It would also overcome the challenge for health care providers and policy makers of determining who should receive palliative care. To achieve such a tailored approach, at clinical and policy levels, measuring individual patient needs and symptoms seems the future course.

One way to determine a patient's needs and symptoms is by asking health care practitioners to estimate them. However, it is known that clinicians are often not very good at estimating patients' needs and suffering, especially in the non-physical domains (51). So, a better way forward might be to ask patients themselves about their needs and symptoms. In older people, multidimensional assessment can indeed reveal problems and is especially beneficial when integrated with long-term follow-ups (52). Measurement can be done using patient-reported outcome measures (PROMs). An outcome can be defined as 'a change in health status attributable to preceding health care' (53). Routine measurement of patients' outcomes allows determination of a baseline measure of their symptoms and needs, as well as changes over time which can then be evaluated against the baseline. By doing this, it becomes possible to determine the effect of the interventions that have taken place between the two (or more) measurement moments.

What makes a good patient-reported outcome measure?

Many PROMs exist, but a good PROM can be characterized by several elements of which some are specifically important to older patients. The European Association of Palliative Care (EAPC) has developed a White Paper on 'Outcome Measurement in Palliative Care', including several key recommendations which a PROM should fulfil (54). These include the use of a measure which:

1 has been validated in palliative populations, is brief, and allows for proxy reports;
2 is multidimensional—capturing the holistic nature of palliative care;
3 assesses the needs of family carers;
4 has sound psychometric properties;
5 is suited for the clinical task and clinical work (e.g. is feasible);
6 is valid and reliable and relevant to the research question while not adding to patient burden;
7 allows for comparisons, is culturally sensitive, and has validated translations.

When focusing on older people, the importance of short PROMs allowing for proxy reports becomes increasingly crucial. When patients are cognitively impaired or frail, it can become difficult for them to complete long measures that risk being seen as burdensome instead of helpful and of producing incomplete information. In addition, for impaired and frail older patients, it is likely that proxies will complete the measures. The validity of such ratings has been discussed, with suggestions that proxies tend to overestimate the patient's experiences (55). To overcome this, simultaneous measurement of patient and proxy reports, when the patient is still able to complete them, might be the way forward. Systematic differences in patient and proxy reports can then be collected and used to adjust proxy reports when patient reports are unavailable (56).

An example of a brief PROM which allows for proxy reports and which also fulfils the other EAPC recommendations, making it a good measure to be used in older populations, is the Palliative care Outcome Scale (POS). POS has ten items which assess physical symptoms, emotional, psychological, and spiritual needs, and provision of information and support. An open question asks patients about their main problems. The mean completion time for patients is seven minutes, which decreases to less than four minutes after repeated measurements (57). Patient, carer, and staff versions have been developed, thus allowing for proxy reports. Lastly, the measure has been used in various settings, disease groups, and languages (visit <www.pos-pal.org> for more information).

However, PROMs are not only relevant from an individual perspective but also from a public health viewpoint. The most important measure of public health is that 'good quality of care is accessible to all, independently of their disease (place of care or income)' (58). Incorporating PROMs into a wider approach of measurement in palliative care seems to be essential to achieving high-quality palliative care.

Measurement from a public health perspective

Measurement is a fundamental aspect of evidence-based medicine and its use has been recommended by the WHO in palliative care provision for older people (9). Measurement can focus on different aspects of care. More specifically, structures (e.g. available budgets), processes (i.e. how resources are used; e.g. given treatments), and outcomes (e.g. patient experiences) can be assessed and should, ideally, be combined.

Expert consensus recommends the development of a minimum set of routinely collected data to measure the quality of end-of-life care for older patients (59). The main reasons underlining this recommendation are that datasets can identify areas in which palliative care improvement is a priority; measurement can determine the effectiveness of interventions, both from patient/provider and economic perspectives; data can help in developing capacity building and funding decisions, and can also provide insights into how demographic trends will affect needs and priorities for future health care delivery. Additionally, public perspectives can be compared against care delivered, and international comparisons allow easy dissemination of findings and a more rapid uptake of successful approaches (59). To achieve such a minimum dataset, measurement of patient outcomes is essential but insufficient on its own. Measurement should also include administrative data (e.g. how many people die in their place of choice), provider-level data (e.g. how many hospices a country has), retrospective data from informal caregivers' perspectives (e.g. their adjustment), and population data (e.g. people's expectations of palliative care) (59). Combining these data would provide insight into palliative care provision in older people and the quality of that care, and develop priorities for development.

The future of measurement of palliative care needs

Achieving such a dataset is still more of an aspiration than a reality and while we can put forward recommendations for measurement in this patient group, more work is needed on both the research and the clinical level.

On a research level, it is essential that more studies specifically focussing on older peoples' needs and symptoms are conducted and that these studies use the same outcome measures to allow for comparisons of the effect of different services and models. As palliative care studies often suffer from low numbers of participants and high attrition rates, setting up multi-centre cross-country studies could achieve more robust numbers and, consequently, more valid and reliable results focused on older patients. A specific focus on non-malignant disease groups, taking into account multi-morbidity, should be a priority. Such efforts can increase the evidence base of palliative care interventions for older people.

On a clinical level, the implementation of routinely collected data and patient outcomes should be achieved. However, clinicians might be reluctant to implement routine PROM measurement in older people for several reasons. Firstly, they might want to protect patients and not overburden them, something often seen in palliative care research (60). Patients themselves are, however, willing to participate in research (61), making it plausible that they have the same attitude to PROM measurement. Secondly, clinicians might fear that it would make consultations longer; however, it can also be argued that it would focus the consultation more on the patient's own priorities. These aspects confirm, however, the importance of short measures allowing for proxy reports among older people. Lastly, the evidence that PROM measurement improves outcomes is just emerging (62), with a present need for evaluating the effects of implementation on older people's outcomes. Successful implementation seems to be easier to achieve when it is well prepared, is strongly led, and has the emotional commitment of the clinicians involved. (63). When achieved, routine measurement of outcomes on a clinical level provides information about the quality of care for individual patients and about the quality of individual service providers and allows for (inter)national comparisons. By comparing sites, as recommended by the EAPC White Paper (54), international standards of quality of care can be determined (56), focused on older people.

Conclusion

This chapter has focused on the symptoms and end-of-life trajectories experienced by older people, the barriers to accessing palliative care, and the importance of measurement to achieve high-quality palliative care. Older people are a heterogeneous group with various needs, differing according to personal, demographic, cultural, clinical, and other characteristics. Symptoms should be interpreted in the light of declining functioning status and multi-morbidities. The widespread assumption that different diseases follow distinct end-of-life trajectories may warrant revision, as several symptoms are common and individual variability in end-of-life trajectories within and between diseases is prevalent. Although older people have high palliative care needs, their access to and use of palliative care is limited. There is an increasing awareness that palliative care should be provided on a needs basis rather than prognosis or diagnosis, which is especially promising to older people. To increase appropriate access to palliative care for older people, screening for problems using PROMs such as the POS is recommended. PROMs should fulfil several criteria. In older people the criteria of brief measures allowing for proxy reports are important, as patients are often cognitively impaired or frail and unable to complete long measures. From a public health perspective, measurement is essential to achieve high-quality palliative care for all. A routinely collected data set should be agreed upon which captures PROM, administrative, provider, and public data. To achieve this, recommendations for patient-reported data measurement in research (e.g. large studies focused on non-malignancies) and clinical care (implementing brief measures and comparing sites) have been made.

In conclusion, it is important to consider and assess individual symptoms, needs, and outcomes of older people, rather than concentrating on discrete diseases and possibly inaccurate expectations about their trajectories. While barriers exist to older people accessing palliative care services, measuring the individual patient's needs could increase access. Integrating these measurements into larger data sets and using (inter)national comparisons has the potential to improve the quality of care provided at individual and public health levels for older people.

References

1 Cai J, Clark J, Croft S, Deakin S, Fowaja G, Hartley A, et al. *Indications of Public Health in the English Regions. 9: Older People*. York: Alcuin Research and Resource Centre University of York; 2008.

2 Seale C, Cartwright A. *The Year Before Death*. Hants, UK: Avebury; 1994.

3 Addington-HalL J, Altmann D, McCarthy M. Variations by age in symptoms and dependency levels experienced by people in the last year of life, as reported by surviving family, friends and officials. *Age Ageing* 1998; 27(2):129–36.

4 Teunissen SC, de Haes HC, Voest EE, de Graeff A. Does age matter in palliative care? *Crit Rev Oncol Hematol* 2006; 60(2):152–8.

5 Hotopf M, Chidgey J, Addington-Hall J, Ly KL. Depression in advanced disease: a systematic review Part 1. Prevalence and case finding. *Palliat Med* 2002; 16(2):81–97.

6 Thompson GN, Chochinov HM. Reducing the potential for suffering in older adults with advanced cancer. *Palliat Support Care* 2010; 8(01):83–93.

7 Public Health England's Knowledge and Intelligence Team (West Midlands Public Health Observatory). *Data for Figures in APHO Indications of Public Health in the English Regions: Older People*. Chapter 7: Quality of life and well-being. Available at: <http://www.wmpho.org.uk/publications/collection.aspx?id=1461> (Accessed on 13-12-2014). Ref. type: online source.

8 Edwards A, Pang N, Shiu V, Chan C. Review: the understanding of spirituality and the potential role of spiritual care in end-of-life and palliative care: a meta-study of qualitative research. *Palliat Med* 2010; 24(8):753–70.

9 Davies E, Higginson IJ. *Better Palliative Care for Older People*. Copenhagen: World Health Organization, Regional Office for Europe; 2004.

10 Gianni W, Madaio R, Di Cioccio L, D'Amico F, Policicchio D, Postacchini D, et al. Prevalence of pain in elderly hospitalized patients. *Arch Gerontol Geriatr* 2010; 51(3):273–6.

11 Wijk H, Grimby A. Needs of elderly patients in palliative care. *Am J Hosp Palliat Care* 2008; 25(2):106–11.

12 Weintraub D, Moberg PJ, Duda JE, Katz IR, Stern MB. Recognition and treatment of depression in Parkinson's disease. *J Geriatr Psych Neur* 2003; 16(3):178–83.

13 Balboni TA, Vanderwerker LC, Block SD, Paulk ME, Lathan CS, Peteet JR, et al. Religiousness and spiritual support among advanced cancer patients and associations with end-of-life treatment preferences and quality of life. *J Clin Oncol* 2007; **25**(5):555–60.

14 Hall S, Petkova H, Tsouros A, Costantini M, Higginson I. *Palliative Care for Older People: Better Practices*. World Health Organization, Regional Office for Europe; 2011.

15 Salive ME. Multimorbidity in older adults. *Epidemiologic Reviews* 2013; **35**(1):75–83.

16 Goldstein NE, Meier DE. Palliative medicine in older adults. In: Hanks G, Cherny NI, Christakis NA, Fallon M, Kaasa S, Portenoy RK (eds). *Oxford Textbook of Palliative Medicine* (4th edn). Oxford: Oxford University Press; 2009.

17 Eurostat. *Causes of Death Statistics—People Over 65—Statistics Explained*. Available at: <http://epp.eurostat.ec.europa.eu/statistics_explained/index.php/Causes_of_death_statistics_-_people_over_65#Further_Eurostat_information> (Accessed February 2014). Ref. type: online source.

18 Van Lancker A, Velghe A, Van Hecke A, Verbrugghe M, Van Den Noortgate N, Grypdonck M, et al. Prevalence of symptoms in older cancer patients receiving palliative care: a systematic review and meta-analysis. *J Pain Symptom Manage* 2013; **47**(1):90–104.

19 Costantini M, Beccaro M, Higginson IJ. Cancer trajectories at the end of life: is there an effect of age and gender? *BMC Cancer* 2008; **8**(1):127.

20 Solano JP, Gomes B, Higginson IJ. A comparison of symptom prevalence in far advanced cancer, AIDS, heart disease, chronic obstructive pulmonary disease and renal disease. *J Pain Symptom Manage* 2006; **31**(1):58–69.

21 Merckaert I, Libert Y, Messin S, Milani M, Slachmuylder JL, Razavi D. Cancer patients' desire for psychological support: prevalence and implications for screening patients' psychological needs. *Psycho-Oncology* 2010; **19**(2):141–9.

22 Roth AJ. Understanding depression in the elderly cancer patient. *J Support Oncol* 2008; **6**(2):84–6.

23 British Heart Foundation, Health Promotion Research Group. *Coronary Heart Disease Statistics. A Compendium of Health Statistics. 2012 Edition*. London: British Heart Foundation; 2012.

24 Selman L, Harding R, Beynon T, Hodson F, Coady E, Hazeldine C, et al. Improving end-of-life care for patients with chronic heart failure: 'Let's hope it'll get better, when I know in my heart of hearts it won't'. *Heart* 2007; **93**(8):963–7.

25 Murray SA, Kendall M, Grant E, Boyd K, Barclay S, Sheikh A. Patterns of social, psychological, and spiritual decline toward the end of life in lung cancer and heart failure. *J Pain Symptom Manage* 2007; **34**(4):393–402.

26 Alzheimer's Disease International. *Dementia Statistics*. Available at: <http://www.alz.co.uk/research/statistics> (Accessed February 2014). Ref. type: online data.

27 Brodaty H, Seeher K, Gibson L. Dementia time to death: a systematic literature review on survival time and years of life lost in people with dementia. *Int Psychogeriatr* 2012; **24**(7):1034.

28 Department of Health. *Living Well with Dementia: A National Dementia Strategy*. London, United Kingdom: Department of Health; 2009.

29 Etters L, Goodall D, Harrison BE. Caregiver burden among dementia patient caregivers: a review of the literature. *J Am Acad Nurse Pract* 2008; **20**(8):423–8.

30 von Kutzleben M, Schmid W, Halek M, Holle B, Bartholomeyczik S. Community-dwelling persons with dementia: What do they need? What do they demand? What do they do? A systematic review on the subjective experiences of persons with dementia. *Aging Ment Health* 2012; **16**(3):378–90.

31 Lunney JR, Lynn J, Hogan C. Profiles of older medicare decedents. *JAGS* 2002; **50**(6):1108–12.

32 Murray SA, Kendall M, Boyd K, Sheikh A. Illness trajectories and palliative care. *BMJ* 2005; **330**(7498):1007.

33 Lunney JR, Lynn J, Foley DJ, Lipson S, Guralnik JM. Patterns of functional decline at the end of life. *JAMA* 2003; **289**(18):2387–92.

34 Teno JM, Weitzen S, Fennell ML, Mor V. Dying trajectory in the last year of life: does cancer trajectory fit other diseases? *J Palliat Med* 2001; **4**(4):457–64.

35 Gill TM, Gahbauer EA, Han L, Allore HG. Trajectories of disability in the last year of life. *NEJM* 2010; **362**(13):1173–80.

36 Higginson IJ, Wade AM, McCarthy M. Effectiveness of two palliative support teams. *J Public Health* 1992; **14**(1):50–6.

37 Bausewein C, Booth S, Gysels M, Kühnbach R, Haberland B, Higginson IJ. Individual breathlessness trajectories do not match summary trajectories in advanced cancer and chronic obstructive pulmonary disease: results from a longitudinal study. *Palliat Med* 2010; **24**(8):777–86.

38 Gott M, Barnes S, Parker C, Payne S, Seamark D, Gariballa S, et al. Dying trajectories in heart failure. *Palliat Med* 2007; **21**(2):95–9.

39 Higginson IJ, Gao W, Saleem TZ, Chaudhuri KR, Burman R, McCrone P, et al. Symptoms and quality of life in late stage Parkinson syndromes: a longitudinal community study of predictive factors. *PloS One* 2012; **7**(11):e46327.

40 Walshe C, Todd C, Caress A, Chew-Graham C. Patterns of access to community palliative care services: a literature review. *J Pain Symptom Manage* 2009; **37**(5):884–912.

41 Catt S, Blanchard M, Addington-Hall J, Zis M, Blizard R, King M. Older adults' attitudes to death, palliative treatment and hospice care. *Palliat Med* 2005; **19**(5):402–10.

42 McIlfatrick S, Hasson F, McLaughlin D, Johnston G, Roulston A, Rutherford L, et al. Public awareness and attitudes toward palliative care in Northern Ireland. *BMC Palliat Care* 2013; **12**(1):1–7.

43 Eurostat. *Major Causes of Death for Persons Under 65 Years and Aged 65 and More—Standardised Death Rates (SDR) per 100,000 Inhabitants*. EU-27, 2009. PNG. Available at: <http://epp.eurostat. ec.europa.eu/statistics_explained/index.php?title=File:Major_causes_of_death_for_persons_ under_65_years_and_aged_65_and_more_%E2%80%93_standardised_death_rates_(SDR)_ per_100_000_inhabitants,_EU-27,_2009.PNG&filetimestamp=20120202142508)> (Accessed February 2014). Ref. type: online data.

44 The National Council for Palliative Care. *National Survey of Patient Activity Data for Specialist Palliative Care Services: MDS Full Report for the Year 2011–2012*. London, United Kingdom: National Council for Palliative Care; 2013.

45 O'Leary N, Tiernan E. Survey of specialist palliative care services for noncancer patients in Ireland and perceived barriers. *Palliat Med* 2008; **22**(1):77–83.

46 Hanratty B, Hibbert D, Mair F, May C, Ward C, Capewell S, et al. Doctors' perceptions of palliative care for heart failure: focus group study. *BMJ* 2002; **325**(7364):581–5.

47 Edmonds P, Hart S, Gao W, Vivat B, Burman R, Silber E, et al. Palliative care for people severely affected by multiple sclerosis: evaluation of a novel palliative care service. *Mult Scler* 2010; **16**(5):627–36.

48 Rabow MW, Dibble SL, Pantilat SZ, McPhee SJ. The comprehensive care team: a controlled trial of outpatient palliative medicine consultation. *Arch Intern Med* 2004; **164**(1):83–91.

49 Temel JS, Greer JA, Muzikansky A, Gallagher ER, Admane S, Jackson VA, et al. Early palliative care for patients with metastatic non–small-cell lung cancer. *NEJM* 2010; **363**(8):733–42.

50 Smith TJ, Temin S, Alesi ER, Abernethy AP, Balboni TA, Basch EM, et al. American Society of Clinical Oncology provisional clinical opinion: the integration of palliative care into standard oncology care. *J Clin Oncol* 2012; **30**(8):880–7.

51 Hladschik-Kermer B, Kierner KA, Heck U, Miksovsky A, Reiter B, Zoidl H, et al. Patients and staff perceptions of cancer patients' quality of life. *EJON* 2013; **17**(1):70–4.

52 Victor CR, Higginson I. Effectiveness of care for older people: a review. *Qual Health Care* 1994; **3**(4):210.

53 **Donabedian A.** *Explorations in Quality Assessment and Monitoring.* Ann Arbor Michigan: Health Administration Press; 1980.

54 **Bausewein C, Daveson BA, Currow DC, Downing J, Deliens L, Radbruch L, et al.** *EAPC White Paper on Outcome Measurement in Palliative Care: Improving Practice, Attaining Outcomes and Delivering Quality Services. Recommendations from the European Association for Palliative care (EAPC) Task Force on Outcome Measurement.* (personal communication)

55 **McPherson C, Addington-Hall J.** Judging the quality of care at the end of life: can proxies provide reliable information? *Soc Sci Med* 2003; **56**(1):95–109.

56 **Bausewein C, Daveson BA, Benalia A, Simon ST, Higginson IJ.** *Outcome Measurement in Palliative Care: The Essentials*; 2011.PRISMA (Reflecting the Positive Diversities of European Priorities for Research and Measurement in End-of-Life Care)

57 **Hearn J, Higginson IJ, Projec PCCA.** Development and validation of a core outcome measure for palliative care: the palliative care outcome scale. *Qual Health Care* 1999; **8**(4):219–27.

58 **Deliens L.** Public health (research) at the end of life. *Prog Pall Care*; **15**(3):103.

59 **Casarett DJ, Teno J, Higginson I.** How should nations measure the quality of end-of-life care for older adults? Recommendations for an international minimum data set. *JAGS* 2006; **54**(11):1765–71.

60 **Hudson P, Aranda S, Kristjanson L, Quinn K.** Minimising gate-keeping in palliative care research. *Eur J Pal Care* 2005; **4**(12):165–9.

61 **Gysels MH, Evans C, Higginson IJ.** Patient, caregiver, health professional and researcher views and experiences of participating in research at the end of life: a critical interpretive synthesis of the literature. *BMC Med Res Methodol* 2012; **12**(1):123.

62 Palliative Care Outcomes Collaboration. *Palliative Care Outcomes Collaboration: Three Years of Progress (2010 to 2013).* Wollongong: University of Wollongong; 2013.

63 **Antunes B, Harding R, Higginson IJ.** Implementing patient-reported outcome measures in palliative care clinical practice: a systematic review of facilitators and barriers. *Palliat Med* 2014; **28**(2):158–75.

Chapter 13

End-of-life decisions for older patients who are approaching death

Agnes van der Heide and Kenneth Chambaere

Introduction to end-of-life decisions for older patients who are approaching death

Around 1900, the average age expectancy in the Netherlands and other Western countries was about 50 years. By 2011, it had increased to something over 80 years (1). Currently, about half the population dies at the age of 80 or over. Previously common causes of death such as infectious diseases and famine have been replaced by heart disease and cancer, diseases that tend to occur at higher ages. Until 1950, these changes were mainly the result of improved living conditions and healthier food patterns. After 1950, and especially after 1970, improvements in health care have resulted in a further increase in average life expectancy (2). The possibilities of postponing death by using medical interventions that change the course of formerly lethal diseases have increased greatly. And this development has not yet come to an end; at the beginning of the twenty-first century, each decade adds two years to our average life expectancy.

It can, therefore, be concluded that public health and health care have been rather successful in postponing death and prolonging our lives. Currently, age by itself is no longer a contraindication for most medical interventions. Advances in medical technology have made it possible to use complex or burdensome life-prolonging interventions for older patients, even those who are frail or have comorbidities. Nevertheless, many health-related factors that are important to take into consideration when making decisions about medical treatment, such as the presence of diabetes or cardiovascular disease, immobility or cognitive decline, are more common in older patients. It has, however, been claimed that these factors are often inappropriately addressed. On the one hand, life-prolonging interventions may be overused in older patients because of an overoptimistic view of their beneficial effects and of the patient's prognosis and a lack of awareness that goals of care need to be adjusted when health conditions deteriorate and death approaches. On the other hand, the lower use of life-prolonging interventions in older compared with younger patients, such as chemotherapy in oncology, are sometimes considered evidence of underuse due to ageism.

Although there are commentators who argue that age-based medical decision making can be ethically justified, the most common attitude seems to be that ageism is not a sound basis for such, including decision making at the end of life. However, application of interventions to prolong life and postpone death is not the preferred option for all patients, even if it might be possible from a medical point of view. Where avoiding premature death has long been the main goal of health care, we are now faced with the problem that death may come too late, or that the pathway towards death is impeded by aggressive, sometimes futile, medical interventions to prolong life at the cost of burdensome side-effects. Medical care that is continued until late in a terminal disease process can stand in the way of a peaceful and dignified last phase of life. Most people prefer to spend their last months or weeks of life in their private environment, surrounded by family and friends, while receiving care that is aimed at providing symptom relief and comfort where possible and needed.

Nowadays, care at the end of life thus sometimes involves making difficult decisions about the use of medical interventions. Patients may, for example, choose to refrain from potentially life-prolonging interventions because such interventions require hospitalization, deprive them of their independence, or involve the risk of burdensome side-effects. Further severe, intractable symptoms may require decisions about the use of medical interventions that involve serious ethical considerations, such as sedation to render patients unconscious of their symptoms, or high dosages of opioids that can decrease the level of breathing and thus risk the shortening of life. Finally, an extremely poor quality of life, suffering due to physical or other symptoms, and the loss of any sense of meaning in living in difficult circumstances without the prospect of improvement may provoke a desire to hasten death, either by stopping all life-prolonging interventions or acts, or by the administration of drugs that hasten the dying process.

End-of-life decisions

End-of-life decisions can be defined as explicit decisions concerning the use of medical interventions at the end of life that can have an impact on the time of death. In end-of-life decision-making research, different types of end-of-life decisions have been distinguished (3). Decisions to refrain from medical interventions aimed at prolonging life have been studied most extensively. These decisions are generally considered to be an acceptable and intrinsic part of medical care at the end of life, which implies that such decision making is subject to general legal and medical-professional regulation. The right of patients to refuse medical interventions, even if that would shorten their life, is recognized in most Western countries. Physicians are allowed to withhold or withdraw treatment if they feel that providing or continuing treatment has no medical value or is not in the best interests of the patient, after due consideration of the patient's preferences.

Another type of decision concerns the use of medication to alleviate severe suffering at the end of life to the extent that death may, unintentionally, be hastened. This category of decisions is, just like decisions to refrain from life-prolonging treatment, generally considered to be part of normal medical practice, which means that decisions should be based on the best interests of patients and that patients, if possible, should be involved in the decision making and give their consent. However, these decisions are often made late in the disease process and patients may be unable to give such consent (e.g. due to unconsciousness), in which case careful communication with and consultation of relatives and health care staff is needed.

End-of-life decision making may also concern palliative or terminal sedation. This practice involves sedating the patient (i.e. lowering the patient's consciousness) at the very end of life, to alleviate severe symptoms which cannot be adequately addressed with conventional symptom treatment. Palliative sedation can be intermittent or continuous and levels of sedation can range from mild to deep. The most far-reaching form of the practice is continuous deep sedation until death, which has stirred up controversy due to its association with intentional hastening of death. For this reason, a number of guidelines have been drafted to support decision making and practices that include, among other issues, stipulations of a limited life expectancy, a lack of alternative treatment options, administration of sedative drugs proportional to symptom severity, and consent of the patient or, if that is not possible, of the relatives (4, 5). Nonetheless, there is still a debate around whether the use of palliative sedation for dying patients may have an impact on the moment of dying.

The most controversial type of end-of-life decision concerns physician assistance in dying. Physician assistance in dying includes euthanasia, which is the administration of lethal drugs upon the explicit request of the patient, and physician-assisted suicide, in which the physician provides the patient with lethal drugs that the patient can self-administer. Euthanasia and physician-assisted suicide are not considered to be part of normal medical practice. A few countries, including the Netherlands, Belgium, and Luxembourg, have adopted specific laws to enable these acts under strict conditions (6–8). Conditions that are included in the law in all three countries are that these acts are only permissible if they are performed at the explicit, well-considered, and voluntary request of the person involved; that they can only be performed by a physician, who is obliged to ask another independent physician for advice; and that physicians providing euthanasia or assistance in suicide have to report their act to a public authority that confidentially assesses whether the physician has complied with the legal regulations.

Frequencies of end-of-life decisions

Refraining from life-prolonging treatment

Most studies that have assessed the occurrence of decisions to refrain from life-prolonging interventions in different age groups have found increasing frequency by age. Frequencies have been studied most extensively in the Netherlands. In this country, end-of-life decision-making practices have been assessed in nationwide surveys, at five-year intervals, since 1990 (9). In these studies, physicians filled in questionnaires about the decision making that had preceded death, for a large representative sample of deaths. About one third of all death cases were found to involve decisions to refrain from life-prolonging treatment, often in combination with decisions to administer potentially life-shortening medication. In 16% to 20% of all deaths, a decision to refrain from life-prolonging treatment is the most important end-of-life decision. Such decisions are most often made for patients dying in the acute hospital setting and they may concern patients dying from cancer as well as those dying from cardiovascular or pulmonary diseases or other illnesses. The estimated amount of time by which life is shortened as a result of decisions to refrain from treatment is typically less than a week, but may extend to more than a month in a minority of cases. The most common interventions that are foregone are artificial administration of hydration and/or nutrition, use of medication such as antibiotic or cardiovascular drugs, artificial ventilation, surgical procedures, and hospitalization (10).

In the Dutch studies, decisions to refrain from life-prolonging treatment were somewhat more likely for patients dying at the age of 80 years or over; about a quarter of all deaths among patients aged 80 or over were preceded by a decision to refrain from life-prolonging interventions, as the most important end-of-life decision, whereas the proportion was found to be 13–19% in younger age groups. About half of all cases in which death was preceded by a decision to either withhold or withdraw treatment concerned patients dying at the age of 80 or over. In 2001, this age distribution was found to be similar in six European countries where an identical study was performed (11). A distinct but comparable study in France, conducted in 2009, found that treatment had been withheld for about 10% of all patients who had died under 70, whereas the percentages were 16.6%, 17.8%, and 22.1%, respectively, for the age groups of 70–79 years, 80–89 years, and 90 or over—a trend stated as being statistically significant (12). A survey among physicians in the United Kingdom demonstrated a frequency of 18.9%, 22.0%, and 23.0% in the age groups of under 60, 60–79 years, and 80 and over, but these differences were not statistically significant (13).

Two comparable Belgian studies on end-of-life decision-making practices, in 1998 and 2007, found no age disparity in the frequency of decisions to refrain from life-prolonging treatment (14–16). In 2007, such decisions had been made in something over half of all death cases in all age categories. Nonetheless, decisions to refrain from life-prolonging treatment are consistently more often the most important end-of-life decision, in terms of possible shortening of life, in older patients: in 2007, the percentage was, respectively, 14.6%, 17.2%, and 18.5% in age groups younger than 65, 65–79 years, and 80 or older. The extent to which patients were involved in making such decisions was also found to be comparable in different age groups; palliative care specialists were more often consulted about the decision when it concerned older patients.

Studies that focused on intensive care settings also found higher frequencies of decisions to refrain from life-prolonging interventions among older patients. An international study comprising over 14,000 patients in 282 intensive care units, in seven regions, found that patients for whom a decision to forgo life-sustaining treatment had been made had a median age of 70, whereas patients without such a decision had a median age of 63—a statistically significant difference (17). A study on patients who had died in a surgical intensive care unit in Germany also found that older age contributed to the likelihood that a decision to withhold or withdraw treatment had been made: an increase of 10 years of age increased this likelihood by 1.66 (18). A study in nine Greek intensive care units, however, found no such effect (19). In this study, physicians self-reported that age had a very limited role in their decision-making practices.

Although not all studies assessing frequencies found statistically significant disparities by age, there seems to be a tendency, in at least some countries, to make such decisions more often for the oldest age groups. It cannot be ruled out that such decision making is partly based on factors that are not medically relevant, such as the patient's high age per se, but medical factors play a role as well. Vrakking et al. compared younger and older patients who had died from comparable diagnoses and found that in both groups similar characteristics, such as comorbidity, quality of life, and wishes of patients, seemed to have determined decisions to limit treatment (20). However, several studies have shown that older patients, more often than younger patients, are not involved in making decisions about their treatment. In a recent review of the literature, it was found that the majority of frail older individuals would appreciate the chance to discuss end-of-life care, but that most are not given this opportunity (21). Whereas early communication about patients' treatment preferences has been shown to result more often in less aggressive care and a timely focus on palliative and comfort care, increased involvement of older patients in making decisions about their medical care is likely to result in a higher frequency of decisions to refrain from life-prolonging interventions.

Alleviation of symptoms with medication that involves a risk of hastening death

Older patients have been found to have less access to palliative care and to receive less treatment to alleviate suffering at the end of life. Research has not demonstrated clear age-based disparities in the provision of medication that may unintendedly hasten death. Until 2005, nationwide studies in the Netherlands had found frequencies of up to 25% of all deceased patients (22). In 2010, the overall frequency had increased to 36%, with the percentage being highest (39%) for the oldest age group of 80 or over (9). These findings contrast with what was found in Belgium, in 2007, where the frequency of intensive alleviation of symptoms was found to decrease by age, although this trend was no longer significant after taking into account differences in causes of death between age groups (13). Studies in the United Kingdom and France and the six-country European End-of-Life Decisions (EURELD) study did not find a significant association between age and intensive alleviation of symptoms either (12, 13, 23). Morphine dosages were lower for the oldest age group in all countries in the EURELD study, but this could also be explained by taking into account different causes of death. The finding in the Belgian study that, independent of other confounders such as cause or place of death, older patients are less often involved than younger patients in the decision-making process and that they less often request intensive alleviation of symptoms is notable (16) but in line with other studies. More communication with older patients about end-of-life care might, thus, also increase the frequency of decisions to alleviate symptoms with medication that may hasten death.

Continuous deep sedation until death

Continuous deep sedation until death was used in 2% to 9% of all deaths in a survey held in 2001 in six European countries (24). Follow-up surveys in Belgium and the Netherlands have found that this percentage has risen significantly, to 14.5% in Belgium in 2007 and 12.3% in the Netherlands in 2010 (9, 25). Because the practice is mostly used in cases of cancer, which affects older people proportionally less frequently, older patients are less likely to be continuously and deeply sedated until death (25–27). Nonetheless, in Belgium, the frequency of its use rose significantly from 4.7% to 11.1%, between 2001 and 2007, in patients older than 80 years (25). Although no large-scale data are available on the characteristics of decision making and practice in older patients, it has been suggested that the practice might be amenable to improvement in Belgian nursing homes (28). Another study showed that in nursing homes, the decision is mostly made at the request of or with consent from the relatives, but without the input of the patient (25).

Euthanasia and assisted suicide

Studies have consistently demonstrated that euthanasia and physician assistance in suicide are relatively rare among the oldest age groups. In 2010, when the last nationwide study in the Netherlands was performed, it was found that the frequency of euthanasia and physician-assisted suicide was 5.6% among persons who were under 65 years of age when dying, whereas it was 4.0% in the age category of 65–79 years and 1.4% in the oldest age group of 80 years and over (9). An interesting finding in the 2010 study was that requests for euthanasia or assistance in suicide were more often granted for younger than for older patients; the percentage of granted requests was 56% for patients under the age of 65, 47% for patients aged between 65 and 79, and 32% for patients aged 80 or over.

In Belgium, the frequency of euthanasia and physician-assisted suicide also declines by age: in 2007, it was used for 4.2% in the under 64 years of age group, for 2.5% in the 65–79 age group, and for 0.8% in the group aged 80 or over (15). This was found to be related to the cause and place of death: whereas physician assistance in dying is most common in patients with cancer and patients dying at home, patients in the oldest age group relatively often die from other causes and in institutional settings. Just as in the Netherlands, older patients (80 and above) were not only significantly less likely to request physician assistance in dying but the rate of their requests being granted was also lower than in younger patient groups (16).

Involvement of older patients in end-of-life decision making

Though existing studies do not shed light on the appropriateness of end-of-life decisions in older patients, it is commonly agreed that their involvement in such important decisions is desirable, if not necessary. In this respect, older patients are often regarded as vulnerable patients, being most at risk of practices that are not in line with their wishes. Older patients are often thought to be less empowered and less assertive than younger people, as having less aspirations towards autonomy and self-determination, and as having more respect for the perceived medical hierarchy and a more 'moral' relationship with their attending physicians (29–31). As a consequence, they are more likely to be excluded from the actual decision making at the end of their own lives. Though under-researched, the lower degree of involvement of older patients has been shown in several studies including a nationwide study in Belgium focused on age-based disparities in end-of-life decision making (15). The older the patient, the less often he or she is involved in decision making, and the less likely it is that he or she will explicitly request a certain action to be taken or treatment to be withheld or withdrawn (16).

In most cases where older patients themselves are not participating in the decision-making process, the family is consulted as proxies (16). However, a few studies have indicated that older patients potentially hold different perspectives about end-of-life treatment decisions from their family members or attending physicians; whereas the latter often focus on the medical indications such as effectiveness of the treatment, older patients tend to consider their personal values and beliefs about life, suffering, and death and to think more in terms of general care goals rather than specific treatments (31–33). Further, there are indications that, in deciding for others, people are less restrictive than in deciding for themselves (34), which underlines the possibility that surrogate decision making may, at times, not be entirely in line with the preferences held by the patient. A Dutch study also found that the preferences of many older people concerning treatment decisions were unknown to their families (35).

Limited decision-making capacity and dementia

Much of the observed age-based disparity in involvement of patients in end-of-life decisions has to do with the patient's decision-making capacity. Decision-making capacity relates to five distinguishable cognitive abilities: understanding the factors relevant to making a decision, appreciating the nature and importance of the decision, understanding the risks as well as the benefits of the decision, ability to communicate about the decision, and deliberation based on personal values (36, 37). Reasons for not discussing end-of-life decisions with older patients, as mentioned by physicians, are very often the lack of capacity and even unconsciousness of the patient (16). Whereas these are obviously acceptable reasons for not consulting with the patient *at the time of the decision*, it is likely that the patient has not always been incapacitated. Indeed, a longitudinal cohort study of older decedents in the Netherlands found that only 27% of people had experienced limited decision-making capacity for longer than one month before death (38). However, two thirds of older decedents had become limited in their decision-making capacity by the last week of life and only a quarter remained lucid until shortly before death, showing that decision-making capacity is reduced or disappears at some point in the majority of older people at the end of life. Older patients often follow an illness trajectory with slow but steady cognitive and functional decline (39, 40). Decision-making capacity may not be limited during a large part of the illness trajectory, but the steady cognitive decline means that, at some time, patients lose capacity, and this moment may be very difficult for health care professionals to pinpoint. Ideally, patient preferences are explored well before the loss of capacity, by addressing possible future treatment decisions through advance care planning, even if such conversations are difficult to initiate and conduct.

The issue is no better illustrated than in people with dementia. Dementia is associated with an often protracted and irreversible period of limited decision-making capacity (38), and patients are often unable to interact cognitively with others in the late stages of the illness, which presents professional caregivers with specific difficulties. Without early discussions with the patient, they are at a loss to know the patient's wishes and, together with the family, need to decide in the patient's best interests. Such decisions, as a Belgian study found, are most often to withhold or withdraw life- prolonging treatment (40.4% of all patients dying with dementia), with the most important considerations not relating to the actual physical suffering of the patient but to the illness prospects and remaining quality of life (41). Arguably, the emotional burden of such a difficult decision could be mitigated if physician and family had some explicit knowledge of the patient's preferences.

Conclusion on end-of-life decisions for older patients who are approaching death

Though there is much concern about either undertreatment or overtreatment of older patients in the last phase of life, there is little evidence suggesting age-based differences in end-of-life decision rates. Differences in end-of-life decisions, whether in refraining from life-prolonging treatment, intensifying symptom treatment, or continuously and deeply sedating until death, are likely to be due mostly to differences in patients' health conditions. There is, however, evidence of less involvement in decision making, which may also partly be due to factors related to age, such as age-specific illness and cognitive deterioration. This is a fairly consistent finding. Current interest in advance care planning is likely to increase older patients' involvement.

It is impossible to make a judgement on the appropriateness of decisions based on an 'optimal' frequency of end-of-life decisions. Assessment of the quality of care and death of older patients should, on the contrary, be based on insight into the characteristics of the decision-making process such as timely and adequate patient involvement, valid and sound medical arguments and reasoning, and good access to available care. If the process of decision making is appropriate, the outcome is very likely to be appropriate too.

References

1 Maddison A. *The world economy. A millennium perspective.* Paris: Organisation for Economic Co-operation and Development; 2001.

2 Mackenbach JP, van der Maas PJ. *Volksgezondheid en gezondheidszorg.* Maarssen: Elsevier Gezondheidszorg; 2008.

3 Van der Maas PJ, van Delden JJM, Pijnenborg L, Looman C. Euthanasia and other medical decisions concerning the end of life. *Lancet* 1991; **338**:669–74.

4 Committee on National Guidelines for Palliative Sedation RDMA. *Guideline for palliative sedation.* Utrecht: KNMG; 2009. [KNMG-richtlijn Palliatieve sedatie. Richtlijn van de Koninklijke Nederlandsche Maatschappij tot Bevordering der Geneeskunst, 2009.]

5 Cherny NI, Radbruch L., the Board of the European Association for Palliative Care. European Association for Palliative Care (EAPC) recommended framework for the use of sedation in palliative care. *Pall Med* 2009; **23**:581–93.

6 *Termination of Life on Request and Assisted Suicide (Review Procedures) Act* 2002. The Hague: Netherlands; 2002. Available at: <http://www.eutanasia.ws/documentos/Leyes/Internacional/Holanda%20Ley%202002.pdf>.(Accessed June 2014). Ref. type: online source.

7 The Belgian Act on Euthanasia of May 28th 2002 [English translation]. *Ethical Perspect* 2002; 9:182–8.

8 Le Gouvernement du Grand-Duché de Luxembourg. Law of March 16, 2009, on euthanasia and assisted suicide [French]. In: *Memorial: legislation.* Luxembourg: Association Momentanée Imprimerie Centrale/Victor Buck 2009; 46:615–9. Available at: <http://www.legilux.public.lu/leg/a/archives/2009/0046/> (Accessed June 2014). Ref. type: online source.

9 Onwuteaka-Philipsen BD, Brinkman-Stoppelenburg A, et al. Trends in end-of-life practices before and after the enactment of the euthanasia law in the Netherlands from 1990 to 2010: a repeated cross-sectional survey. *Lancet* 2012; 380:908–15.

10 Bosshard G, Nilstun T, Bilsen J, et al. Forgoing treatment at the end of life in 6 European countries. *JAMA* 2005; 165:401–7.

11 van der Heide A, Deliens L, Faisst K, et al. End-of-life decision-making in six European countries: descriptive study. *Lancet* 2003; 362:345–50.

12 Pennec S, Monnier A, Pontone S, Aubry R. End-of-life medical decisions in France: a death certificate follow-up survey 5 years after the 2005 act of parliament on patients' rights and end of life. *BMC Palliat Care* 2012; 11:25.

13 Seale C. End-of-life decisions in the UK involving medical practitioners. *Pall Med* 2009; 23:198–204.

14 Deliens L, Mortier F, Bilsen J, et al. End-of-life decisions in medical practice in Flanders, Belgium: a nationwide survey. *Lancet* 2000; 356:1806–11.

15 Chambaere K, Bilsen J, Cohen J, Onwuteaka-Philipsen BD, Mortier F, Deliens L. Trends in medical end-of-life decision making in Flanders, Belgium 1998–2001–2007. *Med Decis Making* 2011; 31:500–10.

16 Chambaere K, Rietjens JA, Smets T, et al. Age-based disparities in end-of-life decisions in Belgium: a population-based death certificate survey. *BMC Public Health* 2012; 12:447.

17 Azoulay É, Metnitz B, Sprung CL, et al. End-of-life practices in 282 intensive care units: data from the SAPS 3 database. *Intensive Care Med* 2009; 35:623–30.

18 Meissner A, Genga KR, Studart FS, et al. Epidemiology of and factors associated with end-of-life decisions in a surgical intensive care unit. *Crit Care Med* 2010; 38:1060–8.

19 Kranidiotis G, Gerovasili V, Tasoulis A, et al. End-of-life decisions in Greek intensive care units: a multicenter cohort study. *Crit Care* 2010; 14:R228.

20 Vrakking AM, van der Heide A, van Delden JJM, Looman CWN, Visser MH, van der Maas PJ. Medical decision-making for seriously ill non-elderly and elderly patients. *Health Policy* 2005, 75:40–8.

21 Sharp T, Mora E, Kuhn E, Barclay S. Do the elderly have a voice? Advance care planning discussions with frail and older individuals: a systematic literature review and narrative synthesis. *Br J Gen Pract* 2013, 63:e657–68.

22 van der Heide A, Onwuteaka-Philipsen BD, Rurup M, et al. End-of-life practices in the Netherlands under the euthanasia act. *NEJM* 2007; 356:1957–65.

23 Bilsen J, Norup M, Deliens L, et al. Drugs used to alleviate symptoms with life shortening as a possible side effect: end-of-life care in six European countries. *J Pain Symptom Manage* 2006; 31:111–21.

24 Miccinesi G, Rietjens JA, Deliens L, et al. EURELD Consortium. Continuous deep sedation: physicians' experiences in six European countries. *J Pain Symptom Manage* 2006; 31:122–9.

25 Chambaere K, Bilsen J, Cohen J, et al. Continuous deep sedation until death in Belgium: a nationwide survey. *Arch Intern Med* 2010; 170:490–3.

26 Seale C. Continuous deep sedation in medical practice: a descriptive study. *J Pain Symptom Manage* 2010, **39**:44–53.

27 Rietjens J, van Delden J, Onwuteaka-Philipsen B, Buiting H, van der Maas P, van der Heide A. The use of continuous deep sedation for patients nearing death in the Netherlands: a descriptive study. *BMJ* 2008; **336**:810–3.

28 Anquinet L, Rietjens JAC, Vandervoort A, et al. Continuous deep sedation until death in nursing home residents with dementia: a case series. *JAGS* 2013; **61**:1768–76.

29 Maddison AR, Asada Y, Urquhart R. Inequity in access to cancer care: a review of the Canadian literature. *Cancer Causes Control* 2011; **22**:359–66.

30 Rurup ML, Onwuteaka-Philipsen BD, Pasman HR, Ribbe MW, van der Wal G. Attitudes of physicians, nurses and relatives towards end-of-life decisions concerning nursing home patients with dementia. *Patient Educ Couns* 2006; **61**(3):372–80.

31 Winzelberg GS, Hanson LC, Tulsky JA. Beyond autonomy: diversifying end-of-life decision-making approaches to serve patients and families. *J Am Geriatr Soc* 2005; **53**:1046–50.

32 Visser A, Dijkstra GJ, Kuiper D, de Jong PE, Franssen CFM, Gansevoort RT, et al. Accepting or declining dialysis: considerations taken into account by elderly patients with end-stage renal disease. *J Nephrology* 2009; **22**:794–9.

33 Gordon M. Ethical challenges in end-of-life therapies in the elderly. *Drugs Aging* 2002; **19**:321–9.

34 Zikmund-Fisher BJ, Lacey HP, Fagerlin A. The potential impact of decision role and patient age on end-of-life treatment decision making. *J Med Ethics* 2008; **34**:327–31.

35 Kaspers PJ, Onwuteaka-Philipsen BD, Deeg DJH, Pasman HRW. Having and discussing preferences on forgoing treatment in the last three months of life of older people with and without an advance directive. In: PJ Kaspers (ed). *End-of-life care and preferences for (non)treatment decisions in older people during the last three months of life.* Amsterdam: Free University; 2013, 75–91.

36 Clore, FC. Decision-making capacity. *J Palliat Med* 2009; **12**:1075.

37 Moye, J, Marson, DC. Assessment of decision-making capacity in older adults: an emerging area of practice and research. *J Gerontology Psychological Sciences* 2007; **62B**:3 11.

38 Kaspers PJ, Onwuteaka-Philipsen BD, Deeg DJH, Pasman HRW. Decision-making capacity and communication about care of older people during their last three months of life. *BMC Palliat Care* 2013; **12**:1–10.

39 Murray SA, Kendall M, Boyd K, Sheikh A. Illness trajectories and palliative care. *BMJ* 2005; **330**:1007–11.

40 Lunney JR, Lynn J, Foley DJ, Lipson S, Guralnik JM. Patterns of functional decline at the end of life. *J Am Geriatr Soc* 2003; **289**:2387–92.

41 Chambaere K, Cohen J, Robijn L, Bailey SK, Deliens L. End-of-life decisions in patients dying with dementia in Belgium. J Am Geriatr Soc 2014 (epub ahead of print).

Chapter 14

Ethical issues in palliative care for older people

Jennifer S. Shaw and Margaret P. Battin

If there were reasons for these miseries, then into limits could I bind my woes.
Shakespeare, Titus Andronicus, Act 3, Scene 1

Introduction to ethical issues in palliative care for older people

Discussions regarding the ethics of palliative care tend to be associated with end-of-life ethics, as these two areas overlap on the health care spectrum and have become, seemingly inextricably, intertwined both in the public mind and among health care providers. When curative care is no longer possible, providers and their patients may think of palliative care, and in many hospitals 'comfort care' is a euphemism for 'dying.' The traditional function of medical care has 'two mutually exclusive goals: either to cure disease and prolong life or to provide comfort care. Given this dichotomy, the decision to focus on reducing suffering is made only after life-prolonging treatment has been ineffectual and death is imminent (1).' In addition to this conceptual paradigm, the relationship between end-of-life care and palliative care is emotional and financial, with palliative care often perceived to reflect an attitude of resignation and 'giving up'. These perceptions of palliative care constitute a particular challenge in the care of older people, raising ethical issues that will be explored in this chapter.

The overlapping relationship between palliative care and end-of-life care has been reinforced and perhaps distorted by issues involving financial reimbursement. Institutional pressures complicate the picture, for instance, when a care facility transfers a dying older person to the hospital rather than spend time coordinating hospice care, only to lose a source of revenue in the process. Similarly, a hospital may pursue aggressive life-prolonging interventions with an older person following surgery so that survival statistics look better. A system has inadvertently been created that asks older patients nearing the end of their lives to make an artificial and sometimes gut-wrenching choice between palliative care, with the option of hospital-based interventions, or hospice care, with an emphasis on optimal comfort measures at home. In an ideal world, this would not be an either/or choice but a matter of emphasis and proportionality. There is something unsettling about asking a family to choose between prolonging life so that 'Mum' might live until a son can arrive from out of town and doing everything possible to reduce suffering, but that is exactly what families are sometimes asked to do.

Separating palliative care from other areas of health care, in an attempt to discern ethical issues unique to palliative care, can be a meaningless exercise. In the practical application of bioethical concepts across the health care spectrum, concerns tend to be discussed in terms of normative principles ('What is at stake here?'), and when that fails to enlighten, in terms of formal decision-making procedures ('Who gets to decide?' and 'How do we approach this issue in order to feel good about our decisions?'). The language that emerges from such discussions can be impoverished and lack the ability to describe in detail the richness of the issue at hand. Rather than asking which concepts are more or less prominent in palliative care with the older population, perhaps we should ask how to best re-conceptualize the language in more helpful and multidimensional ways.

Imagine that health care professionals know an older patient is unhappy. That knowledge, while helpful, does not enable them to be optimally responsive to that person's needs. In order to be truly helpful, they need to understand why he or she is unhappy. Is it related to loneliness, anxiety, pain, loss, physical difficulties, spiritual distress, or all of these?

The same situation arises when discussing ethical issues. For example, it has been said that the 'ascendancy of autonomy over other medical ethical principles is the centre for most of the ethical dilemmas encountered in palliative care (2).' It is not enough to suspect that autonomy is threatened by a series of treatment decisions unfolding in a health care facility, and providers need to know more to best serve their patients. An individual's disease, personality, circumstances, wishes, values, family members, religious affiliations, and cognitive abilities are just the beginning of an almost inexhaustible list of things health care providers should understand in order to grasp the situation at hand. Therefore, the label given to the ethical issue involved (e.g. 'autonomy', 'paternalism', 'informed consent') represents just the tip of an iceberg, and an understanding of what is beneath the surface is needed if health professionals want to use their understanding of ethical issues to best respond to their patients' needs. For this reason, the discussion of ethical concerns that arise when providing palliative care to older people must involve an in-depth and individualized understanding of the situation at hand. The conversation cannot be scripted, and the decisions reached may be varied.

Palliative care programmes can address the needs of many older patients with an emphasis on communication and decision making guided by the individual patient and negotiated by health care providers with an attitude of respect, kindness, and compassion. An ageing population has a variety of chronic conditions which may not be life-threatening but have significant and cumulative symptom burdens (3). An illness may be accompanied by the small daily insults of arthritis and mobility problems, visual and hearing deficits, or bowel and bladder problems that arise with ageing. The relative insignificance of these issues to the medical community stands in contrast to their functional significance in everyday life, and 'palliative care offers an opportunity to thoughtfully pursue only those treatments that match the patient's values and goals of care' (4).

Few would argue that palliative care should be reserved for the dying. After all, nausea is nausea, whether one is terminally ill or not. Both ageing and terminal illness are universal experiences for most people, unless they die an early or sudden death, and it feels fundamentally unnecessary to ask patients to wait until they are within earshot of death to receive care that is intended to reduce suffering. The symptomatic burden of many chronic illnesses is heavy in terms of both physical and emotional suffering, and ignoring this, or waiting until the weeks preceding death to address this, is rarely in a patient's best interests.

Some might suggest that comfort is a less legitimate goal than cure. Although an ancient goal of medicine, and a central one of nursing, comfort has become eclipsed in the past century by our increasing ability to manage, or even cure, one's illness. As a culture, humans have had a love affair with curative possibilities, and this suggests that something is seriously amiss when, and if, the trajectory of an illness is not altered by the good doctors at hand. When physical health is threatened, western culture demands a fight, regardless of age. People expect sicknesses to be cured and discomforts eased.

Expanding palliative care to older people, whether they are terminally ill or not, may best unfold by revamping the ethical landscape with an emphasis on attempts to construct patient-specific ethical narratives. These narratives provide flexible tools and helpful guidance to physicians and nurses in a wide variety of settings, from the hospital to the care facility to the home, whether early or late in the course of a patient's illness, which may be acute or chronic, slowly progressive or terminal. The ability to negotiate this terrain is limited if our understanding stops once a uniform ethical vocabulary has been established. Individualized narratives also make room for shared medical decision making, a model which becomes more relevant as people age, and the decisions reached are based not on generalizable principles but on individually negotiated goals (5, 6). When narratives are constructed, ethical vocabulary becomes richer and, hence, more able to embrace uncertainty and change as circumstances unfold. What was thought to best serve a patient last year may indeed be different this year, and health care institutions should have the ability to recognize ethical issues unfolding in dynamic ways over time.

Health care decisions affect the older population and those who are terminally ill differently, as they are seen through different lenses, yet this distinction is also problematic. There is little agreement on when someone living with a progressive illness becomes 'terminal'. Is it when they have a six-month life expectancy? Does it occur only when professionals and patients have convinced themselves that there are no further treatment options likely to extend one's life expectancy? Or can all those people diagnosed with a progressive and life-limiting illness be safely called 'terminal' because their illness will eventually contribute to their death? For most people, being told they have a terminal illness changes their life journey, and they proceed inexorably toward an end, whether that end is welcome, feared, or both. This is not so for people who are simply old and whose list of symptomatic woes extends indefinitely toward the final horizon of their lives.

This chapter explores common ethical themes that arise when providing palliative care for older people. While one-on-one conversations, occurring over time, and the subsequent construction of individualized narratives will, in practice, provide a road map of sorts for ethical decision making, it is important to acknowledge that this takes time and will require a shared ethical vocabulary to facilitate discussion between and among clinicians and patients.

Beneficence as an ethical issue

First, albeit controversially, the very essence of palliative care is beneficence—the principle that one ought to act and do good. Many practitioners in the field go home at the end of a busy work day and review whether or not they have truly helped another person and made a positive difference in someone's life. In palliative care, as in other domains of health care, ethical uneasiness arises if one suspects that what is offered is not helping, that efforts to do good may in fact be causing harm (7). Questions concerning beneficence may well be of this form: 'Am I solving a short-term problem but creating a long-term one?' or 'Am I neglecting a short-term problem in order to avoid a long-term one?'

For example, it is clear that pain is widely undertreated among older people, especially if they have cognitive impairments (8). The question for palliative care specialists is how to weigh the obligation to provide effective pain management against the potential risks, which include safety concerns and the possibility of drug diversion. The continued and long-term use of opioids by older people has the potential for compromised cognitive function, constipation, and increased fall risk, while changing liver and kidney function affects drug metabolism.

Autonomy as an ethical issue

Autonomy is sometimes used as a trump card in ethical discussions. Though routinely prioritized over beneficence in theoretical discussions, autonomy takes a decided second place to beneficence, non-maleficence, and other principles in the actual practice of palliative care. Single-minded appeals to autonomy, for example, may not be helpful during the fuzzy transition period to shared decision making that characteristically accompanies ageing. Autonomy is not always absolute, and a person's decision-making capacity can be temporarily clouded by medications or intoxication, an acute change in health, existential despair, cognitive deficits, or cultural practices that do not prioritize autonomy. Perceptions of patient wishes may also be distorted by the values and emotions of the surrogate decision maker. As one son might say to his father who no longer wants renal dialysis: 'But you have to fight, Dad. Be strong for us." Conversely, another son might say to another father who may have wanted to continue dialysis: 'It's alright, Dad, if you've had enough. We understand and don't want to see you suffer any more.' These kinds of exchanges often prompt feelings of discomfort for clinicians and hospital staff, and what might have been the autonomous choices of the patient may be lost in the process. How to balance the relative weight of autonomy and beneficence is an ongoing concern in palliative care for older people.

Promise-keeping as an ethical issue

Promises are slippery things that can roll off the tongue casually when wanting to reassure patients. Health professionals sometimes say things like 'We'll make sure you don't suffer' or 'You'll have a little discomfort but be up and at 'em before long' or 'We'll help your mother have a peaceful death'. Comments like these often represent empty promises—ones that health carers can influence but not actually control, despite their training and expertise. A practitioner can promise to pay close attention to a patient's discomfort and suffering, but he or she cannot promise that there will not be pain or distress. These promises represent not malicious or intentionally misleading behaviour, but a certain linguistic laziness and, perhaps, an inflated sense of self-importance or a desire to provide reassurance.

Failing to keep promises is an obvious breach of trust between health care provider and patient, and while promises are occasionally broken by an individual, there are times when the system is to blame. Failures in promise-keeping may be particularly problematic in the care of older people, where not only is competence diminished but the patient's recollection of promises given may also be impaired—and yet, they were promises, robustly made.

One area in which this can come into play with older adults involves living wills and advanced directives. Patients are frequently encouraged to articulate their wishes for life-prolonging interventions both verbally and in writing, with assurances that their health care providers will respect those wishes should the time come when they become critically ill and no longer have decision-making capacity. In an emergency, however, many physicians will not search the labyrinth of a patient's medical records to discover whether that person has written directives in their file. Although advanced directives are supposed to be readily accessible, it often takes time and energy to conduct initial and subsequent searches for documents. Especially if a patient's condition is deemed treatable, aggressive life-saving interventions will be provided by default. While this is both an understandable and easily defensible decision for physicians to make when facing a rapid and critical change in a patient's health, it does come as a surprise to patients who honestly believed that they would not be resuscitated once legal paperwork to that effect was completed. As an older woman told one of us, 'It was Easter. I had a good day and looked forward to going to bed. The next thing I knew there were fire-fighters looking down at me and I woke up in the ICU on a breathing machine. I never wanted that to happen and thought I had done what I needed to prevent it. What else am I supposed to do?'

Informed consent as an ethical issue

Informed consent is a common issue among older people, especially those who interact with health care providers in institutional settings. Let us imagine that a woman in her late 60s was diagnosed with ovarian cancer a number of years ago. While she received the utmost in treatment for that cancer, within five years she learns that it has spread and the burden of related symptoms becomes considerable: she struggles with daily nausea and her tumours interfere with normal digestion and bowel function. After several months, she and her oncology team decide to try surgery to see if anything can be done to reduce her tumours and unblock her intestines. She formally consents to the surgery. All goes well during the surgery, but she does not bounce back afterward. She continues to experience nausea and have signs of a bowel obstruction. Her appetite is poor and she does not feel like eating, so she eats very little. She has told her team upfront that she does not want to be dependent on machines or tubes to keep her alive, and although she was willing to try surgery and felt the potential benefits were worth the risk, she was adamant that she did not want a feeding tube.

The surgical team, however, had a different perspective: she had agreed to surgery and that meant she agreed to all interventions needed to help her recover from surgery. They insisted that she have a feeding tube because they felt it was necessary for an optimal outcome surgically. They did not believe she had the right to refuse their recommended treatment, or to say 'no' half-way through the recovery process, or to change her mind for spurious reasons. Additionally, they recognized the ways in which feeding tubes are often maligned in the public imagination and believed she misunderstood how the tube would contribute to her recovery.

Speaking ethically and not merely legally, did her consent to surgery include consent to all appropriate post-operative treatment? There is no easy answer to this question.

Futility, non-maleficence, and proportionality as ethical issues

These terms have helped many providers frame ethical discussions in ways that facilitate conversation and decision making, but it may be time to move beyond them. The term 'futility' implies that an effort is made for naught, with a high suspicion that it would not accomplish anything meaningful, either physiologically or in terms of quality of life (9, 10). In geriatrics, it may be futile to fill pillboxes thinking that an older person's ability to adhere to a recommended medication schedule will improve, knowing that he or she does not have the dexterity to open the pillboxes or make sense of what is inside. Similarly, handing an older person a mobile phone and feeling better about their ability to call in an emergency sounds nice, but even if the emergency number is pre-programmed into the phone, it may be futile if he or she cannot remember to keep the thing charged. We sometimes suspect we are offering medically futile interventions if we are doing so because someone wants to make sure that 'everything is done'.

The term 'non-maleficence', in contrast, captures the principle of 'do no harm' as enshrined in the Oath of Hippocrates. It can be understood narrowly to mean that the clinician should avoid directly and intentionally causing harm, or it can be understood more broadly to prohibit causing harm whether intentionally or not, whether by commission or omission.

Both terms are important but they represent a relatively static interpretation of a patient or provider's ethical dilemma: Is a recommended treatment futile? Are we causing harm, and if so, is it justifiable? Yes, no, or maybe? Such discussions can continue at great length, but they represent a limited interpretation of a patient's more complicated reality.

Some bioethicists are reframing these issues in terms of 'proportionality'—a term often associated with Catholic moral theology or, in layman's terms, balancing benefits and risks, pros and cons, ways we help and ways we hurt. Rather than spending time and energy trying to define futile interventions, both patients and their providers are better served by focusing 'on communication and negotiation at the bedside' (9). This is an individualized approach, based on an in-depth reading of a patient's situation and geared towards assessing, at this moment in time, the predicted benefits of a certain procedure, drug, or recommendation, and balancing these against the predicted costs or drawbacks. One person may reach a different decision than another. One patient may be willing to tolerate nausea for a few days after treatment, and another, not. And that same person may reach a different decision at different times in his or her life. This, now, is truly flexible medical decision making, grounded in an individualized approach—but still dependent upon informed consent and the ability to communicate, something potentially problematic among older people.

Proportionality represents a model that shifts the physician role from one of authoritative decision maker to one of educator and advisor. One common example involves the trade-off when a patient has moderate to severe pain. Do we offer opioids, knowing that they may cloud a patient's mental status while offering effective pain relief? How do we balance the burden and the benefit? Ideally, these questions can be answered only by knowing the patient and family well, because some people want to sleep through a painful experience and others want to be awake and interactive at all costs.

This shifting role asks providers to have sophisticated communication skills in addition to clinical expertise. Of note, this model takes time, is best practiced by providers who know a patient well over time, and is not favoured by rule-oriented work environments. It also asks physicians to broaden their view of the 'burdens' accompanying clinical recommendations and to consider non-medical concerns as legitimate considerations in the medical decision-making process. For example, factors affecting patient decisions may be influenced in legitimate ways by the financial cost of a new drug, the guilt of family members if they do not try "everything", or providers' fear of potential litigation (11).

Uncertainty and guilt are often behind-the-scenes forces when there are differences of opinion regarding the medical benefit of a given intervention, and it takes skilled communicators to negotiate these emotions with patients and caregivers. 'Patients are uncomfortable with uncertainty about diagnoses and prognoses and often request tests to help alleviate those anxieties' (12). Moreover, patients and caregivers feel guilty if they do not pursue all care options available.

Decisions regarding life-sustaining measures

This area of bioethics has innumerable examples of ethical decision-making dilemmas in palliative care for older people. Among those that arise with regularity are:

Tube feeding and dementia

As people age, so does the likelihood that they will experience cognitive deficits of some sort. And as dementia progresses, so does the inability to swallow. Swallowing is an extraordinarily complex process requiring well-coordinated muscles; late-stage dementia takes a toll on muscle coordination and, eventually, this leads to both the decreasing ability to maintain adequate nutrition and the increased risk of aspiration pneumonia when these patients eat.

When patients reach this point, they and their families have the option of allowing the disease process to unfold naturally, which means that the patient will eat less and less over time, get thinner and cachexic, and be at risk for aspiration pneumonia. Or, they may consider having a feeding tube placed so that the patient can be fed artificially for an indefinite period of time. This decision is more complicated than one might initially believe, in part because the effect of a feeding tube on life expectancy and quality of life is not clear-cut (13, 14). Inevitably, powerful cultural issues around feeding and starvation surface.

Since the severely demented patient is not capable of informed consent and, hence, has already lost some measure of autonomy, decision-making now been shared or displaced onto others. Because the patient can no longer clearly and consistently articulate his or her wishes, the caregivers' feelings, values, and expectations become more prominent. Antecedent wishes of the patient, even those clearly documented in advanced directives, may be ignored or overridden; the underlying philosophic issue is whether the precedent autonomy of the previously competent person should govern treatment of the now-compromised person (and indeed, whether this is the "same" person) or whether the demented person's current experiential preferences should be followed. When balancing the benefits and burdens of an intervention like tube feeding, non-medical concerns often outstrip medical ones in the final outcome. From a medical perspective, feeding tubes are recommended mostly as a bridge to recovery, or a way to move from illness to wellness. However, this is not so with advanced dementia, a disease process in which feeding tubes 'are associated with considerable harm and do not provide a mortality benefit' (15). Moreover, decisions regarding feeding tubes are often informed by moral, religious, and legal issues, not to mention reimbursement considerations, rather than scientific ones (16).

Implantable devices in heart failure

Millions of older people live with heart disease, from heart arrhythmias to advanced heart failure (17). In addition to transplants or artificial hearts, implantable devices are increasingly being used and can eventually be deactivated, raising ethical concerns surrounding decisions to withdraw life-sustaining or life-saving interventions that may lead to death.

Other ethical questions involving the initial decision to implant and/or deactivate mechanical devices to support the circulatory system include the importance of informed consent, balancing benefits and burdens, and the need for clear and ongoing communication between the medical team and the patient regarding advanced directives, patient wishes, and the point at which quality of life becomes unacceptable (10, 18, 19). The treatment of advanced heart failure offers a unique challenge to integrate palliative care and life-prolonging care, and it raises questions of distributive justice (18).

Cardiopulmonary resuscitation and mechanical ventilation

To the extent that palliative care nurses and physicians help patients articulate their wishes regarding potentially life-saving efforts, there can be a schism between what a patient hopes will happen and what providers feel is reasonable. For example, a patient may want resuscitation but not intubation and ventilation, which, in a critical care setting, sounds inconsistent and impractical. Others may want resuscitation if they have a heart attack, but not if they are dying from cancer. Many want practitioners to give on-the-spot predictions of survival and ask for resuscitation only if it will return them to a previous level of health and well-being. 'You can try,' says one older woman, 'only if I won't be disabled once you bring me back.' This request overestimates the accuracy of clinical prognostication. Patients may request 'Do not resuscitate' orders when they are not terminally ill, but physicians look askance at making this decision before the nature of an illness or the medical facts are understood.

Refusal of care as an ethical issue

A number of ethical issues arise when providing palliative care to older people who refuse care. Physicians and nurse practitioners are accustomed to having their recommendations followed, despite widespread evidence of non-adherence with treatment recommendations, especially in chronic diseases like diabetes, depression, and heart disease. Sometimes this is simple non-compliance: the patient dislikes the side-effects of a medication, turns to 'natural' therapeutics, or just forgets. Sometimes refusal is based in mistrust of the physician or the wish to let nature take its course. It should not come as a surprise when patients or their families refuse a recommended therapy, although for many clinicians it does. Emotionally, refusal of care can feel like rejection, and professionals may respond with a feeling that the patient deserves to suffer the consequences of an ill-advised choice.

Conflicts over refusal of care between provider and patient may reflect egos, decision-making control, proportionality, or simple misunderstandings. Clinicians may fail to perceive or value a patient's priorities, and patients may fail to understand the value of a recommendation that does not contribute meaningfully to daily quality of life. A classic example of this involves the pharmacological management of patients at risk of developing a blood clot. Imagine a woman in her late 70s who has a certain heart rhythm, atrial fibrillation, that predisposes her to developing a blood clot and increases her risk of having a stroke. Palliative care providers recommend that she take a blood thinner to help prevent this potentially disabling complication. She, however, feels fine and does not want to take any more medicines. She refuses because her assessment of the risk is small and her negative feelings about the side-effects of medication are great. Plus, her closest friend developed a bleed in her brain after falling down stairs while taking a blood thinner, and she never wants to be in that situation. In a clinical setting, a friend's tragedy often trumps medical advice. In the internet age, a patient does not even need to know a friend who has experienced an adverse complication; all he or she needs to do is read a sensational story online.

Refusal of care may represent a patient's wish not to prolong life, especially in situations where quality of life is experienced as poor and a patient fears disability. In the minds of some older people, preventing a major life-ending stroke in order to live with the mobility deficits of a lesser stroke is not a desirable outcome.

End-of-life decision making

When patients are unable to understand the nature of medical decisions being made on their behalf, either because of a temporary or permanent lack of decision-making capacity, surrogate decision makers are asked to help. Typically, but not always, these decision makers are next of kin. In an ideal situation, the patient has already contemplated the possibility of this situation and has designated a medical power of attorney in writing. But often a patient's family finds itself trying to make weighty decisions of considerable clinical importance with little preparation, during a time of heightened emotions. When a patient is incompetent or lacks decision-making capacity, families are asked what the patient would have wanted if able to speak for him or herself, and also what they think is in the patient's best interests. These are not simple decisions, often involving internal tension between the patient's presumed antecedent preferences and his or her presumed current best interests. Families being families, the dynamics are often difficult.

Among the most controversial decisions for palliative care clinicians and their older patients are those involving the withdrawal or withholding of treatment that will hasten death, including renal dialysis, the provision of antibiotics, artificial nutrition and perhaps hydration, or blood transfusions.

The practice of terminal sedation, in which a patient with intractable suffering and nearing death is purposely sedated, typically to unconsciousness, while withholding artificial nutrition and hydration, is considered by some to be an appropriate response to suffering. From one perspective, tacit appeal to the principle of double-effect obviates questions about the direct causing of death: death is foreseen, but not intended. Others, noting the various alternative locutions that omit any reference to terminality—'palliative sedation,' 'continuous deep sedation,' 'primary deep continuous sedation' (20)— reply that terminal sedation by any name, where artificial nutrition and hydration are not provided, deliberately brings about death (21).

Still greater controversy surrounds such practices as physician-assisted suicide (as opponents call it) or physician aid-in-dying (as proponents do). Legal, as of early 2015, in four American states and in a number of European countries, the average age of terminally-ill patients receiving assistance to end their lives, in both Oregon and the Netherlands, is about 70, and the most frequent diagnosis is cancer (22). Palliative care organizations have generally been opposed to these practices, though views may be changing. Proponents of the legalization of aid-in-dying, on the other hand, point out that the provision of palliative care and direct assistance in dying need not be incompatible. Data from Oregon for 2013 show that 85.7% of those who died under the Death With Dignity Act were enrolled in hospice care either at the time the prescription was written or at the time of death (23).

The discussion of patient and family wishes concerning the ending of life requires deft communication skills, even in the absence of language or cultural differences. Open discussion exploring whether or not a patient wants to hasten death is not easily undertaken. 'Negotiation' of the circumstances of dying is often accomplished via hints, innuendo, and indirect implication. What can be a crucially important element of palliative care in terminal illness—discussion of the question 'how do you want your death to go, given that, unfortunately, we cannot find any way to prevent it?'—is often undertaken hesitantly and with great difficulty, especially in jurisdictions where assisted dying is not legal.

Conclusion: quality of life issues

Successful care of the ageing involves an ongoing process of assessment and reassessment of treatment decisions and goals of care. Clinicians often ask if a recommendation that made sense five or ten years ago continues to make sense now. Part of this process involves a sometimes subtle shift away from a curative paradigm, looking instead at managing illness in ways that optimize quality of life. The success of medical interventions is now measured on the basis of optimizing comfort, functioning, and 'normalcy'. Patients themselves also ask whether a past treatment decision continues to make sense. These questions raise the issue of whether quality of life is to be assessed subjectively or objectively, or both, and in both cases, how assessment should proceed.

Competing views of suffering arise as an issue with older adults, especially if competence is questionable. One perspective, characteristic of palliative care, holds that suffering is bad and almost always to be prevented, even at the cost of cognitive functioning. On the other hand, a quite different and often religiously-based view holds that suffering can have deep spiritual meaning and that it can, or should, be a fitting conclusion to life in this world, a prelude to reward in the afterlife. Ethical analysis cannot resolve such disparate views; these are a function of deeply different metaphysical commitments. Palliative care providers, however, must be able to respond to patients with widely different views and to their nearly universal searches for meaning in suffering and death.

The ethical issues that arise with the geriatric population are familiar but nuanced. Models relevant to palliative care will both acknowledge the inevitability of death while not becoming preoccupied by it. They will reflect one-on-one conversations with an individual who is perceived as something other than a generic 'patient'. The best palliative care models will be flexible, dynamic, and useful in different settings across the health care spectrum. They will accept uncertainty and embrace humility, since we do not know what is best for all ageing adults who are, after all, as diverse as their younger counterparts. The nonmedical concerns of patients and families will be valued and the sometimes problematic influence of financial reimbursement structures, acknowledged. Learning to talk and listen with understanding, respect, and compassion will take valuable time from a clinician's busy practice, but we will all benefit.

References

1 Morrison RS, Meier DE. Palliative care. *NEJM* 2011; **350**(25):2582–90.

2 Cimino JC. A clinician's understanding of ethics in palliative care: an American perspective. *Crit Rev Oncol Hemato* 2003; **46**(1):17–24.

3 Ritchie CS. Palliation in the care of older adults. In: Yennurajalingam S, Bruera E (eds). *Oxford American Handbook of Hospice and Palliative Medicine*. New York: Oxford University Press; 2011, 349.

4 Henson DM. Toward a theology of palliative care: faith, reason, praxis, and love. *The Heythrop Journal* 2012; Published online 29 October 2012, pp 1–13; doi: 10.1111/j.1468-2265.2012.00778.x.

5 Lanoix M. The ethics of imperfect cures: models of service delivery and patient vulnerability. *J Med Ethics* 2013; **39**(11):690.

6 Lorenzl S. End of one's life–decision making between autonomy and uncertainty. *Geriatric Mental Health Care* 2013; **1**:63–6.

7 Dawson KA. Palliative care for critically ill older adults: dimensions of nursing advocacy. *Crit Care Nur Q* 2008; **31**(1):19–23.

8 Goldstein NE, Meier DE. Palliative medicine in older adults. In: Hanks G, Cherny NI, Christakis NA, Fallon M, Kassa S, Portenoy RK (eds). *Oxford Textbook of Palliative Medicine* (4th edn). Oxford: Oxford University Press; 2010, 1386–99.

9 Burns JP, Truog RD. Futility: a concept in evolution. *CHEST Journal* 2007; **132**(6):1987–93.

10 Fins JJ, Nilson EG. Withholding and withdrawing life-sustaining care. In: Hanks G, Cherny NI, Christakis NA, Fallon M, Kassa S, Portenoy RK (eds). *Oxford Textbook of Palliative Medicine* (4th edn). Oxford: Oxford University Press; 2010, 320–9.

11 Kirk TW, Luck GR. Dying tax free: the modern advance directive and patients' financial values. *J Pain Symptom Manage* 2010; **39**(3):605–9.

12 Liepert AE, Leichtle SW, Santin BJ. Surgery at the end of life. *Bull Am Coll Surg* 2012; **97**(8):36–40.

13 Congedo M, Causarano RI, Alberti F, Bonito V, Borghi L, Colombi L, et al. Ethical issues in end of life treatments for patients with dementia. *Eur J Neurol* 2010; **17**(6):774–9.

14 Widera E, Covinsky K. What are appropriate palliative interventions for patients with advanced dementia? In: Goldstein N, Morrison RS. *Evidence-Based Practice of Palliative Medicine*. Philadelphia, PA: Elsevier Saunders; 2013, 295–9.

15 Quill TE, Bower K, Holloway RG, Shah M S, Caprio TV, Olden A, et al. *Primer of Palliative Care* (6th edn). Chicago, IL: American Academy of Hospice and Palliative Medicine; 2014, 66.

16 Gillick MR, Volandes AE. The standard of caring: why do we still use feeding tubes in patients with advanced dementia? *JAMDA* 2008; **9**(5):364–7.

17 Johnson MJ. Extending palliative care to patients with heart failure. *Brit J Hosp Med* 2010; **71**(1):12–5.

18 Tanner CE, Fromme EK, Goodlin SJ. Ethics in the treatment of advanced heart failure: palliative care and end-of-life issues. *Congestive Heart Failure* 2011; **17**(5):235–40.

19 Brush S, Budge D, Alharethi R, McCormick AJ, MacPherson JD, Reid BB, et al. End-of-life decision making and implementation in recipients of a destination left ventricular assist device. *J Heart Lung Transpl* 2010; **29**(12):1337–41.

20 Vena C, Kuebler K, Schrader SE. The dying process. In: Kuebler KK, Mellar PD, Moore CD. *Palliative Practices*. St. Louis, MO: Elsevier Mosby; 2005, 342–6.

21 Battin MP. Terminal sedation: pulling the sheet over our eyes. *Hastings Center Report* 2008; **38**(5):27–30.

22 Battin MP, van der Heide A, Ganzini L, van der Wal G, Onwuteaka-Philipsen BD. Legal physician-assisted dying in Oregon and the Netherlands: evidence concerning the impact on patients in 'vulnerable' groups. *J Med Ethics* 2007; **33**(10):591–7.

23 <Http://public.health.oregon.gov/ProviderPartnerResources/EvaluationResearch/DeathwithDignityAct/Documents/year16.pdf>, page 2 of 7, accessed 2/8/15.

Chapter 15

Cultural issues in palliative care for older people

Marjolein Gysels

Introduction to cultural issues in palliative care for older people

Ageing populations across the world are increasingly presenting challenges to health systems. Living longer generally brings debilitating chronic diseases, from which people will eventually die (1–3). This leads to a greater need for palliative care (4) and governments are becoming more aware of the necessity to include palliative care as an essential part of their health care systems (5, 6). However, there are challenges regarding the integration of palliative care into particular health systems. Its expansion and ways of organization differ extensively across countries, due to the various ways in which health and social care is funded and delivered.

In order to understand the progress of palliative care in different countries, mapping exercises have been undertaken documenting, comparing, and ranking levels of service development (7, 8). These provide essential evidence for the further advancement of palliative care practice, research, and policy making. However, other factors such as cultural attitudes towards ageing, health, illness, and dying are also powerful forces that shape the way communities arrange care. There is little research on cultural issues in palliative care and these issues are, therefore, a lot less understood (9).

This chapter first clarifies the concept of culture, informed by decades of research in anthropology. To find out what is known about cultural issues in palliative care, it turns to the literature produced in this field, which focuses mainly on the disparities in the use of health care services. The notion of cultural competence, which has been promoted to address these problems, is explored and its assumptions are critically considered in the context of palliative care. The chapter then considers palliative care in an historical and international perspective as it has developed through time and place, and how that has influenced its meaning. The value of palliative care for the needs of older people will be discussed.

The concept of culture in palliative care

The lack of attention to cultural issues in palliative care is in part due to the complexity of the concept of culture (9). Without taking into account the theoretical knowledge on culture, there is the risk that research reaches results which are, at best, simplistic and, at worst, careless or harmful to the people in question (10).

Culture is defined as 'presupposed, taken-for-granted models of the world, that are widely shared (although not necessarily to the exclusion of other, alternative models) by the members of a society, and that play an enormous role in their understanding of that world and their behaviour in it' (11). Cultural models are, in other words, systems of shared ideas, and rules and meanings, that underlie and are expressed in the ways that people live (12). These shared meanings are learned and sustained through shared practice. People do not simply act routinely in everyday life, choosing between appropriate alternatives, but attach meaning to social interactions and interpret one another. Cultural meaning is negotiated, questioned, or confirmed in social processes and is shaped by specific circumstances and histories (13). Understanding prevailing attitudes about illness, dying, and care, and how that is distributed across time and place, is an interpretive task.

Studies enquiring about differences between people often use categories such as ethnicity, which is often confused with cultural variation. Ethnicity refers to the heritage that people share in a particular society, based on a common language or religion and leading to a sense of identity or group awareness (14). People with the same ethnicity can, however, differ vastly in terms of world-view and values, and these are highly variable according to changing circumstances (15). In quantitative analyses, ethnicity is often used as a demographic variable for the prediction of specific behavioural characteristics. However, culture is infinitely more complex.

The evidence on culture in palliative care research: the focus on minority ethnic groups

Although the equation of culture with ethnicity is criticized here, ethnicity is a useful part of culture that can shed light on the low use of palliative care services by people from ethnic minorities (16, 17). Disparities between ethnic minority groups' estimated need of palliative care services and their actual service use have been reported (16, 17). Therefore, it is not surprising that the research literature addressing diversity issues in palliative care approaches these from a perspective of ethnicity, and this is especially the case in the United Kingdom. A recent systematic review identified 13 literature reviews on ethnic minorities and palliative care in the United Kingdom, which is related to the growing attention to this issue by policy makers in palliative care (18). A subsequent systematic review which synthesized the primary research on this topic unearthed another 45 original studies (19). Together, these reviews give a comprehensive view of the evidence concerning ethnic minorities' use of palliative care in the United Kingdom. The syntheses revolve around the same themes:

Structural inequalities surfaced as services were acknowledged to be disproportionately absent in areas of social deprivation.

Inequality by disease group appeared from the studies. The focus on cancer in palliative care provision was cited as a major source of inequality due to the greater importance of non-malignant diseases among ethnic minority groups.

Referrals were problematic due to limited knowledge of services and the referral process among physicians who are not palliative care or cancer specialists.

Place of death and care: a number of reviews highlighted the perceived preference among minority ethnic groups for home care. However, other sources found that the preferred place of death depended on multiple factors, and this could vary across different groups.

Awareness and communication were identified as barriers to service use. There was a lack of information in appropriate formats, negative perceptions, and low awareness of services. Problems persisted once services had been accessed.

Cultural competency was called for in the reviews as negative perceptions towards services were considered significant impediments to utilization and some services were identified as culturally insensitive (19, 20, 26). A common recommendation was the need for training in care that is sensitive to cultural differences. In contrast to the frequent recognition that services need to provide culturally competent care, few reviews provided recommendations about how to achieve this. Cultural differences were said to lead to uncertainty, even when staff were trained in 'cultural competency' issues. The importance of monitoring service users' ethnicity was frequently stressed. However, data were said to be inadequately collected and rarely used to influence service provision.

Cultural competence in palliative care

Studies which showed that patients who came from similar socio-economic backgrounds and had similar language abilities and health care needs received different treatment and had differential health care outcomes related solely to their ethnicity, led to the development of expertise in cultural competence (21). Cultural competence was a response to the wish of health professionals to provide appropriate care—care that takes 'cultural' differences into account (21). This has developed into a movement which has had substantial impact on the organization of health care and which focuses especially on training health professionals in the development of a body of knowledge, skills, attitudes, and behaviour to ensure that they are able to work in a sensitive way with patients from diverse backgrounds (22). Originally coming from the United States, these ideas also gained popularity elsewhere and were attributed with normative power. In palliative care, however, they have only found resonance relatively recently.

The idea of cultural competence has remained relatively untouched by anthropological insights into culture. It is based on questionable assumptions and has, therefore, received a number of important criticisms. The most prominent one is an uncritical view of culture as ethnicity, referring to groups of people with homogeneous characteristics and clearly distinguishable boundaries. Such an approach would provide clinicians with a well-delineated body of knowledge that they were required to become competent in. However, the attempt to classify ethnic beliefs and practices under the label of 'culture'—also referred to as the 'fact-file' or 'cookbook' approach—risks reinforcing the stereotypes it purports to overcome (23, 24).

Recent research, especially from the United Kingdom, critically analysed the conceptual framework of cultural competence and found it to represent an overly rationalist model emphasizing competence at the expense of the relational and emotional dimensions of care and professional vulnerability, uncertainty, and doubt (25, 26). It can distract from what matters to the person, him or herself, and their family, and obfuscate change and diversity.

Palliative care in a cultural perspective

Palliative care, itself, is a culture-specific phenomenon. It developed within the context of the prevailing norms of the time regarding the management of advanced illness and dying. The early ideas on which palliative care is based are related to the contested approaches that existed towards pain. Several perspectives—philosophical, theological, and medical—were responsible for the inadequate treatment of pain (27). Cicely Saunders was actively researching pain in terminal illness. Her work had significant consequences for future pain control as she showed that pain was incorrectly treated, due to health professionals' prejudices and restrictive rules impeding the use of effective drugs. These insights led her to develop the concept of 'total pain' which she saw as not only a physical phenomenon but which also entailed psychological, social, and spiritual dimensions, requiring 'total care' (28). For such an integrated approach she did not consider the hospital environment suitable and instead developed the idea of hospice to fulfil this task.

The term 'palliative care' only started to be used later in its current sense. This was when Balfour Mount, in 1975, opened a palliative care unit in Montreal in a hospital setting where the name 'hospice' was not suitable. This marked a significant moment in the development of the palliative care movement as from then on, this type of care was no longer restricted to a special institution, the hospice. Palliative care could be integrated into the care provided in other settings, including hospitals. It formed a response to the cure-centred vision, pursued to the extreme in the then newly created intensive care units (29).

With this approach, which goes beyond the understanding of culture in terms of ethnicity, it is possible to understand the significance of palliative care amidst the contextual forces that frame it. A narrower perspective of culture takes biomedicine as its basis and studies different cultural expressions as they come into contact with biomedicine, which is itself seen as neutral and not part of culture. This is called the 'culture *in* medicine' approach. Here, we adopt the 'culture *of* medicine' approach which sees medicine as one of many cultural perspectives on health, illness, and dying (30). In this way, we can get a better view of the assumptions underlying this type of care and how it relates to other ways of caring. It throws light, for example, on palliative care's position vis-à-vis other fields of care, such as family, nursing, spiritual, and medical care. Palliative care is a partial integration of these fields which were previously conceived as separate, whereby it influenced them and eventually led to their redefinition (29). Such understandings still underlie the contemporary division of the specialty of palliative medicine with palliative care and how they differ from other forms of health care.

Palliative care as a developing notion

As the field of palliative care has evolved over time, its concept has undergone several changes. These are reflected in the terms and definitions that have been used to describe care for people with life-limiting illness, which changed from care of the dying to terminal care, hospice care, palliative care, and, in some contexts, to supportive care (31).

Definitions of palliative care have broadened considerably over time (31). The concept has changed in relation to when it is considered appropriate, from the last phase of illness to the moment when illness is first diagnosed. It has also expanded in terms of the clinical conditions that it focuses on; palliative care was initially directed towards cancer patients but now, all illnesses with a life-threatening character fall under its remit. Palliative care has become increasingly secularized and universal bioethical principles have replaced its original religious values.

Unlike other medical specialties, palliative care is not concerned with a specific condition (such as oncology), bodily organ (nephrology), or system (gastroenterology) (32). It is a multidimensional concept with a distinctive moral philosophy, which makes its definition immensely complex.

Currently, a multiplicity of terms and definitions referring to the concept of palliative care exist alongside each other. An analysis of the term 'palliative care' showed 37 different English language definitions in the specialist literature (33). This lack of consistency in the use of terms and definitions can lead to confusion (34). It reflects a discipline that is still emerging and coming to terms with its identity. This is visible from the recently updated definition from the World Health Organization (WHO), which is based on current insights into pain and symptom management and the growing awareness of the relevance of palliative care to the rest of the world (35). With its global expansion, palliative care is coming into contact with new formal health systems (36) and cultural views on illness, suffering, and dying.

It is important to keep track of its self-understanding now that palliative care has moved into new territories. For this purpose, a web-based survey among experts in palliative care was undertaken, which enquired about the remit of palliative care as defined in different countries (37). The analysis of the findings on the definitions that are in use in a variety of cultural contexts confirmed that, in practice, there is no consensus on the terms for palliative care nor on the components of its definition.

Common elements of the definitions concern the goals of the optimization of quality of life and the prevention and relief of suffering through a holistic approach that requires multidisciplinary attention to those who are affected by advanced illness. However, even at this level, there is a lot of ambiguity and each element is open to interpretation. These ambiguities become especially apparent when attempting to delineate this type of care. For example, at what point does care need to take over from cure? In response, specific time- frames for palliative care are drawn. These are mostly uncertain and lacking in evidence of reliable prognostication (38, 39), which was reflected in the diversity of participants responses; time-frames ranged from years to the final minutes before death.

This argues for an integrated rather than divisive approach to palliative care. In this way, by thinking inclusively, it becomes possible to break through conventional categories, which are generally disease-specific and cure versus care oriented. Such a broad view is consistent with the current broadening of the remit of palliative care to non-cancer conditions where prognoses are very difficult to establish (38). Different transitions, such as the transition between the curative and the palliative care settings, become apparent (40) and need to be well coordinated. This also leads to a broadening on other levels, such as the expertise required to work with the complexities of this field.

A broad approach to palliative care can also facilitate understanding of the variety of meanings attached to it. Palliative care did not maintain its original position as a separate approach to care for the incurably ill, but was most often integrated into the existing health care structures of particular countries (36). Together with pre-existing care traditions, this has brought about changes to the original concept of 'palliative care'. One example is the concept of 'integral palliative care' in Belgium, which is radically different from the original concept of palliative care as it embraces the option for euthanasia (41).

Differences in palliative care between countries

There are few studies that have attempted to address directly the socio-cultural issues in palliative care in particular countries. Therefore, a large scoping review (851 articles) of the research literature of seven European countries—Germany, Norway, Belgium, the Netherlands, Spain, Italy, and Portugal—was conducted to provide a view of the socio-cultural issues that shape palliative care (42). The themes that were covered in the literature, which facilitated cross-cultural comparison, could be categorized into the following areas: setting, caregivers, communication, medical end-of-life decisions, minority ethnic groups and knowledge, attitudes, and values surrounding death and care. From the frequency with which the themes were addressed in the evidence and the different issues that characterized these themes, culture-specific concerns in particular countries could be discerned.

The reviews confirm that there are clearly distinguishable national cultures of palliative care. There are distinct approaches between countries that are the result of different institutional forms of health care and a variety of ways of organizing the professions in charge of care provision at the end of life.

From the evidence, the clearest contrast was visible between the United Kingdom and other European countries. In the United Kingdom, research has focused predominantly on the care needs of ethnic minority groups. In contrast, very little attention has been paid to cultural issues of ethnic minorities in the European countries. In the Netherlands, we found that some pioneering work has started in this area and, in the other countries, there were a few scattered exceptions. Instead, European countries wrote about their 'own' cultural traditions and practices. This focus on cultural identity may be due to self-reflection as a consequence of the process in which palliative care is incorporated into national health systems.

Place of care and death appeared as a prominent theme in the literature in the different countries, with evidence produced from the various different settings where people received care in the last phase of life. Practices around medical decision making regarding the end of life varied radically between countries, motivated by religious commitment or more secular values regarding death and dying. This was most apparent from the diverging ideas about life-shortening interventions between the Low Countries, where euthanasia is legal, and the other countries, which expressed different reasons for opposition to the hastening of death. Norms around end-of-life decision making were complex, interrelating with, for example, conservative attitudes regarding medical authority and the law in Norway, or the collective emotions of the Nazi past evoked by the term euthanasia in Germany. The theme of communication contained mostly studies on the use of advance directives and persistent difficulties in talking about death, and, especially in the Mediterranean countries, issues around disclosure featured prominently, relating to close family involvement in the care of people in Spain and Italy and leading to practices that contradict the obligation to open information about diagnosis.

Palliative care for older people

The role of palliative care is now increasingly recognized as applicable to older people who are suffering from chronic conditions and who will eventually die from them. This is a new development; specialist palliative care services have not traditionally extended to older people. In the United Kingdom, for example, the chance of dying in a hospice declines with age (43).

The inclusion of older people in palliative care raises the question of what their particular needs are and how palliative care can best attune its expertise to the realities in which older people are living, especially in the currently rapidly changing service and policy contexts. Ageing is generally immediately associated with bodily decline, evoking images of grey hair, wrinkled skin, and physical frailty. These are the opposite attributes to what is desirable in contemporary Western consumer culture, which strives after youth and optimal health and relates this to beauty and success (44). These bodily characterizations carry moral judgements whereby older people are considered as ugly, unproductive, or old-fashioned. These negative stereotypes form the basis of ageism—the systematic discrimination against people on the basis of age. Ageism pervades daily life and occurs in all countries and cultures, though differently expressed. Its consequences can be felt on various levels, through direct disrespect or actions based on covert assumptions, adversely influencing people's care (45).

The internalization of ageist understandings are embedded and reinforced by cultural models and institutions that legitimize practices and knowledge relating to ageing. Biomedicine considers ageing as a biological process of bodily deterioration, establishing it as a natural process, which strengthens its persuasive force (46). This raises questions regarding the status of disease and ageing, where the former is an inherent part of ageing, while the latter cannot, unproblematically, be considered as pathological (47). The view of ageing as inevitable decline is reflected in social policies, which imply progressive worsening of health, disengagement from work and social life, and growing needs for support. The ageing of the population has been conceived in terms of the burden it places on the limited resources available for care. Policy making has direct consequences for older people as it establishes the scope and conditions of the services and practices of care. Although the welfare state traditionally cared for the needs of older people, its policies also contributed to their marginalization. Disengagement was, in fact, realized by policies excluding older people from employment and separating them from society by housing them in institutional care facilities (48, 49). Images of physical and mental decline also appear in the media, which strengthen the effect of exclusion of older people from society (48).

Appropriate responses to the needs of older people require an understanding of the meanings of ageing and the contexts in which they are produced. Gerontology has already accomplished major insights, by pointing at the large diversity that exists in age-related experiences. Ageing involves a lot more than declining health, which is only one aspect of growing older. Recent restructurings of care systems have introduced new arrangements to meet the needs of older people, with a greater emphasis on their own resources and individual responsibility (50). As palliative care extends its remit to the needs of older people, it needs to work more closely with the disciplines which have developed expertise in the management of age-related problems, such as geriatrics, general practice, and social care. Equally important are the different ways that older people themselves interpret the process of ageing, their responses to dominant representations, and reasons for accepting, rejecting, or transforming those.

Among older people, there is a high prevalence of dementia (51). Dementia carries the stigma of both ageing and mental illness. It is often represented as an illness more frightening than death (52). It is characterized as the emptying out of the self and, therefore, the removal of what makes one human (53, 54). These views have a devastating effect on the self-esteem, social life, and care of those involved (55, 56). Throughout history, dementia has been variously interpreted, with implications for the social position and the clinical treatment of people who are affected (57). Whereas it was originally considered as a part of normal ageing (58), the dominant biomedical understanding has reduced this condition into a single universal disease category, known as 'Alzheimer's disease' (59). This was originally intended to raise awareness about dementia and incite commitments to research funding. However, medicine's exclusive focus on cure reinforces the negative images and prejudicial views of dementia and exacerbates already detached attitudes and practices (60).

The personhood concept is a recent reaction to the fatalist assumptions about dementia, leading to a new ethics in dementia (61). Kitwood, one of its most influential proponents, opposes the view of dementia as a 'death that leaves the body behind' and proposes an alternative notion of personhood as being social and made through relationships rather than based on memory and cognition alone (62). Those who do not possess memory and cognition are left to a life without value, a social death (63); the personhood model extends personhood to include those human beings who lack these capacities (64).

Whereas dementia did not traditionally fall under the remit of palliative care, there is increasing recognition that people with dementia have palliative care needs (65). Growing evidence shows that dementia imposes the greatest burden on carers, whether at home or in nursing homes, and on health systems, as they incur the highest costs of any life-limiting conditions, higher than heart disease and cancer together (66, 67). People with dementia are among the most vulnerable to social exclusion of those who are already disadvantaged on the basis of their age, gender, ethnicity, or class background because of their cognitive impairment (68).

The value of palliative care for dementia exists in its expanding knowledge base concerning the management of pain and symptoms and the growing expertise in multi-morbidity affecting people with progressive illness. The distinctive moral philosophy of palliative care promotes a holistic approach comprising symptom control, psychosocial and spiritual care, and including the carer in the unit of attention.

At the same time, it embraces a person-centred approach closely linked with the arguments developed in the personhood movement. Experiences from palliative care could help operationalize personhood models further. Its original concern with death and dying has enabled the development of moral dispositions towards people when they are most vulnerable and the realization that care never becomes futile. Dementia presents palliative care with a whole new set of challenges due to its long trajectory of cognitive and functional decline. However, its tradition of multidisciplinary working can bring together models, practices, and technologies from a diversity of disciplines, (such as neurology, psychiatry and psychology, nursing, and allied health professions) which have acquired expertise in dementia. The benefits of collaboration between these different areas of expertise are increasingly recognized. The incorporation of the challenges posed by older people and those with dementia will inevitably further change the field of palliative care.

Conclusion on cultural issues in palliative care for older people

This chapter presents the state of the evidence on culture and palliative care in the light of its growing expertise regarding older people. It considers the continuous broadening of the remit of palliative care as it developed historically and spread geographically, whereby its original notions adapted to the various cultural contexts and circumstances in which it was practiced. The literature on culture and palliative care only provides a partial perspective on this field. Therefore, to cover the field it has been necessary to widen the scope of sources, and this provides insight beyond inequalities in the use of palliative care services; it also covers perspectives on current differences in understandings and practices regarding palliative care internationally.

As palliative care is increasingly found to offer new solutions to the needs of older people, it is important to evaluate these experiences. The distinctive contribution which palliative care is able to make to the care of older people will help to further improve services for this group. In turn, the questions regarding the ethical issues and conceptual notions this raises, and how this changes the nature of palliative care, need on-going analysis. This will help palliative care to continue to respond adequately to the diverse needs of changing societies.

References

1 **Giannakouris K.** *Regional Population Projections EUROPOP2008: Most EU Regions Face Older Population Profile in 2030.* Luxembourg: European Commission; 2010.

2 **Gomes B, Cohen J, Deliens L, Higginson IJ.** International trends in circumstances of death and dying amongst older people. In: Gott M, Ingleton C (eds). *Living with Ageing and Dying: Palliative and End of Life Care for Older People.* Oxford: Oxford University Press; 2011, 3–18.

3 **Mathers CD, Loncar D.** Projections of global mortality and burden of disease from 2002 to 2030. *PLoS Med* 2006; **3**(11):e442.

4 **Stjernsward J, Clark D.** Palliative medicine—a global perspective. In: Doyle D, Hanks G, Cherny N, (eds). *Oxford Textbook of Palliative Medicine.* New York: Oxford University Press; 2004, 1199–224.

5 **Foley K.** How much palliative care do we need? *European Journal of Palliative Care* 2003; **10**:5–7.

6 **Singer PA, Bowman KW.** Quality end-of-life care: a global perspective. *BMC Palliat Care* 2002; **1**(1):4.

7 **Centeno C, Clark D, Lynch T, Rocafort J, Flores LA, Greenwood A, et al.** *EAPC Atlas of Palliative Care in Europe.* Houston: International Association for Hospice and Palliative Care Press; 2007.

8 **Clark D, Centeno C.** Palliative care in Europe: an emerging approach to comparative analysis. *Clinical Medicine* 2006; **6**(2):197–201.

9 **Gysels M, Meñaca A, Andrew E, Bausewein C, Gastmans C, Gomez-Batiste X, et al.,** on behalf of Project PRISMA. Culture is a priority for research in end-of-life care in Europe: a research agenda. *J Pain Symptom Manage* 2012; **44**(2):285–94.

10 **Koenig BA, Gates-Williams J.** Understanding cultural difference in caring for dying patients. *West J Med* 1995; **163**(3):244–9.

11 **Holland D, Quinn N.** Culture and cognition. In: Holland D, Quinn N (eds). *Cultural Models in Language and Thought.* Cambridge: Cambridge University Press; 1987, 3–40.

12 **Keesing RM, Strathern AJ.** *Cultural Anthropology. A Contemporary Perspective.* New York: Rinehart & Winston; 1998.

13 **Geertz C.** *The Interpretation of Cultures.* New York: Basic Books; 1973.

14 **Wimmer A.** The making and unmaking of ethnic boundaries: a multilevel process theory. *Am J Sociol* 2008; **113**:987–1022.

15 **Cornell S, Hartmann D.** *Ethnicity and Race: Making Identities in a Changing World.* London: Pine Forge Press; 1998.

16 **Hill D, Penso D.** *Opening Doors: Improving Access to Hospice and Specialist Palliative Care Services by Members of the Black and Ethnic Minority Communities.* London: National Council for Hospice and Specialist Palliative Care Services; 1995.

17 **Rees W.** Immigrants and the hospice. *Health Trends* 1986; **18**(4):89–91.

18 **Evans N, Meñaca A, Andrew EV, Koffman J, Harding R, Higginson IJ, et al.** Appraisal of literature reviews on end-of-life care for minority ethnic groups in the UK and a critical comparison with policy recommendations from the UK end-of-life care strategy. *BMC Health Serv Res* 2011; **11**:141.

19 **Evans N, Andrew E, Meñaca A, Koffman J, Higginson I, Harding R, et al.** Systematic review of the primary research on minority ethnic groups and end-of-life care from the UK. *J Pain Symptom Manage* 2012; **2**:261–86.

20 *Palliative Care Fourth Report of the Session*. House of Commons; 2004. Available at: <http://www. publications.parliament.uk/pa/cm200304/cmselect/cmhealth/454/45402.htm>. (Accessed April 2014). Ref. type: online source.

21 Betancourt JR. Cultural competence: marginal or mainstream movement? *NEJM* 2004; **351**(10):953–5.

22 Fox RC. Cultural competence and the culture of medicine. *NEJM* 2005; **353**(13):1316–9.

23 Good-DelVecchio MJ, Good JCB, Becker AE. *The Culture of Medicine and Racial, Ethnic,and Class Disparities in Health*. Russell Sage Foundation Working Paper 199; 2002. Available at: <https://www. russellsage.org/sites/all/files/u4/Good,%20James,%20Good,%20%26%20Becker_Culture%20of%20 Medicine%20and%20Racial,%20Ethnic,%20%26%20Class%20Disparities%20in%20Healthcare. pdf>. (Accessed April 2014). Ref. type: online source.

24 Hunt LM, de Voogd KB. Clinical myths of the cultural 'Other': implications for Latino patient care. *Academic Medicine* 2005; **80**(10):918–24.

25 Gunaratnam Y. *Culture is Not Enough: A Critique of Multiculturalism in Palliative Care*. London: Routledge; 1997.

26 Gunaratnam Y. Intercultural palliative care: do we need cultural competence? *Int J Pall Nurs* 2007; **13**(10):470.

27 Donovan MI. An historical view of pain management: how to get where we are! *Cancer Nursing* 1989; **12**(4):257–61.

28 Saunders C. The need for institutional care for the patient with advanced cancer. *Cancer Institute, Madras* 1964; Anniversary Volume:1–8.

29 Garcia D. Palliative care and the historical background. In: ten Have H, Clark D (eds). *The Ethics of Palliative Care: European Perspectives*. Buckingham: Open University Press; 2002, 18–33.

30 MacDonald ME. Understanding what residents want and what residents need: the challenge of cultural training in pediatrics. *Medical Teacher* 2007; **29**(5):465–71.

31 Clark D, Seymour J. *Reflections on Palliative Care: Sociological and Policy Perspectives*. Buckingham: Open University Press; 1999.

32 Billings BA. What is palliative medicine? *J Palliat Med* 1998; **1**:73–81.

33 Pastrana T, Junger S, Ostgathe C, Elsner F, Radbruch L. A matter of definition: key elements identified in a discourse analysis of definitions of palliative care. *Palliat Med* 2008; **22**:222–32.

34 Walshe C. What do we mean by palliative care? In: Preedy VR (ed). *Diet and Nutrition in Palliative Care*. Boca Raton, Fl: Taylor & Francis Group; 2011, 17–29.

35 Sepulveda C, Marlin A, Yoshida T, Ullrich A. Palliative care: the World Health Organization's global perspective. *J Pain Symptom Manage* 2002; **24**(2):91–6.

36 Clark D, ten Have H, Janssens R. Common threads? Palliative care service developments in seven European countries. *Palliat Med* 2000; **14**(6):479–90.

37 Gysels M, Evans N, Meñaca A, Higginson IJ, Harding R, Pool R, et al. Diversity in defining end of life care: an obstacle or the way forward? *PLoS One* 2013; **8**(7):doi:10.1371/journal.pone.0068002.

38 Shipman C, Gysels M, White P, Worth A, Murray SA, Barclay S, et al. Improving generalist end of life care: national consultation with practitioners, commissioners, academics, and service user groups. *BMJ* 2008; **337**:a1720.

39 Coventry PA, Grande GE, Richards DA, Todd CJ. Prediction of appropriate timing of palliative care for older adults with non-malignant life-threatening disease: a systematic review. *Age Ageing* 2005; **34**(3):218–27.

40 Lynn J, Adamson DM. *Living Well at the End of Life. Adapting Health Care to Serious Chronic Illness in Old Age*. Washington: Rand Health; 2003.

41 Bernheim JL, Deschepper R, Distelmans W, Mullie A, Bilsen J, Deliens L. Development of palliative care and legalisation of euthanasia: antagonism or synergy? *BMJ* 2008; **336**(7649):864–7.

42 Gysels M, Evans N, Meñaca A, Andrew EVW, Toscani F, Finnetti S, et al. Culture and end of life care: a scoping exercise in seven European countries. *PLoS One* 2012; 7(4):e34188

43 Lock A, Higginson IJ. Patterns and predictors of place of cancer death for the oldest old. *BMC Palliat Care* 2005; 4(6):doi:10.1186/1472–684X–4–6.

44 Turner B. *The Body and Society*. London: Sage; 1996.

45 Nolan M. Ageism: what's in a word! *J Adv Nurs* 2003; 41(1):8–9.

46 Tulle-Winton E. Old bodies. In: Hancock P, Hughes B, Jagger K, Paterson R, Russel E, Tulle-Winton E, et al. (eds). *The Body, Culture and Society: An Introduction*. Buckingham: Open University Press; 2000, 64–83.

47 Katz S. *Disciplining Old Age: the Formation of Gerontological Knolwedge*. Charlottesville: University Press of Virginia; 1996.

48 Bond J, Peace S, Dittman-Kohli, Westerhof G. *Ageing in Society: European Perspectives on Gerontology*. London: Sage Publications; 2007.

49 Walker A. Public policy and the construction of old age in Europe. *Gerontologist* 2000; 40(3):304–8.

50 Tulle E. *Old Age and Agency*. New York: Novascience; 2004.

51 Hall S, Petkova H, Tsouros AD, Constantini M, Higginson IJ. *Palliative Care for Older People: Better Practices*. Copenhagen: WHO; 2011.

52 Gubrium J. *Oldtimers and Alzheimer's: The Descriptive Organisation of Senility*. Greenwich, Connecticut: JAI Press; 1986.

53 Fontana A, Smith RW. Alzheimer disease victims: the unbecoming of self and the normalisation of competence. *Sociological Perspectives* 1989; 32:35–46.

54 Morris D. *Culture and Pain*. Berkeley, CA: University of California Press; 1999.

55 Morgan K. Diagnosis in dementia: a personal view. *Dementia* 2011; 10(3):281–2.

56 Beard RL, Knauss J, Moyer D. Managing disability and enjoying life: how we reframe dementia through personal narratives. *J Aging Stud* 2009; 23: 227–35.

57 George DR, Whitehouse PJ, Ballenger J. The evolving classification of dementia: placing the DSM-V in a meaningful historical and cultural context and pondering the future of 'Alzheimer's'. *Cult Med Psychiatry* 2011; 35(3):417–35.

58 Cohen L. *No Aging in India: Alzheimer's, the Bad Family, and Other Modern Things*. Berkely: University of California Press; 1998.

59 Engstrom EJ. Researching dementia in imperial Germany: Alois Alzheimer and the economies of psychiatric practice. *Cult Med Psychiatry* 2007; 31(3):405–12.

60 Ballenger JF. The biomedical deconstruction of senility and the persistent stigmatisation of old age in the United States. In: Leibing A, Cohen L (eds). *Thinking About Dementia: Culture, Loss, and the Anthropology of Senility*. New Brunswick: Rutgers University Press; 2006, 106–19.

61 Leibing A. Divided gazes: Alzheimer's disease, the person within, and death in life. In: Leibing A, Cohen L (eds). *Thinking About Dementia: Culture, Loss and the Anthropology of Senility*. New Brunswick: Rutgers University Press; 2006, 240–59.

62 Kitwood T. *Dementia Reconsidered: The Person Comes First*. Buckingham: The Open University Press; 1997.

63 Sweeting H, Gilhooly M. Dementia and the phenomenon of social death. *Sociol Health Ill* 1997; 19:93–117.

64 Fleischer TE. 'The personhood wars: body, soul, and bioethics' by Gilbert C. Meilaender; and 'What is a person? An ethical exploration' by James W. Walters. *Theor Med Bioeth* 1999; 20(3):309–18.

65 van der Steen JT, Radbruch L, Hertogh CM, de Boer ME, Hughes JC, Larkin P, et al. White paper defining optimal palliative care in older people with dementia: a Delphi study and recommendations from the European Association for Palliative Care. *Palliat Med* 2014; 28(3):197–209.

66 **Callahan CM, Arlain G, Wanzhu Tu, Stump TE, Arling GW.** Cost analysis of the geriatric resources for assessment and care of elders care management intervention. *JAGS* 2012; **57**(8):1420–6.

67 **Hurd MD, Martorell P, Delavande A, Mullen KJ, Langa KM.** Monetary costs of dementia in the United States. *NEJM* 2013; **368**:1326–34.

68 **Graham R.** Cognitive citizenship: access to hip surgery for people with dementia. *Health* 2004; **8**(3):295–310.

Chapter 16

Spirituality and spiritual palliative care for older people

Marie-José H.E. Gijsberts

Introduction to spirituality and spiritual palliative care for older people

Spiritual care is increasingly recognized as an integral part of palliative care alongside physical and psychosocial care. However, this change in perception has taken several decades. In 1988, Cicely Saunders first introduced spirituality in relation to palliative care. She published an article on spiritual pain (1) in which she started to develop the concept of total pain. She described how, in the care of the individual in pain, there must be attention to the patient's inner life. This requires an ability to make sense of the inner concerns and values of the person. She proposed that there is a need to engage with 'the whole area of thought concerning moral values throughout life'. This is what she defined as 'the spiritual' and refers to a desolate sense of meaninglessness encountered by the person at the end of life that is the essence of 'spiritual pain'. In the 1990 Report on Cancer Pain Relief and Palliative Care by the World Health Organization, the dimensions of palliative care were introduced, including care for *spiritual needs* (2). In 1998, The World Health Organization introduced the concept of patient-centred care, in which emphasis is placed on the need for individual treatment plans that take into account the psychological, social, physical, as well as spiritual (3). The current definition of palliative care by the World Health Organization dates from 2002:

> Palliative care is an approach that improves the quality of life of patients and their families facing the problem associated with life-threatening illness, through the prevention and relief of suffering by means of early identification and impeccable assessment and treatment of pain and other problems, physical, psychosocial *and spiritual* (4).

In 2010, the European Association of Palliative Care instituted a taskforce on spiritual care, to promote recognition, education, and implementation of spiritual caregiving at the end of life (5).

Although spiritual care has been recognized as a dimension of palliative care, and the attention given to spirituality has clearly increased (6), the spiritual dimension of palliative care is still the least developed (7–9). This is illustrated by the fact that ageing is still often described as an increase of disabilities that cannot be cured and, therefore, much emphasis is put on symptom management and training (10). In addition, 'successful ageing' is promoted to support older people to engage in society and in physical and psychosocial activities (11). A third approach is described by MacKinlay, in which life is regarded as a 'spiritual journey' with challenges that continue across the later years— a journey that aims to find hope and meaning in life for people living with increasing disability (including physical and cognitive decline), allowing them to flourish, even in the face of uncertainty (12).

In this chapter, the importance of spirituality at the end of life will be discussed, with an emphasis on spiritual care in older people and the importance of attention to spiritual well-being in this group. Further, the dimensions of spirituality at the end of life, the assessment of spiritual needs, and the importance of multidisciplinary (spiritual) palliative care will be discussed, with special attention given to the challenges of spiritual caregiving in dementia.

The importance of spirituality and spiritual care at the end of life

Spiritual care at the end of life is important because it contributes significantly to quality of life, the most important outcome measure in palliative care (13, 14). Patients often experience spiritual distress at the end of life and alleviation of this contributes to spiritual and psychosocial well-being (15, 16). In a Dutch study on palliative care consultation, new consultations mostly concerned psychosocial and spiritual needs (17). Spirituality is considered to be a resource in maintaining psychological well-being in frail and non-frail older adults, and the use of this resource is more significant to individuals with greater levels of frailty (18).

Spirituality and spiritual care in older people with dementia are issues that will be a concern to many people; in 2010, about 35.6 million people were living with dementia, and this number will almost double by 2030 (19, 20). A quarter (25%) of people aged 85 years and older die with dementia (21). As literature shows, spiritual caregiving in dementia is still an understudied topic (22, 23) and spiritual care and nursing measures may be less developed than medical care (24). Patients with dementia who are admitted to hospital were asked significantly less often about their spiritual needs and religion than patients without dementia (25). An internationally introduced booklet to inform families of advanced dementia patients on comfort care did not include spiritual issues (26). In 'Supportive Care for the Person with Dementia', spiritual issues are described as: acknowledging and supporting spirituality, giving regard to overall quality of life, and promoting dignity, and include support for grieving, the importance of communication, and issues of maintaining the self (27). In the EAPC White Paper on palliative care in dementia (22), the lowest research priority ratings overall were for 'societal and ethical issues' and 'psychosocial and spiritual support', and one of the recommendations was that 'spiritual caregiving in dementia should include at least assessment of religious affiliation and involvement, sources of support and spiritual wellbeing; in addition, referral to experienced spiritual counsellors such as those working in nursing homes may be appropriate', and 'religious activities, such as rituals, songs, and services may help the patient because these may be recognized even in severe dementia' (22). Further study is needed on spirituality and spiritual care in older people with dementia at the end of life; recent studies show that a patient-centred approach may be a good way through which to address these needs (28–30).

Spirituality at the end of life and its dimensions

Spirituality is a complex concept; a review restricted to health care literature counted 92 separate definitions (31). In a recently performed systematic review, a conceptual model of spirituality at the end of life was constructed which distinguished dimensions of spirituality and their associations (see Figure 16.1) (32).

The aim of constructing this model was to make the concept of spirituality more comprehensive, thus contributing to a better understanding of this concept at the end of life. In this model, three dimensions of spirituality were distinguished: spiritual well-being, spiritual coping, and the spiritual cognitive behavioural context. Spiritual well-being comprises several aspects (e.g. peacefulness, a sense of purpose and meaning, and completion of life) and this may be regarded as the aim/outcome of spiritual care giving, to which spiritual coping and the spiritual cognitive behavioural context (spiritual beliefs, spiritual activities, and spiritual relationships) may contribute. Spiritual coping was regarded as all behaviour and cognitions aimed at the decreasing of perceived distress and the increasing of spiritual

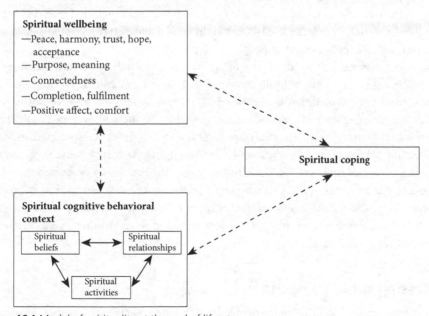

Figure 16.1 Model of spirituality at the end of life

Reprinted with permission from *Journal of Palliative Medicine*, volume 14, 2011, published by Mary Ann Liebert, Inc., New Rochelle, NY.

well-being. The dimension of spiritual coping appears to be understudied. Further exploration of this dimension may be important to understanding how people at the end of life cope with spiritual distress. The model shows that the concept of spirituality is broader and more inclusive than religion, which may be recognized as part of the spiritual cognitive behavioural context. This was emphasized by other studies; one systematic review showed that most spirituality items concerned the meaning or purpose of life (33). The model and its dimensions may help caregivers to better understand the needs of their patients and may help researchers to plan studies and choose appropriate outcome measurements.

Other concepts of spirituality at the end of life place emphasis on the different dimensions and categories. In a recent study, cognitive appraisal is an essential component of the concept (34) with categories such as 'self-transcendence' and 'transcendence with a higher being'. According to this approach, cognitive capacities are significant in experiencing spirituality and may exclude many older patients with mild or more severe cognitive impairment from experiencing spirituality and spiritual well-being and receiving spiritual care (35). This concept, therefore, appears to be less appropriate in a part of the older population, especially older people suffering from dementia. Another study on spirituality at the end of life distinguishes two different measures, 'functional' and 'substantial' (36). A substantial measure 'explores areas such as spiritual beliefs, spiritual experiences or spiritual orientation, focusing on the content or the substance of people's religious or spiritual beliefs' which is in accordance with the dimension of 'spiritual cognitive behavioural context' of the model just described. A functional measure 'is concerned with how a person finds meaning and purpose in life and with the behaviour, emotions, relationships and practices associated with that meaning and purpose'. The 'functional measure' accords with the dimension of spiritual well-being in the model, but also represents aspects of the 'spiritual cognitive behavioural context'.

The concept of spirituality at the end of life is considered to be culturally sensitive. In a systematic review of cross-culturally validated instruments measuring spirituality, a conceptual model of spirituality was developed (37). Most dimensions and categories in the model shown in Figure 16.1 can also be recognized in the model developed in the cross-cultural study. Interestingly, this study had 'a central individual experience of illness of the patient', but did not have a dimension of spiritual coping. As this systematic review only included cross-culturally validated instruments, and the previously described model was limited to cultures within the English language, the more active dimension of spiritual coping may be a specifically culturally sensitive dimension of spirituality at the end of life and, therefore, may not be emphasized or recognized in other cultures as a dimension of spirituality at the end of life.

Assessing spiritual needs

How can we explore whether older people have spiritual needs and spiritual resources at the end of life and whether those spiritual needs require professional support? In literature, 'taking a spiritual history' is promoted to assess a patient's beliefs and values, spiritual strength (e.g. hope, meaning, purpose), and spiritual distress (e.g. meaninglessness, hopelessness), and to identify patients who need referral to a board-certified chaplain/spiritual care provider (7). The information from the spiritual history allows the health care practitioner to understand how spiritual concerns could either complement or complicate the patient's overall care. Screening instruments are available, most of which include questions on religious affiliation and spiritual practices and also touch upon aspects of spiritual well-being (e.g. meaning, importance of belief, sources of hope) (7).

The Faith, Importance and Influence, Community, and Address (FICA) spiritual history tool is the most used screening instrument (38–40). A recent European study showed that the questions in the FICA instrument could be feasible for the assessment of spirituality by general practitioners, provided that physicians could bring these questions into a natural conversation with the patient (41). Questions in the FICA instrument include: 'What things do you believe in that give meaning to your life? How have your beliefs influenced your behaviour during this illness? Is there a person or group of people you really love or who is really important to you? How would you like me, your health care provider, to address these issues in your health care?'. Another instrument that has useful questions is the HOPE instrument (42) which includes the following concepts for discussion: H—sources of hope, strength, comfort, meaning, peace, love, and connection; O—the role of organized religion for the patient; P—personal spirituality and practices; E—effects on medical care and end-of-life decisions. Additionally, the SPIRIT instrument (43) is a guide to identifying important components of the spiritual history.

Spiritual caregiving to older people

Spiritual issues are not often discussed at the end of life; studies show that spiritual and existential issues were the least frequently discussed (44) and that, in the last weeks of life, 90% of patients received care for physical needs but, respectively, only 25% and 54% for spiritual and psychosocial needs (45). Spiritual caregiving by nursing home staff is related to a better family evaluation of end-of-life care for nursing home residents (46).

How can spirituality, as a resource for well-being, be supported in older people? For nursing home residents, the religious affiliation of a nursing home may be important to support them in their spiritual needs. There are indications that religious affiliation of a nursing home is positively associated with provision of spiritual care (47); this applies also to dementia (48).

Other interesting approaches are focused on supporting spiritual well-being and spiritual coping, in which group counselling is considered important. Harvey Chochinov has been concerned with dignity at the end of life, and ways to recognize, assess, and address psychological, existential, and spiritual needs (49). He describes the overlap and reciprocity between spirituality and dignity: 'spirituality has to do with respecting the inherent value and dignity of all persons' (50). He developed an assessment of dignity at the end of life (51, 52), the Patient Dignity Inventory, and an intervention, Dignity Therapy (53), in which patients are invited to discuss what matters most to them and how they would most want to be remembered (54). After participating in a Dignity Therapy group, patients report a higher sense of dignity and significantly more purpose and meaning in life—both aspects of spiritual well-being. A follow-up study of feasibility in long-term care indicates an increased sense of meaning in older people in such care (55). William Breitbart developed 'spirituality- and meaning-centred group psychotherapy', in which patients at the end of life are also encouraged to find meaning and purpose in living until their death (56, 57). With this therapy, he aims to integrate meaning and spirituality in end-of-life care. Elizabeth MacKinlay developed 'spiritual reminiscence', helping frail old people to 'reflect and reframe aspects of their life journey in the process of ageing and coming to final meanings in life'. She considers spiritual care giving and spiritual reminiscence as an integral part of end-of-life care, with a specialist aged care chaplain as a part of the care team (58). She describes the goal of the spiritual aspect of the process of ageing as finding 'ultimate meaning in life', and this goal is related to finding 'final meanings in life, finding hope, finding intimacy with God and/or others, and to transcend loss and disabilities'.

The role of the *health care chaplain* in supporting older people in their spiritual needs is underlined in several publications. MacKinlay promotes spiritual care giving and 'spiritual reminiscence' as an integral part of end-of-life care: 'having a specialist aged care chaplain employed in the facility makes it easier to engage the chaplain as an integral part of the care team. In this case, pastoral care becomes readily recognized as a part of 'wholistic' aged care, rather than an add on, optional component of care.' (58) Puchalski et al. (7) expressed a specific opinion on the multidisciplinary teamwork in health care settings, in which clinically trained board-certified chaplains should play a key role as the team member most directly responsible for spiritual care. Their responsibility in health care organizations should be to 'focus directly on the significance and incorporation of cultural, spiritual, and religious practices into the plan of care.' (7) All members of the inter-professional team should be respected and valued as integral participants in the care of the patient. Finally, patients and family members also have roles to play as members of the palliative care team.

Documentation (of spiritual needs and spiritual care) in the patient record is considered essential to communicate spiritual concerns. Thus, the trained board-certified chaplains are co-equal professionals in the multidisciplinary team. The Dutch guideline on spiritual care in palliative care also states that palliative care is, by definition, multidisciplinary, and close multidisciplinary cooperation is of fundamental importance for spiritual care, but the various disciplines each have their own expertise, role, and task, the health care chaplain being the trained professional in spiritual care (59). This opinion accords with the work of McSherry, who thinks that health care workers who master communicative skills such as listening and 'presence and facilitation' can meet many spiritual needs, but some needs require referral to a specialist/health care chaplain (60). A recent ethnographic study in Dutch nursing homes among residents with and without dementia found that physicians did not actively address spiritual issues, nor was it part of the official job of care staff. There was no communication between physicians and the spiritual counsellor. When a resident (either suffering from dementia or with physical disabilities) was about to die, the nurses started an informal care process aimed at spiritual well-being, including cuddling, rituals, and music. This was not mentioned in the care plan or the medical chart. The nurses even supported the residents outside of their professional role, in their spare time. The goal of the spiritual caregiving activities by the nurses appeared to be to help the resident die peacefully, to complete his or her life and his or her relationships with loved ones (29). The role of the health care chaplain in the multidisciplinary team concerned with *patient-centred* spiritual caregiving to older people in nursing homes may need improvement to best address spiritual needs in older people at the end of life.

Conclusion on spirituality and spiritual palliative care for older people

The spiritual dimension has been represented in the definition of palliative care since 1990. Despite this, spirituality remains understudied in older people. Recently, specific attention has been given to spiritual care at the end of life in dementia, an important topic since the number of people living with dementia will double in the coming 20 years.

The concept of spirituality at the end of life is complex and culturally sensitive. A recently developed model includes the dimensions of spiritual well-being, spiritual coping, and spiritual cognitive behavioural context. The model shows that the concept of spirituality is broader and more inclusive than religion, and aims to contribute to a better understanding of spirituality at the end of life by distinguishing three dimensions of spirituality and their associations.

The spiritual resources and spiritual needs of older people can be assessed, as can the question of whether those spiritual needs require professional support. Screening instruments provide useful questions that may help the health care practitioner to understand how spiritual concerns could either complement or complicate the patient's overall care. Different approaches are described to support spirituality and spiritual well-being at the end of life and these include the religious affiliation of the nursing home, various methods of supporting spiritual well-being and spiritual coping, patient-centred care by a multidisciplinary team, and the inclusion of a health care chaplain with a distinct role within the multidisciplinary team.

References

1 Saunders C. Spiritual pain. *Journal Palliative Care* 1988; **4**(3):29–32.

2 World Health Organization. *Cancer Pain Relief and Palliative Care, Report of a World Health Organization Expert Committee* 1990. Technical Report Series No 804. Available at: <http://apps.who.int/bookorders/anglais/detart1.jsp?codlan=1&codcol=10&codcch=804> (Accessed March 2014). Ref. type: online source.

3 World Health Organization. *Symptom Relief in Terminal Illness*. Geneva: World Health Organization; 1998. Available at: <http://apps.who.int/bookorders/anglais/detart1.jsp?codlan=1&codcol=15&codcch=455> (Accessed March 2014). Ref. type: online source.

4 World Health Organization. *Defining Palliative Care*, 2002. Available at: <http://www.who.int/cancer/palliative/definition/en/> (Accessed March 2014). Ref. type: online source.

5 European Association for Palliative Care. *EAPC Taskforce on Spiritual Care in Palliative Care*. Available at: <http://www.eapcnet.eu/Themes/Clinicalcare/Spiritualcareinpalliativecare.aspx> (Accessed March 2014). Ref. type: online source.

6 Sinclair S, Pereira J, Raffin S. A thematic review of the spirituality literature within palliative care. *J Palliat Med* 2006; 9(2):464–79.

7 Puchalski C, Ferrell B, Virani R, et al. Improving the quality of spiritual care as a dimension of palliative care: the report of the Consensus Conference. *J Palliat Med* 2009; 12:885–904.

8 Doyle D, Hanks G, Cherny N, Calman K. *Oxford Textbook of Palliative Medicine*. Oxford: Oxford University Press; 2005; 3.

9 Puchalski CM, Kilpatrick SD, McCullough ME, Larson DB. A systematic review of spiritual and religious variables in Palliative Medicine. *J Palliat Support Care* 2003; 1(1):7–13.

10 Hall S, Petkova H, Tsouros A, Costantini M, Higginson I. *Palliative Care for Older People: Better Practices*. World Health Organization, Regional Office in Europe; 2011. Available at: <http//www.euro.who.int/en/health-topics/noncommunicable-diseases/cancer/publications/2011/palliative-care-for-older-people-better-practices> (Accessed March 2014). Ref. type: online source.

11 Rowe J, Kahn R. *Successful Aging*. New York: Random house; 1999.

12 MacKinlay EB, Trevitt C. Spiritual care and ageing in a secular society. *Med J Aust*. 2007; 186(10 Suppl):S74–6.

13 Scobie G, Caddell C. Quality of life at end of life: spirituality and coping mechanisms in terminally ill patients. *The Internet Journal of Pain Symptom Control and Palliative Care* 2005; 4(1):2.

14 Hills J, Paice JA, Cameron JR, Shott S. Spirituality and distress in palliative care consultation. *J Palliat Med* 2005; 8(4):782–8.

15 Brown AE, Whitney SN, Duffy JD. The physician's role in the assessment and treatment of spiritual distress at the end of life. *Palliat Support Care* 2006; 4:81–6.

16 Block SD. Perspectives on care at the close of life. Psychological considerations, growth, and transcendence at the end of life: the art of the possible. *JAMA* 2001; 285:2898–905.

17 Vernooij-Dassen MJ, Groot MM, van den Berg J, Kuin A, van der Linden BA, van Zuylen L, et al. Consultation in palliative care: the relevance of clarification of problems. *Eur J Cancer* 2007; 43:316–22.

18 Kirby S, Coleman P, Daley D. Spirituality and well-being in frail and nonfrail older adults. *The Journals of Gerontol Series B, Psychol Sci and Soc Sci* 2004; 59(3):P123–9.

19 World Health Organization. Dementia: A Public Health Priority. Geneva: WHO; 2012. Available at: <http://whqlibdoc.who.int/publications/2012/9789241564458_eng.pdf> (Accessed March 2014). Ref. type: online source.

20 Alzheimer's Disease International. *World Alzheimer Report* 2010. *The Global Economic Impact of Dementia*. Available at: <www.alz.org/documents/national/world_alzheimer_report_2010.pdf>. (Accessed March 2014). Ref. type: online source.

21 Mitchell SL, Teno JM, Miller SC, Mor V. A national study of the location of death for older persons with dementia. *J Am Geriatr Soc* 2005; 53:299–305.

22 van der Steen JT, Radbruch L, Hertogh CMPM, de Boer ME, Hughes JC, Larkin P, et al., on behalf of the European Association for Palliative Care (EAPC). White Paper defining optimal palliative care in older people with dementia: a Delphi study and recommendations from the European Association for Palliative Care. *Palliat Med* 2014 Mar; 28(3):197–209.

23 Bonelli RM, Koenig HG. Mental disorders, religion and spirituality 1990 to 2010: a systematic evidence-based review. *J Relig Health* 2013 Jun; 52(2):657–73.

24 van der Steen JT. Dying with dementia: what we know after more than a decade of research. *J Alzheimers Dis* 2010; 22(1):37–55.

25 Sampson EL, Gould V, Lee D, Blanchard MR. Differences in care received by patients with and without dementia who died during acute hospital admission: a retrospective case note study. *Age Ageing* 2006 Mar; 35(2):187–9.

26 van der Steen JT, Arcand M, Toscani F, de Graas T, Finetti S, Beaulieu M, et al. A family booklet about comfort care in advanced dementia: three-country evaluation. *JAMDA* 2012; **13**(4):368–75.

27 Hughes C, Lloyd Williams M, Sachs G. *Supportive Care for the Person with Dementia*. Oxford: Oxford University Press; 2010.

28 MacKinlay EB, Trevitt C. *Finding Meaning in the Experience of Dementia*. London: Jessica Kingsley Publishers; 2012.

29 Gijsberts MJ, van der Steen JT, Muller MT, Hertogh CM, Deliens L. Spiritual end-of-life care in Dutch nursing homes: an ethnographic study. *JAMDA* 2013 Sep; **14**(9):679–84.

30 Odbehr L, Kvigne K, Hauge S, Danbolt LJ. Nurses' and care workers' experiences of spiritual needs in residents with dementia in nursing homes: a qualitative study. *BMC Nurs* 2014; **13**:12.

31 Unruh AM, Versnel J, Kerr N. Spirituality unplugged: a review of commonalities and contentions, and a resolution. *Can J Occup Ther* 2002; **69**(1):5–19.

32 Gijsberts MJ, Echteld MA, van der Steen JT, Muller MT, Otten RH, Ribbe MW, et al. Spirituality at the end of life: conceptualization of measurable aspects—a systematic review. *J Palliat Med* 2011; **14**(7):852–63.

33 Albers G, Echteld MA, de Vet HC, Onwuteaka-Philipsen BD, van der Linden MH, Deliens L. Content and spiritual items of quality-of-life instruments appropriate for use in palliative care: a review. *J Pain Symptom Manage* 2010; **40**(2):290–300.

34 Vachon M, Fillion L, Achille M. A conceptual analysis of spirituality at the end of life. *J Palliat Med* 2009; **12**:53–9.

35 van der Steen JT, Gijsberts MJ, Echteld MA, Muller MT, Ribbe MW, Deliens L. Defining spirituality at the end of life. *J Palliat Med* 2009; **12**(8):677.

36 Vivat B, Young T, Efficace F, Sigurðadóttir V, Arraras JI, Åsgeirsdóttir GH, et al. Cross-cultural development of the EORTC QLQ-SWB36: a stand-alone measure of spiritual wellbeing for palliative care patients with cancer. EORTC Quality of Life Group. *Palliat Med* 2013; **27**(5):457–69.

37 Selman L, Harding R, Gysels M, Speck P, Higginson IJ. The measurement of spirituality in palliative care and the content of tools validated cross-culturally: a systematic review *J Pain Symptom Manage* 2011; **41**(4):728–53.

38 Puchalski C, Romer AL. Taking a spiritual history allows clinicians to understand patients more fully. *J Palliat Med* 2000; **3**:129–37.

39 Puchalski CM. Spiritual assessment in clinical practice. *Psychiatr Ann* 2006; **36**:150.

40 Puchalski CM. The FICA spiritual history tool #274. *J Palliat Med* 2014; **17**(1):105–6.

41 Vermandere M, Choi YN, De Brabandere H, Decouttere R, De Meyere E, Gheysens E, et al. GPs' views concerning spirituality and the use of the FICA tool in palliative care in Flanders: a qualitative study. *Br J Gen Pract* 2012; **62**(603):e718–25.

42 Anandarajah G, Hight E. Spirituality and medical practice: using the HOPE questions as a practical tool for spiritual assessment. *Am Fam Physician* 2001; **63**:81–9.

43 Maugans TA. The SPIRITual history. *Fam Med* 1996; **5**:11–6.

44 Evans N, Costantini M, Pasman R, Van den Block L, Donker G, Miccinesi G, et al. End-of-life communication: a retrospective survey of representative GP networks in four countries. *J Pain Symptom Manage* 2014; **47**(3):604–6.

45 Van den Block L, Deschepper R, Bossuyt N, Drieskens K, Bauwens S, Van Casteren V, et al. Care for patients in the last three months of life: findings from the nationwide SENTI-MELC study in Belgium. *Arch Intern Med* 2008; **168**(16):1747–54.

46 Daaleman TP, Williams CS, Hamilton VL, Zimmerman S. Spiritual care at the end of life in long-term care. *Med Care* 2008; **46**(1):85–91.

47 Hamilton VL, Daaleman TP, Williams CS, Zimmerman S. The context of religious and spiritual care at the end of life in long-term care facilities. *Sociol Relig* 2009; **70**(2):179–95.

48 Gijsberts MJ, van der Steen JT, Muller MT, Deliens L. End-of-life with dementia in Dutch antroposofic and traditional nursing homes. *Tijdschr Gerontol Geriatr* 2008; **39**(6):256–64.

49 Chochinov HM. Dying, dignity, and new horizons in palliative end-of-life care. *CA Cancer J Clin* 2006; **56**(2):84–103.

50 Puchalski CM. Spirituality and end-of-life care: a time for listening and caring. *J Palliat Med* 2002; **5**(2):289–94.

51 Chochinov HM, Hassard T, McClement S, Hack T, Kristjanson LJ, Harlos M, et al. The patient dignity inventory: a novel way of measuring dignity-related distress in palliative care. *J Pain Symptom Manage* 2008; **36**(6):559–71.

52 Chochinov HM, McClement SE, Hack TF, McKeen NA, Rach AM, Gagnon P, et al. The Patient Dignity Inventory: applications in the oncology setting. *J Palliat Med* 2012; **15**(9):998–100.

53 Chochinov HM, Hack T, Hassard T, Kristjanson LJ, McClement S, Harlos M. Dignity therapy: a novel psychotherapeutic intervention for patients near the end of life. *J Clin Oncol* 2005; **23**(24):5520–5.

54 Chochinov HM, Cann B, Cullihall K, Kristjanson L, Harlos M, McClement SE, et al. Dignity therapy: a feasibility study of elders in long-term care. *Palliat Support Care* 2012; **10**(1):3–15.

55 Hall S, Goddard C, Opio D, Speck P, Higginson IJ. Feasibility, acceptability and potential effectiveness of Dignity Therapy for older people in care homes: a phase II randomized controlled trial of a brief palliative care psychotherapy. *Palliat Med* 2012; **26**(5):703.

56 Breitbart W, Gibson C, Poppito SR, Berg A. Psychotherapeutic interventions at the end of life: a focus on meaning and spirituality. Can J Psych. *Can J Psychiatry* 2004; **49**(6):366–72.

57 Breitbart W. Spirituality and meaning in supportive care: spirituality- and meaning- centered group psychotherapy interventions in advanced cancer. *Support Care Cancer* 2002; **10**(4):272–80.

58 E. MacKinlay. *Spiritual Growth and Care in the Fourth Age of Life*. London: Jessica Kingsley Publishers; 2006.

59 Integraal Kankercentrum Nederland. *Dutch Guideline: Spiritual Care in Palliative Care*. Available at: <http://www.oncoline.nl/index.php?pagina=/richtlijn/item/pagina.php&id=36581&richtlijn_id=907> (Accessed March 2014). Ref. type: online source.

60 McSherry W. *Making Sense of Spirituality in Nursing and Health Care Practice, an Interactive Approach*. London: Jessica Kingsley Publishers; 2006.

Part IV

Use of and access to palliative care for older people

Chapter 17

Use of generalist and specialist palliative care for older people

Thomas M. Carroll and Timothy Quill

Introduction to use of generalist and specialist palliative care for older people

Palliative care is many things to many people, evoking a wide range of emotions depending on one's point of view. For our purposes, palliative care is a philosophy of health care that focuses on individuals, and their families, who are experiencing suffering from serious medical conditions that limit their quality and/or expected length of life. The aims of palliative care are to help relieve uncomfortable symptoms, to assist with difficult medical decision making, and to provide added support for patients and their families. Comprehensive palliative care is ideally delivered by an interdisciplinary team, focusing on the relief of suffering from all causes, including physical, emotional, and spiritual sources. This philosophy is compatible with any plan of care, whether the goals involve disease-modifying treatments, be they curative or palliative, or whether the exclusive focus is on palliation of symptoms and suffering without disease modification. The medical specialty of palliative care has established expertise in at least two categories of patient care: the management of the suffering associated with complex or refractory symptoms, and resolution of conflict, generally related to medical decision making (patient–clinician, patient–family, etc.).

Palliative care is a relatively new field that has yet to gain official specialty status in many countries. This newness, in combination with the fact that it is a field not defined by an organ system or set of diseases, has made the distinction between what sort of palliative care skills should be mastered by a generalist versus a specialist particularly difficult to define. This distinction is important because, at some level, all seriously ill patients would benefit from a palliative care approach, and it is neither feasible nor desirable for a specialist to be involved with every case. Rather, the palliative care skill sets that potentially distinguish a specialist from a generalist must take into account the potential benefits and burdens of having yet another clinician or team involved in a patient's care. The specialized field of palliative care must thoughtfully consider which interventions should be taught to all clinicians, which might be provided in relatively brief consultation after which follow-up occurs with the primary referring team, and which types of clinical problems might require ongoing management by the palliative care specialized team. This is particularly important in the case of older adults, as more clinicians often mean more medications, more side-effects, more potentially conflicting recommendations, and, generally speaking, lower quality of life.

In this chapter, we will briefly review the history of palliative care, discuss the developing problem of providing high-value care to an expanding and ageing population of patients with serious illness, and suggest a method to distinguish between the roles of generalists versus specialists in providing palliative care.

Further, although palliative care has been frequently associated with the end of life, we will argue that such care (mainly generalist, but sometimes specialist) should be part of the treatment plan for all seriously ill patients rather than based on specific diagnosis or arbitrary thresholds of expected survival. Finally, we will suggest a general framework for ensuring the provision of sufficient palliative care services in the face of an ageing worldwide population.

A brief history of palliative care

The philosophical origins of hospice and palliative care can arguably be traced back to the Crusades and the Knights Hospitallers who, in the eleventh century AD, established houses of rest and healing for travellers making the arduous journey between Europe and the Middle East (1). These houses, though primarily for weary travellers, are notable for providing care to the incurably dying who, at the time, were a group often shunned out of fear that their presence was a detriment to the healing of others. This tradition persisted through the fifteenth century before fading from the historical record, only to be reborn in the seventeenth century, in Paris, through the efforts of the Sisters of Charity, founded by St. Vincent de Paul. Ensuing centuries saw similar efforts undertaken around Europe including the Our Lady's Hospice in Dublin, founded by the Irish Sisters of Charity. This same order founded St. Joseph's Hospice in South London in 1902, in part to complement their ongoing ministry of visiting the sick in their homes. It was at this hospice, nearly 60 years later, that Cicely Saunders would begin her work as a physician. Dr. Saunders, widely considered the founder of the modern hospice movement, was an early advocate for a number of concepts that have become mainstays in the field of palliative care. In 1967, she and her colleagues opened St. Christopher's Hospice; the first hospice facility built specifically for this purpose. The hospice movement officially made its way west across the Atlantic in 1971 with the founding of Hospice Inc. in New Haven, Connecticut. Home care services began two years later and a 44-bed in-patient facility was opened in 1980, the first of its kind in the United States and still functioning today.

Palliative medicine gained the status of a certified medical specialty in the United Kingdom in 1987 (2), with similar recognition in Ireland in 1995 (3) and in the United States in 2006 (4). Other European countries have recognized palliative medicine as a sub-specialty, meaning that certification in a primary specialty is also required. These include: Poland in 1999, Romania in 2000, Slovakia in 2005, Germany in 2006, and France in 2007 (3).

A number of other European countries provide official certification without having established specialty or sub-specialty status (3). A review of palliative care's emergence around the world shows a wide range of developmental stages, largely in line with countries' general economic development (5).

The earliest roots of hospice and palliative care provided services to 'the sick,' without distinction among diseases (such as they were understood at the time). Ironically, the modern incarnation of hospice has largely been designed to accommodate people suffering from cancer, which has often made it difficult to provide hospice-level care to people suffering from other diseases, generally related to organ failure. Fortunately, this is beginning to change with the growth of palliative care programmes around the world, leading to the creation of interdisciplinary teams to focus on people with non-cancer illnesses in a more flexible way than hospices often allow. Additionally, in the United States, there are signs that the Centers for Medicare Services (CMS) may relax the current requirement that patients forgo disease-altering or curative treatments to be eligible for hospice enrolment (6). While these developments certainly represent improvements, the next steps towards creating an effective and sustainable model for providing such care will be discussed later in the chapter. These changes may also make palliative care and hospice care more available to our ageing population who may be suffering with multiple co-morbid conditions rather than a single disease entity such as cancer.

Distinctions among hospice care, palliative care, and palliative medicine are a relatively recent, country-specific development. The term 'palliative care' was coined in 1974 by Balfour Mount who was a surgeon working at The Royal Victoria Hospital in Montreal, Canada. He chose this term in part to avoid the negative connotations associated with the term 'hospice' within the local French-speaking community (7). Today, hospice care in the United States is a federally-defined Medicare benefit for patients with an expected survival of six months or less who meet additional, disease-specific enrolment criteria that include a clear decision to forgo disease-directed therapies (8, 9). This separate hospice insurance benefit covers some added home care services, and can supplement care in a nursing facility if that is where the patient resides (though the custodial part of the care would require a separate payment source).

There is a distinction, in the United States, between hospice care and palliative care, where palliative care refers to a type of care given, regardless of formal hospice enrollment or prognosis, no matter what other disease-directed therapies are simultaneously offered. Palliative care in the United States generally refers to a consultative service that addresses pain and symptom management and goals of treatment, and that provides added support, but it is not part of a comprehensive system of care. Palliative care consultations are paid for much like consultations by other medical sub-specialists, and their input is entered into the mix of all other specialty inputs. Patients seen by palliative care specialists may or may not be terminally ill. This distinction unfortunately leads to much confusion among patients and medical professionals alike. An additional subtle distinction is sometimes made between 'palliative care', which refers to any and all care provided by an interdisciplinary team to alleviate suffering, and 'palliative medicine,' where the latter refers to such care that is delivered by clinicians who have prescribing authority. This distinction has developed somewhat organically and is illustrated by the fact that many hospitals have 'Palliative Care' programmes, while certification programmes are generally labelled with some variation on 'Palliative Medicine' (e.g. Hospice and Palliative Medicine). This is in contrast to the United Kingdom and Canada, where 'hospice' generally refers to a building or institution ('a hospice') which specializes in palliative care and where seriously ill, generally 'terminal' patients reside and are cared for regardless of prognosis, disease type, or treatment plan. Outside of the United States, there is generally not such sharp division of terminology or funding, and palliative care would refer to all palliative treatment regardless of prognosis.

The field of palliative care in the twenty-first century continues to grow and evolve at an almost frantic pace. Unlike organ system- or disease-defined specialties, palliative care transcends such boundaries—a quality that can be invoked as both its greatest strength and its Achilles heel (2). How the field will change with time is anyone's guess, but what is certain is that the need for comprehensive, coordinated focus on the alleviation of suffering and improved medical decision making for patients with serious illness has been recognized and is advancing.

The developing problem of providing palliative care for older people

Since its inception, the field of palliative care has become integral to many aspects of the practice of medicine around the world. Growing recognition of the value added to patients' care by palliative care teams has led to increased demand for their services, and in a growing number of instances, has even resulted in requirements that palliative care clinicians be a part of institutional programmes as a condition of accreditation (10). A question remains about which of these skills should be developed in all clinicians who care for seriously ill patients (generalist palliative care skills), and which should be generally reserved for palliative care specialists who have had added training and interest. Unfortunately, many generalists have never been properly trained in providing basic palliative care, so there may be considerable training requirements to ensure competence in this domain. The floor for such training would be the management of pain and other common symptoms. In this group, there may also be a general discomfort and lack of training about how to conduct difficult discussions, especially related to death and dying. Compounding the problematic effects of this general discomfort is the reality that such difficult discussions are time intensive, a commodity for which clinicians have traditionally been poorly reimbursed. Finally, extrinsic factors play a role as well including, but certainly not limited to, the toxic and adversarial environment created in many jurisdictions with respect to the prescription of controlled substances, especially opioids.

Factors contributing to the growth of palliative care from the specialist point of view include an increasing recognition of value provided by palliative care consultation and management. This added value takes a number of forms including expertise in the diagnosis and management of complex symptoms and an ability to work with complex family dynamics, as well as a growing body of literature supporting improvements in symptom burden, overall quality of life, and, perhaps, even survival (11). Finally, palliative care clinicians have the advantage of both bringing these considerable assets to a patient's care and of providing a fresh perspective on a patient's condition. When a team of clinicians has been involved with a patient's 'battle' against a disease process, it can be difficult for them to recognize when the time has come to change focus, and it may feel like doing so would be perceived as capitulation or even abandonment. One of the most powerful roles a palliative care team can play is to help patients and their care teams re-internalize the distinction between the goals (e.g. living better and, hopefully, longer) and the strategies (e.g. proper mix of disease-modifying and symptom-modulating treatment).

Coincident with the rise of palliative care as an independent specialty has been the much discussed ageing of the population in developed nations. In the United States, for example, it is estimated that from 2011 through 2030, approximately 10,000 Americans will turn 65 years old each day (12), with similar projections for western European countries (13, 14). This demographic phenomenon will likely be transformative in ways that are both predictable and unpredictable. One likely consequence is a vast increase in the worldwide burden of chronic and life-limiting disease. This dramatic growth of the number of seriously ill older persons will place drastic stresses on the health care systems of the Western world.

The generation currently entering their retirement years, the so-called 'baby boomers', is different from the prior generation for sociological reasons. This generation was born into, and matured with, the modern world in a very real sense, witnessing exponential growth and radical change in wide-ranging fields including technology, medicine, and the scope of governmental services. These, and other factors, have combined to create a 'perfect storm' wherein a large cohort of ageing individuals will begin to require the services of the medical system while bringing with them an expectation that every problem can be fixed. Where the field of palliative care fits into this transition from the generation of the Second World War, with their generalized stoicism and tendency to accept their fate, to the baby boomers, with their highly individualistic focus on fixing each problem as it arises, remains an open question. We will not attempt to answer such lofty questions but, rather, will offer some possible solutions to the problems and tensions that may arise as a function of this generational transition in the setting of a relatively fixed supply of specialist palliative care services and increasing pressure to control overall medical spending.

Defining generalist and specialist palliative care

Before considering how palliative care can best serve our ageing population, it is important to define the boundary between two complimentary groups who provide palliative care services: generalists and specialists. Distinguishing between a generalist and a specialist is certainly not a new concept in the medical world. It is the very nature of a new diagnostic or therapeutic modality that initially requires a specialist to assume nearly monopolistic control for some period of time, only to eventually cede some or all of that monopoly to the generalist. Despite serial losses of monopoly, far from becoming extinct, specialists have grown dramatically in number and power within medicine such that it is not uncommon to have a different specialist managing aspects of each organ system of a complex patient without anyone overseeing the entire enterprise. The primary care physician is currently an endangered species, and palliative care sometimes steps into this central decision-making role, along with the patient/family, when no one else has done so.

Palliative care differs from many other specialties in that it is not defined by a given organ system or set of procedures, and it tends to focus patients, families, and other treating clinical teams on the overarching goals of treatment. For this reason, the field may follow a different developmental path. The development of geriatrics may, to some extent, provide a template to help understand and possibly predict the future of palliative care. The two are similar in their explicit patient-centred focus and lack of disease/organ specificity. However, geriatrics does have a more concrete inclusion criterion, namely age, whereas palliative care is potentially directed at patients with 'serious illness' in any age group.

A number of authors have provided their perspectives as to what sort of palliative care related skills should be considered primary (15) or generalist (16), and which might reasonably be reserved for the designation of specialist. Figure 17.1 represents our conception of how the palliative care skills might be divided between the generalist and the specialist on a continuum, rather than attempting to rigidly define discrete skill categories. We have chosen to designate symptom diagnosis/management, end-of-life care, assistance with medical decision making, and, to a lesser extent, conflict resolution as categories of palliative care that fall more heavily within the generalist's purview. At the opposite end of the spectrum, it is appropriate for a specialist to be involved only with a minority of cases involving aspects from these categories, and generally once the complexity and/or severity have reached the point where the generalist feels assistance is necessary. Additionally, the specialist end of the spectrum contains issues and skill sets that have sufficiently low prevalence and high complexity as to almost universally require involvement, if not direct management, by a specialist. These include, but are not limited to, evaluation of cases of near futility, consideration and management of palliative sedation, managing requests for

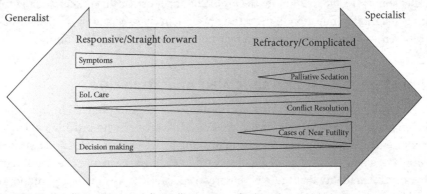

Figure 17.1 Generalist versus specialist palliative care: finding the right balance

assisted death, helping address highly conflicted decision making, and helping manage intractable symptoms.

Thinking about the designation of generalist and specialist on a spectrum will, we hope, allow for a more nuanced discussion about how the field of palliative care should evolve over time. It may drive the kinds of training programmes needed to ensure basic competence of generalists (both primary care and specialists in other domains), as well as clarify common situations where referral to a palliative care specialist might be indicated. Some non-palliative care clinicians may develop expertise in all generalist domains and some specialist domains. So, potentially, each clinician may find his or her own, personalized set of palliative care skills and threshold for referral. In most circumstances, at least in the United States, palliative care should be considered a consultation service to help answer clinical questions, with the patient returning to the main treating physician/clinical team for ongoing care, though referral for ongoing treatment is also possible for particularly challenging cases. These distinctions would need negotiation between the referring clinician and the consultant but, ideally, the consultation model will avoid further fragmentation of the care of these seriously ill patients.

Determining the optimal time for specialist palliative care referral

The literature on palliative care referral reflects confusion around the issue of who needs palliative care treatment, and who needs specialty palliative care referral. If the primary treating clinicians do not provide basic palliative care treatments, then the need for referral would be virtually unlimited (all seriously ill patients.) If such clinicians do possess these skills, then the need for consultation and/or referral would be much less. A body of literature has developed around the definition and recognition of optimal timing for specialist palliative care referral, though it generally does not consider this background issue. Instead, such studies focus on intrinsic patient characteristics (e.g. age, diagnosis), measures of function (e.g. Palliative Performance Scale, Karnofsky Scale), and predictors of survival (e.g. Seattle Heart Failure Model, the surprise question).

A number of investigators have tried to determine to what extent patients in need of specialist palliative care are receiving it, often generating conflicting data. For example, a systematic review, for which only retrospective primary studies were available, found increasing age to be associated with a lower likelihood of appropriate involvement of specialist palliative care (17), while another group of investigators, using a prospective study design, found no effect of age on likelihood of specialist involvement (18). Work attempting to understand what drives palliative care referral in the United Kingdom suggested that the decision to refer depends on a complex and fluid relationship among a number of factors both intrinsic and extrinsic to the potential referrer (19). Specifically, decisions about referral are based on a combination of the referrer's perception of their rightful role in providing primary palliative care and their perception about the services for which they might refer. These studies lead to a number of conflicting conclusions and, more than anything else, illustrate the need for commonly accepted definitions of generalist and specialist palliative care.

Our approach when addressing this issue involves considering three categories of patients who are certainly appropriate for at least a generalist palliative care focus and may be appropriate for specialist consultation or referral: 1) cases in which the referring clinician has a question and needs help (consultation only); 2) patients with predicted survival shorter than an agreed-upon threshold (consultation or referral); and 3) diagnosis-specific early involvement (referral and co-management). We fully recognize that any generalized thresholds that are set for referral should be a function of the relative value added by such referral, which in turn is a function of the relative skill sets of the generalist and the specialist, as well as local practice patterns and palliative care specialist availability. Therefore, the extent to which any educational programme expands the palliative care skill set of generalists will necessarily alter the thresholds for each of these categories of potential referrals.

Of these three categories, the first is the most difficult to address systematically, simply because it is entirely dependent upon an individual clinician's knowledge and skill set as they relate to a particular patient and clinical situation. This category is associated with the highest risk of both under- and over-utilization of specialist palliative care consultation— the former due to clinical 'blind spots' (i.e. being unaware of what one does not know) and the latter due, for example, to the short-term ease of having the palliative care specialist handle all opioid pain management (which the generalist could capably do but prefers not to). The solution to most under- or overutilization is education. In thinking about such educational efforts, it is instructive to consider where we are starting. Several studies have attempted to address this starting point, including one utilizing semi-structured interviews of medical professionals (primarily generalists) in Northern Ireland who had significant difficulty defining palliative care (20). The health care professionals studied generally agreed on the overarching definition of palliative care, but strongly associated the field with cancer and active dying rather than a philosophy of care ideally implemented further upstream in all seriously ill patients. Even more telling was a study done in the United Kingdom, also using semi-structured interviews, that explored clinicians' experiences regarding barriers to accessing palliative care services for people with dementia (21). Published in 2011, these data revealed significant barriers to making the transition to a palliative approach for people with dementia, in part because dementia was viewed as not 'a disease— it's just something that happens to people' and 'not terminal'. Interestingly, the first comment was extracted from a specialist palliative care focus group, while the second was from a general practice focus group.

These and other similar data suggest that there may be a general knowledge deficit with respect to both what palliative care is in general and what added value specialist palliative care clinicians can provide to patient care. Given this confusion, it is not surprising that there is difficulty in recognizing patients who might benefit from palliative care. While this should not be viewed as an indictment of any group (lay or professional), it does present a challenge in terms of effectively utilizing available specialist palliative care resources. At our institution, the palliative care division has begun to attend various oncology tumour board conferences to both provide clinical input as well as general information/education regarding the specific skill set of our division's clinicians. This is generating useful discussions about which patients can be well managed by non-palliative care clinicians, which might benefit from a brief consultation, and which would be best referred for co-management. Although there are few available data to provide guidance as to whether this practice is effective, it is hoped that through these efforts, a more consistent and, hopefully, accurate view of specialist palliative care will begin to take shape, at least within our institution.

Predicted survival thresholds comprise a second category of patient-specific criteria that have been suggested as a mechanism to prompt, or even mandate, when aspects of palliative care should be addressed, whether or not a specialist in palliative care is consulted. In the United States, the primary eligibility criterion for hospice enrolment is that the patient is expected to live six months or less if the primary life-limiting disease runs its usual course. This criterion works reasonably well for patients with cancer, the set of diseases for which the Medicare hospice benefit was originally designed, but does not accommodate diseases of organ failure nearly as well, given their very different trajectories (22). In an attempt to provide added support for patients with any type of life-limiting disease, cancer or otherwise, some authors have suggested that patients should be considered for palliative care involvement if clinicians would not be 'surprised' if the patient survived less than twelve months. This broader prognostic net is especially important because of clinicians' tendencies to overestimate, rather than underestimate, survival, for those who want to include this domain in referral decisions. Furthermore, threshold levels of unrelieved suffering generally make a lot more sense than survival thresholds, since there is widespread agreement that palliative care interventions should not be reserved for the very end of life. However, our view is that survival thresholds should not specifically drive specialist palliative care consultation, for at least two reasons. First, there is not (and likely never will be) a sufficient workforce of specialist palliative care clinicians to help care for every patient who appears to be nearing the end of life; and, second, standardized consultation based on expected survival would likely lead to further fragmentation of patient care.

Finally, the third category of patients sometimes suggested as automatically appropriate for specialist palliative care involvement is defined by specific life-limiting disease. The landmark study by Temel and colleagues (11), perhaps the single most cited research article in the palliative care literature to date, was a single-centre randomized controlled trial of early specialist palliative care referral for patients newly diagnosed with metastatic (stage IV) non-small-cell lung cancer versus usual care, with the primary outcome being the difference in quality of life between the two groups. While the study found a higher quality of life among patients randomized to the palliative care intervention arm, the finding that made the study famous was that patients who were randomized to receive early specialist palliative care lived a median of 2.7 months longer than those in the control arm. This magnitude of difference, if confirmed, would appear to place early specialist palliative care involvement in this particular disease on the same level as standard successful chemotherapy regimens. These data have sparked numerous publications and intense speculation as to whether this effect might apply to other cancers and even other categories of disease. While this result is intriguing, the trial, involving a total of 152 patients, should be analysed with appropriate caution given its status as the first of its kind. Additionally, although potential mediating factors for this apparent effect have been suggested, there are yet no data supporting any one of the many possible mechanisms. Therefore, as well as confirming this survival benefit in other settings/institutions, a top research priority should be to elucidate the mechanism of this effect so that rational decisions can be made regarding whether, and if so to what extent, early specialist palliative care involvement is the critical ingredient. And so, in our view, the question remains as to whether all such patients would need specialized palliative care if the standard of oncology care included first-rate primary palliative care—but such questions await further research.

Developing a more sustainable model of palliative care

Estimates of demand for physicians trained in hospice and palliative medicine in the United States indicate that there is already an acute shortage, which is likely to worsen in the coming years (23). These estimates suggest that there were, as of 2010, 4400 specialist palliative care physicians in the United States, providing between 1700 and 3300 full-time equivalents (FTEs) of specialist services. The estimated concurrent demand of physician FTEs was approximately 15,000, leaving a deficit of 3000 to 7500 FTEs, which would be equivalent to 6000 to 18,000 physicians, depending on percentage time devoted to specialist palliative care. A similar situation has been documented in western Europe (24). However, these shortfalls in the United States and western Europe are dwarfed by the situation in central and eastern Europe (25), as well as around the developing world (5). Assuming that these estimates are in the right ballpark, training of specialist palliative care clinicians by fellowship training programmes, and even including future alternative pathway certification options for practicing physicians, is unlikely to overcome this shortfall in supply. Therefore, the only alternative, to avoid underservicing patients in need, is to decrease demand for specialist palliative care services by expanding the scope of generalists in the provision of palliative care. Any strategy that successfully expands access to palliative care services should focus on training both generalists and specialists in palliative care, including physicians and other health care professionals.

Although formal fellowship training programmes, following the typical western model, are efficacious in training highly skilled clinicians, they are often less effective than desired in terms of increasing the overall workforce, given their logistical complexity and high overheads. Much more effective, particularly in resource-limited environments, are training programmes aimed at establishing first a minimum generalist palliative care competence level among all health care professionals, and then providing further tiered educational and practice opportunities for those interested in developing more specialized palliative care skills while maintaining their primary practice specialties.

There are already a number of robust and well-designed web-based programmes that provide tiered instructional levels, suitable for a wide range of learners. Two of special note are Education in Palliative and End-of-life Care (26) and Oncotalk (27). Both appear to be effective in providing instruction in some of the skill sets necessary to deliver high- quality generalist palliative care. Education in Palliative and End-of-life Care, in particular, is widely applicable in that it provides both a general curriculum as well as tailored curricula for specific groups, including clinicians in geriatrics, emergency medicine, long-term care, oncology, and paediatrics, with additional curricula aimed at caregivers, veterans, and Roman Catholics.

Conclusions on the use of generalist and specialist palliative care for older people

When considering how best to improve the provision of palliative care services for older adults, it is the effectiveness of those services, and not the specialty of those providing the care, that ultimately matters. All health care professionals who plan to care for seriously ill patients have an obligation to develop and maintain basic palliative care skill sets that allow for effective palliation of suffering, planning for the future, and compassionate care at the end of life. Where the specialist in palliative care fits into a given patient's care depends very much on the interplay between the patient's needs and the generalist's skill set. It is our hope that effective educational efforts are undertaken to expand the delivery of palliative care to everyone in need and, in doing so, improve not only the quality, but perhaps even the quantity, of life among patients suffering from serious diseases.

References

1 Connor S. *Hospice, Practice, Pitfalls, and Promise*. Washington, D.C.: Taylor & Francis; 1998.

2 Fordham S, Dowrick C, May C. Palliative medicine: is it really specialist territory? *J R Soc Med* 1998; **91**(11):568–72.

3 Centeno C, Noguera A, Lynch T, Clark D. Official certification of doctors working in palliative medicine in Europe: data from an EAPC study in 52 European countries. *Palliat Med* 2007; **21**(8):683–7.

4 American Board of Medical Specialties. 'ABMS Establishes New Subspecialty Certificate in Hospice and Palliative Medicine' [press release]; 2006. Available at: <http://www.abms.org/News_and_Events/downloads/NewsubcertPalliativeMed.pdf> (Accessed March 2014). Ref. type: online source.

5 Lynch T, Connor S, Clark D. Mapping levels of palliative care development: a global update. *J Pain Symptom Manage* 2013; **45**(6):1094–106.

6 American Academy of Hospice and Palliative Medicine. *Medicare Care Choices Model Will Test Effectiveness of Curative and Palliative Care for Certain Beneficiaries*; 2014. Available at: <http://amc-aahpm.informz.net/InformzDataService/OnlineVersion/Individual?mailingInstanceId=3143453&subscriberId=819305926> (Accessed March 2014). Ref. type: online source.

7 Loscalzo MJ. Palliative care: an historical perspective. *Hematology Am Soc Hematol Educ Program* 2008; 465. doi: 10.1182/asheducation-2008.1.465.

8 Ross JS, Sanchez-Reilly S. *Hospice Criteria Card*; 2013. Available at: <http://geriatrics.uthscsa.edu/gerifellowship/documents/updated_08_2013/Hospice%20Card%20%20JSR%20SSR%202013.07.10.pdf> (Accessed March 2014). Ref. type: online source.

9 Centers for Medicare & Medicaid Services. *Medicare Hospice Benefits*. Baltimore: Centers for Medicare & Medicaid Services; 2013.

10 American College of Surgeons. *Cancer Program Standards 2012*; 2011. Available at: <http://www.facs.org/cancer/coc/programstandards2012.html> (Accessed March 2014). Ref. type: online source.

11 Temel JS, Greer JA, Muzikansky A, Gallagher ER, Admane S, Jackson VA, et al. Early palliative care for patients with metastatic non-small-cell lung cancer. *NEJM* 2010; **363**(8):733–42.

12 Cohn DV, Taylor P. *Baby Boomers Approach 65—Glumly*; 2010. Available at: <http://www.pewsocialtrends.org/2010/12/20/baby-boomers-approach-65-glumly/> (Accessed November 2013). Ref. type: online source.

13 Cracknell R. *The Ageing Population*; 2010. Available at: <http://www.parliament.uk/business/publications/research/key-issues-for-the-new-parliament/value-for-money-in-public-services/the-ageing-population/> (Accessed November 2013). Ref. type: online source.

14 Carone G, Costello D. Can Europe afford to grow old? *Finance and Development* 2006; **43**(3):28.

15 von Gunten CF. Secondary and tertiary palliative care in US hospitals. *JAMA* 2002; **287**(7):875–81.

16 Quill TE, Abernethy AP. Generalist plus specialist palliative care—creating a more sustainable model. *NEJM* 2013; **368**(13):1173–5.

17 Walshe C, Todd C, Caress A, Chew-Graham C. Patterns of access to community palliative care services: a literature review. *J Pain Symptom Manage* 2009; **37**(5):884–912.

18 Burt J, Plant H, Omar R, Raine R. Equity of use of specialist palliative care by age: cross-sectional study of lung cancer patients. *Palliat Med* 2010; **24**(6):641–50.

19 Walshe C, Chew-Graham C, Todd C, Caress A. What influences referrals within community palliative care services? A qualitative case study. *Soc Sci Med* 2008; **67**(1):137–46.

20 McIlfatrick S. Assessing palliative care needs: views of patients, informal carers and health care professionals. *J Adv Nurs* 2007; **57**(1):77–86.

21 Ryan T, Gardiner C, Bellamy G, Gott M, Ingleton C. Barriers and facilitators to the receipt of palliative care for people with dementia: the views of medical and nursing staff. *Palliat Med* 2012; **26**(7):879–86.

22 Murray SA, Kendall M, Boyd K, Sheikh A. Illness trajectories and palliative care. *BMJ* 2005; **330**(7498):1007–11.

23 Lupu D, American Academy of H, Palliative Medicine Workforce Task F. Estimate of current hospice and palliative medicine physician workforce shortage. *J Pain Symptom Manage* 2010; **40**(6):899–911.

24 Lynch T, Clark D, Centeno C, Rocafort J, de Lima L, Filbet M, et al. Barriers to the development of palliative care in Western Europe. *Palliat Med* 2010; **24**(8):812–9.

25 Lynch T, Clark D, Centeno C, Rocafort J, Flores LA, Greenwood A, et al. Barriers to the development of palliative care in the countries of Central and Eastern Europe and the Commonwealth of Independent States. *J Pain Symptom Manage* 2009; **37**(3):305–15.

26 Education in Palliative and End-of-life Care. Available at: <http://www.epec.net/s> (Accessed November 2013). Ref. type: online source.

27 Back AL, Arnold A, Baile W, Tulsky J, Fryer-Edwards K. *Oncotalk*. Available at: <http://depts.washington.edu/oncotalk/> (Accessed December 2013). Ref. type: online source.

Chapter 18

Compassionate communities: caring for older people towards the end of life

Allan Kellehear

Introduction to compassionate communities

Compassionate communities are community development experiments dedicated to encouraging *all people* to take some active responsibility for end-of-life care. They are public health models of care that recognize that living with a life-threatening or life-limiting illness, grief and bereavement, and caregiving, have their own personal and social costs in terms of associated morbidity and mortality. Compassionate communities recognize that ageing, dying, and the occurrence of death and bereavement can cause a host of other problems—from anxiety, depression, social withdrawal, and suicide, to social isolation, stigma, discrimination. and job loss, among many other consequences. The adoption of a community development approach to these troubles is recognition that most of these troubles, indeed if not all of them, are amenable to prevention, harm reduction, and early intervention. In other words, compassionate communities are public health approaches to end-of-life care.

In this chapter, I will begin briefly by describing the particular sense in which I am using the phrase 'public health'. I will then trace the rise of the compassionate community idea to the earlier idea of the healthy community as developed by the World Health Organization. Following this, I will describe three examples of compassionate community programmes that enhance the health and well-being of older people at the end of life, before concluding with some remarks about the challenges that these type of practices face now and in the future.

The meaning of public health

The broadest meaning of public health is the system-wide efforts of any society to prevent disease, injury, and unnecessary death and to promote health and well-being. However, the historical realities have been that early public health efforts focused mainly on disease and injury prevention and especially infectious diseases (the 'old' public health). Health and medical services have historically been designed as troubleshooters and problem solvers. This understanding of 'public' health was basically a crisis management model that emphasized an acute care, clinical (face-to-face) approach to health care. It is this approach and emphasis that has historically been responsible for the development of our acute care services such as hospitals, sanitariums, and, later, hospices. Concepts of prevention and harm reduction were also integral to this approach, but the onus of prevention efforts was largely with health or other professional services. So, for example, doctors and nurses led inoculation schemes for the prevention of childhood or adult infections; engineers and local government authorities led the establishment of building codes, clean sewerage disposal, and the purification of drinking water, and this, in turn, led to the prevention of injuries and diseases at home or work.

In the mid-twentieth century, this twin emphasis on professional authorities on the one hand, and disease and injury on the other hand, shifted to include a far greater role for communities—and the emphasis shifted to health and well-being (the 'new' public health). The best prevention of disease and illness was a healthy community. A healthy community was one where its peoples were well informed about basic ideas about good nutrition, the benefits of exercise, and ways to enhance health protection and safety. In this approach, 'being healthy' would be more than visiting the local doctor or dentist. People could take more responsibility for their own health and this, in turn, would complement the efforts by public services to keep them healthy. At the same time, these efforts might help people to use services less or to work in partnership with services for their own health and ill-health experiences. Local communities—schools, workplaces, churches/temples, trade unions, the local media, and recreational clubs and societies—were all asked to take some role in their community's health and safety. It is exactly these kinds of efforts and this kind of emphasis from which compassionate communities derive.

'Healthy Cities', 'Compassionate Cities'

Compassionate Cities was an idea derived from the Healthy Cities movement initiated by the World Health Organization (WHO). Healthy Cities—a phrase coined by the psychiatrist and public health worker Leonard Dahl—was one main way that WHO thought it might achieve the aims of the Ottawa Charter for Health Promotion in the mid-1980s (1). Whole communities might be enlisted to examine how they could make an active contribution to their own members—from local governments and health services to workplaces, schools, and local media. The idea of the Healthy 'City' originally had little to do—at least in inspirational terms—with urban areas. Rather the word 'city' was chosen to emphasize the fundamental etymological origins of the term, that is, an assembly of citizens enjoying certain limited rights, but especially equality, work, and health, and enjoying that social solidarity despite social differences related to gender, race, class, or religion, for example (2).

Thus, Healthy Cities were communities, both urban and rural, that strived, by their own civic efforts, to raise the standard of health and safety in partnership with their 'official' health services and professionals. In Healthy Cities, health becomes everyone's business. In exactly this way, Compassionate Cities were envisioned to be healthy communities that understood and aspired to make end-of-life care everyone's responsibility (3, 4). With its theoretical roots in a parallel health promotion tradition in palliative care (5), compassionate communities were communities that understood that contributing to the care of those living with a life-threatening/limiting illness, bereavement, and caregiving was an absolutely intrinsic part of the health and well-being responsibilities of all 'healthy communities'.

In this way, the morbidities and mortalities associated with dying, death, bereavement, and caregiving—such as loneliness, social isolation, depression, anxiety, job loss, suicide, stigma, or excessive burdens of care, to name only a few examples—could be identified by communities as targets for prevention, harm reduction, and early intervention. These aspirations would be achieved by similar, and sometimes the same, methods that had been shown to work in healthy communities—health promotion, community development, education, social marketing, participatory relations, and service partnerships (6). These methods, and any achievements hard won by them, would be developed with an eye to their sustainability, owned and nurtured as part of a community's assets similar to any other important amenity under its protection.

The rise of compassionate communities

Although originally an Australian public health idea, compassionate communities have now been widely adopted in the United Kingdom and Ireland (7). There have also been parallel social developments almost identical to these practice models but without the label of 'compassionate community', such as the numerous community development projects in Africa (8) and the world renowned community development palliative care model in Northern Kerala in India (9). In fact, much of what passes for dementia-friendly community practice is also driven by modern health promotion ideas and practices, although of course, often confining itself to a specific disease group rather than the end of life more broadly conceived.

In recent years, there have been numerous articles in the British medical and palliative care periodic literature that have documented the rise of compassionate communities (10–14). Paul and Sallnow (13), for example, found that over 200 palliative care services in the United Kingdom were 'prioritizing' community engagement initiatives and many were attempting to do so along compassionate community guidelines. Barry and Patel (14), on behalf the (UK) National Council for Palliative Care, conducted an in-depth examination of what some of these 'compassionate communities' were actually doing under this overarching concept. They found there was great diversity among those who were attempting to facilitate community 'engagement' in end-of-life care but that, most commonly, many were rethinking their use of community volunteers as simply adjuncts to their service and, instead, were re-orienting these community members to be active agents for change, support, and advocacy within their own communities. This approach seems to be a core effort in British compassionate communities, though it is not the only model of practice.

Care for (only) older people?

Although it is true that dying, death, bereavement, and long-term caregiving may occur at any age, the historical and epidemiological reality of modern affluent societies points starkly to the fact that most of this occurs to older people. Most people who die every year in Europe, North America, Canada, Australia, Japan, Taiwan, or South Korea do so over the age of 65 (15). Moreover, this means that most of the burden of long-term care is shouldered by older people, especially, but not exclusively, by spouses. With ageing come the chronic diseases of age—cancers, serious neurological disorders, organ failure, frailty, and the dementias. In this precise epidemiological way, palliative care services primarily deal with older people with cancer, while conversely, aged care services who cater for long-term, chronic conditions often encounter significantly higher mortality rates than other health services who commonly deal with a cross-section of the community.

In modern, affluent societies, end-of-life care is, therefore, often synonymous with care for older people and their social networks. So, although compassionate communities are communities responsive to *all* individuals and groups experiencing dying, death, bereavement, and caregiving, including care of dying children and their families, most of the efforts of compassionate communities are geared towards care of older people. However, unlike dementia-friendly community practices, compassionate communities attempt to embrace a wide variety of people in an equally wide variety of end-of-life experiences and circumstances. A compassionate community might deploy special volunteers to help particular families experiencing a life-limiting illness or bereavement, but it might also encourage schools to adopt bereavement policies for its teachers, students, or parents. A compassionate community may also recognize and adopt practices that support those who experience grief from the death of animal companions or may assist the frail aged or those living with dementia to make care and support plans for their animal companions. Compassionate communities are communities that recognize that end-of-life care is mostly care for older people, but that recognition must sit alongside the equally important insight that dying, death, bereavement, and caregiving can and does occur to almost anyone and that its population presence, and therefore its care, is complex and diverse.

National case examples of compassionate communities

In Japan, a national committee of academics, government officials, trade unions, and business interests, as well as private charities, lead and facilitate a dementia-friendly community programme. Calling themselves 'The 100-Member Committee', this Japanese innovation well illustrates the system-wide approach possible in such public health initiatives as compassionate or dementia-friendly communities (16). National prizes are advertised and awarded to the most innovative community support models for people living with dementia and their caregivers.

Among the hundreds of major projects considered each year is a project that changes the way respite care is delivered. People living with dementia arrive at a day care centre and are asked to brainstorm a set of ideas for their lunch that day. After a group decision has been made about the menu, staff and clients go shopping to buy the ingredients. When they return, everyone cooks and shares the meal. This programme allows the local town people to familiarize themselves with those living with dementia and to deepen their understanding and their communication skills in dealing with people with these kinds of disability. They are sharing the care. At the respite centre, staff are able to enter a collegial set of relations with their clients rather than positioning themselves as carers only and clients as passive recipients and consumers of care. Relations became more participatory.

In another part of Japan, the major school in one town has formed a regular relationship with the local aged care centre which has a large proportion of residents living with dementia. Children from the school visit the centre some four times a year, while the residents themselves visit the school several times a year for special events such as sports days. A report on this school even describes residents in wheelchairs participating in tug-of-war games with the students (which the residents tend to lose!). In this project, young people are able to deepen their understanding of ageing and disability and also to form friendships with an older generation.

In the United Kingdom, St Christopher's Hospice has developed a similar set of projects (17) including a schools programme where young children visit several times a year to spend time with in-patients and out-patients with advanced life-limiting illness. Joint activities familiarize students with chronic illness, dying, disability, and loss and facilitate friendships outside the formal programme. The residents, on the other hand, are able to exercise their own usual desire to care for others and to feel active and useful, rather than falling back to a sense of being simply a passive patient. Relationships become 'health and well-being' promoting for both parties and, similar to the Japanese examples just described, permit different sections of the community to care for one another at the end of life when conventional professional services would normally divide and hide.

In Shropshire, Birmingham, and Weston-Super-Mare (18), hospices and community-based charities have developed compassionate communities by soliciting volunteers to work with the frail, vulnerable, and chronically ill. Volunteers are drawn from all walks of life—retired as well as workers—who are able to dedicate a portion of their week to visiting others at home. These programmes are about raising awareness of the need for every community member to become actively involved in the care of the frail and vulnerable in their own locality, despite not necessarily 'knowing' these people. Often called 'compassionate friends' or 'compassionate companions', these volunteers frequently meet together and help problem solve social and practical problems encountered by their frail or isolated neighbours. They are, therefore, actively involved in end-of-life care, whether this is imminent (as in an explicit life-limiting illness) or expected during the course of advanced age (where end of life refers simply to life during the 'end times').

The evidence base for the effectiveness of these kinds of initiatives has a considerably long history, especially in health care contexts more broadly. For example, a recent systematic review of over 130 community engagement programmes initiated since 1990 in the United Kingdom (19) found that there was 'solid evidence that community engagement interventions have a positive impact on health behaviours, health consequences, self-efficacy and perceived social support outcomes, across various conditions'. Early evaluations of the aforementioned compassionate community projects have supported these findings. In the Shropshire compassionate community project, for example, evaluations have described significant drops in unscheduled (i.e. emergency) use of local health services (4).

Conclusion—the future

As the demography of ageing and dying increases over the next decade, reflecting the impact of the ageing baby-boomer generation (15), and as governments worldwide attempt to contain health service costs, there is a growing need for more innovative models of health care that can extend access while maintaining quality of care. Community development models such as compassionate communities are able to meet these criteria by asking modern populations to think in terms of community-wide responsibility actions, partnerships, and alternatives. In these ways, compassionate communities can improve access to end-of-life care more broadly conceived and executed, and are able to address the many barriers encountered by health services, to provide a seamless experience of continuity of care.

However, the challenges remain significant (20). There is a pressing need for greater evaluation of the effectiveness of these programmes, ensuring that the evidence base for their effectiveness (or otherwise) is more publicly available. At present, much of this evidence remains buried in the grey literature—conference proceedings, doctoral work, health service reports, etc.

Furthermore, community development models require that we understand and accept that there are serious limits to direct service provision. For cultures of health and social care, such as those found in the United Kingdom, this might mean reluctant acceptance that all of us must make some contribution to each other's care. Modern industrial cultures are accustomed to creating individuals who are socialized to think of themselves as offering a specialized set of skills and to purchasing, from others, the skills they do not have—including health care. Although we have come a long way in changing attitudes and behaviour towards our own health, to include personal and social responsibility, this process of change for end-of-life care has only just commenced.

References

1 Aicher J. *Designing Healthy Cities: Prescriptions, Principles and Practice*. Malabar, Florida; Krieger; 1998.

2 Turner BS (ed). *Citizenship and Social Theory*. London: Sage; 1993.

3 Kellehear A. *Compassionate Cities: Public Health and End of Life Care*. London: Routledge; 2005.

4 Kellehear A. Compassionate communities: end of life care as everyone's responsibility. *Quarterly Journal of Medicine* 2013; **106**(12):1071–6.

5 A. Kellehear. *Health-Promoting Palliative Care*. Melbourne: Oxford University Press; 1999.

6 O'Mara-Eves A, Brunton G, McDaid D, Oliver S, Kavanagh J, Jamal F, et al. Community engagement to reduce inequalities in health: a systematic review, meta-analysis and economic analysis. *Public Health Research* 2013; **1**(4).

7 Conway S. *Governing Death and Loss Empowerment, Involvement and Participation*. Oxford: Oxford University Press; 2011.

8 Downing J, Gwyther L, Mwangi-Powell F. Public health and palliative care: a perspective from Africa. In: Sallnow L, Kumar S, Kellehear A (eds). *International Perspectives on Public Health and Palliative Care*. Abingdon: Routledge; 2012, 69–84.

9 Kumar S. Public health approaches to palliative care: the neighborhood network in Kerala. In: Sallnow L, Kumar S, Kellehear A (eds). *International Perspectives on Public Health and Palliative Care*. Abingdon: Routledge; 2012, 98–109.

10 Scottish Government. *Living and Dying Well—A National Action Plan for Palliative and End of Life Care in Scotland*. Edinburgh: Scottish Government; 2008.

11 Haraldsdottir E, Clark P, Murray SA. Health-promoting palliative care arrives in Scotland. *Eur J Pall Care* 2010; **17**(3):130–2.

12 Abel J, Bowra J, Walter T, Howarth G. Compassionate community networks: supporting home dying. *BMJ Support Palliat Care* 2011; **1**(2):129–33.

13 Paul S, Sallnow L. Public health approaches to end of life care in the UK: an online survey of palliative care services. *BMJ Support Palliat Care* 2013; **3**(2):196–9.

14 Barry V, Patel M. *An Overview of Compassionate Communities in England*. London: Murray Hall Community Trust and National Council for Palliative Care; 2013.

15 Kellehear A. *A Social History of Dying*. Cambridge: Cambridge University Press; 2007.

16 The 100-Member Committee. The campaign to build a dementia-friendly community. In: Sallnow L, Kumar S, Kellehear A (eds). *International Perspectives on Public Health and Palliative Care*. Abingdon: Routledge; 2012, 123–38.

17 Hartley N. 'Let's talk about dying': changing attitudes towards hospices and end of life care. In: Sallnow L, Kumar S, Kellehear A (eds). *International Perspectives on Public Health and Palliative Care*. Abingdon: Routledge; 2012, 156–71.

18 The Irish Hospice Foundation (eds). *Abstracts of the 3rd International Public Health and Palliative Care Conference*. Limerick: Milford Care Centre, University of Limerick; 2013.

19 O'Mara-Eves A, Brunton G, McDaid D, Oliver S, Kavanagh J, Jamal F, et al. Community engagement to reduce inequalities in health: a systematic review, meta-analysis and economic analysis. *Public Health Res* 2013; **1**(4).

20 Abel J, Walter T, Carey L, Rosenberg J, Noonan K, Horsfall D, et al. Circles of care: should community development redefine the practice of palliative care. *BMJ Support Palliat Care* 2013; **3**(4):436–43.

Chapter 19

Palliative care for older people with dementia

Ladislav Volicer, Noorhazlina Binte Ali, and Joyce Simard

Introduction to palliative care for older people with dementia

Alzheimer's disease and other progressive dementias are becoming one of the most important issues in public health. Prevalence of these diseases increases with age and extended life expectancy results in a rising number of people suffering from them. The number of people living with dementia worldwide is currently estimated at 35.6 million. This number will double by 2030 and more than triple by 2050 (1). The percentage of deaths attributed to Alzheimer's disease, which is the most common cause of progressive dementia, is increasing, while other causes of death (e.g. breast and prostate cancers, heart disease, and stroke) are decreasing (2). The estimated annual worldwide cost to society of dementia, US$604 billion, highlights the enormous impact that dementia has on socio-economic conditions. In the United Kingdom, the societal costs of dementia (£23 billion) almost match those of cancer (£12 billion), heart disease (£8 billion), and stroke (£5 billion) combined (1). Increasing prevalence of dementia may lead to the collapse of health care systems worldwide.

This chapter explains why palliative care as a person-centred approach to care is needed for people with dementia and their families. It stresses the maintenance of quality of life and the importance of family involvement and education of health care teams.

Applicability of palliative care in dementia

Alzheimer's disease and other progressive dementias (vascular, dementia with Lewy bodies, frontotemporal dementia) lead to gradual loss of independence that cannot be prevented or stopped by current treatments. Therefore, the care of people with these conditions should follow the principles of palliative care—providing relief from symptoms, pain, and stress, with the goal of improving quality of life for both the patient and their family. Recommendations for optimal palliative care for older persons with dementia were recently developed by the European Association for Palliative Care (3). This paper was prepared using a five-phase Delphi study involving 64 experts from 23 countries. It consists of 57 recommendations covering 11 domains important in providing palliative care for persons with dementia.

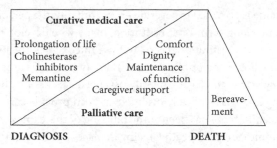

Figure 19.1 Types of care for persons with dementia

Palliative care principles apply from the time of diagnosis of Alzheimer's disease or other progressive degenerative dementias because both the patient and his/her family need the care provider's support to maintain their quality of life. Palliative care does not exclude concomitant curative treatment of comorbid diseases in earlier stages of dementia (Figure 19.1) and may include hospice care. Both of these strategies should be available at the same time and their use should be directed by the goals of care described in this chapter.

A person-centred approach and continuity of care for older people with dementia

Palliative care can be considered as a person-centred approach to caregiving. Tom Kitwood first introduced the concept of a person-centred approach to care in dementia and emphasized the importance of the preservation of personhood through social interaction with others (4). People's reaction or response towards those with dementia will determine the preservation of their personhood despite their cognitive and neurological impairment. As dementia progresses in tandem with an increasing burden of care and worsening neurological deficits, the focus has always been on the complications of the illness rather than the person behind the diagnosis.

There is no consensus about the actual definition of person-centred care in dementia. Brooker (5) summarized the various definitions and concepts and came up with an equation to explain what it embodies. There are four elements to person-centred care (PCC), namely, valuing persons with dementia and the people who care for them (V), treating people as individuals (I), seeing things from the perspective of the person with dementia (P), and creating a positive social environment (S). Thus:

$$PCC = V + I + P + S$$

These elements have been applied to the management of behavioural symptoms in dementia. One study that evaluated the effect of person-centred dementia care on nursing home residents reported that such an approach helps to reduce agitation and improve depressive symptoms among the residents (6). By understanding the person behind the diagnosis of dementia, we can more easily interpret their behaviour or bodily expressions and tailor care according to them, so that resistance to care is diminished.

Care for people with dementia is provided in several venues. Initially, the person may be living at home or already be in a long-term care institution; many who develop dementia at home will eventually require such institutional care. In the United States, the institution may be either an assisted living home or a nursing home. These two settings differ in their main emphasis: assisted living strives to provide mainly psychosocial care in a home-like environment, while a nursing home is medically oriented and can provide care for complex medical issues. More recently, there has been some blurring of these lines with some assisted living facilities providing care until death ('ageing in place'), while nursing homes are trying to become less medical and more residentially orientated ('culture change') (7).

Continuity of care in an institution is adversely affected by high staff turnover. The family members often feel that they have to monitor care and provide feedback to the staff. Different physicians may be involved in care—the general practitioner at home, a hospitalist/consultant in a hospital, and different physicians in nursing homes. A Rapid Assessment Interface and Discharge service was recently developed in the United Kingdom to improve continuity of care (8). This service uses a multi-skilled team that provides comprehensive assessment of a person's physical and psychological well-being in a hospital setting, and it is effective in reducing the length of stay and avoiding readmissions. If a person with dementia enrols in a hospice, they may have to face a new set of caregivers, although they could maintain their original physician.

Maintaining quality of life for older people with dementia

The main goal of palliative care is to improve the quality of life of the patient and his or her family members. In people with dementia, quality of life can be maintained in different ways: prognostication and timely recognition of the dying process; avoiding aggressive and burdensome treatments; providing meaningful activities and psychosocial and spiritual support; and through managing behavioural and psychiatric symptoms—all of which will now be described in more detail.

Prognostication and timely recognition of dying

It is very difficult to estimate prognosis in an individual with advanced dementia because death is not caused by the dementia itself but by intercurrent diseases and infections, making it thus almost impossible to predict. In addition, some infections resolve, while others lead to early death, again with little advance notice. Therefore, many persons may live with very advanced dementia for several years. The difficulty of prognostication was demonstrated by a study that followed 1,609 residents with advanced dementia who died in New York State nursing homes. While only 1.1% of them were identified on admission as likely to die within six months, 71% actually died during that time (9).

Prognostication is important for family members but, in the United States, it also affects the setting of care as a free hospice programme is available for persons whose prognosis is six months or less. Current criteria for hospice enrolment of people with dementia are not research-based and are correctly predicting survival in only half of patients. However, an even more complex mortality risk score using many clinical parameters was only moderately accurate, and the authors concluded that care provided to these residents should be guided by their goals of care rather than their estimated life expectancy (10).

Avoiding overly aggressive and burdensome treatment

Before any medical treatment is initiated, its compatibility with goals of care should be evaluated. The goals of care may change during the course of a progressive degenerative dementia. There are basically three main goals of care: survival, maintenance of function, and comfort (11). The problem is that these goals cannot be achieved simultaneously and there is a need for prioritization. In mild dementia, the main goal may be survival but achieving this goal may require hospitalization in an intensive care unit, which decreases comfort and leads to loss of function. In moderate dementia, the main goal of care may be maintenance of function and that may include avoidance of hospitalization. In severe and terminal stages of dementia, the main goal of care may be comfort and that goal would exclude some aggressive medical interventions that cause discomfort. Knowledge of benefits and burdens of different medical interventions is necessary for decisions about which should be used or excluded, based on the goal of care.

Cardiopulmonary resuscitation

Cardiopulmonary resuscitation is a stressful experience for those who survive, often associated with injuries such as broken ribs and frequently necessitating mechanical respiration. The intensive care unit environment produces additional confusion and, almost invariably, delirium. The immediate survival after cardiopulmonary resuscitation is lower in nursing homes than in other settings (10.4% versus 18.5%) and, in one study, no nursing home patients survived to hospital discharge, while 5.6% patients from other settings survived (12). In the presence of dementia, successful cardiopulmonary resuscitation is three times less likely—almost as low as in metastatic cancer. Therefore, cardiopulmonary resuscitation is not recommended unless the primary goal of care is survival at all costs with maintenance of function and comfort a distant second and third.

Transfer to an acute care setting

Transfer of older people to an emergency room or hospital exposes them to serious risks. Shortly after hospital admission of older people, deterioration can occur in mobility, transfer, toileting, feeding, and grooming, with few, if any, of these functions improving significantly by discharge (13). Transfer from a long-term care facility to an acute-care setting is most often due to an infection and/or breathing difficulties, but it may not be optimal for management of infections and other conditions. Immediate survival and mortality rates from pneumonia are comparable, regardless of whether the treatment is received in the long-term care facility or the hospital. Long-term outcomes are, in fact, better for residents treated in a nursing home since, two months after the onset of pneumonia, a greater proportion of hospitalized individuals had declined in their functional status or died (14). Therefore, transfer to an emergency room or hospital should be used only when it is consistent with the overall goals of care and not as a default option.

Artificial nutrition and hydration

Eating difficulties are common in individuals with dementia. Apraxia prevents patients from using utensils correctly and ultimately disrupts their ability to eat unassisted. In addition, patients intermittently refuse food. Eating apraxia can be managed by hand feeding, and food refusal may be improved by administration of antidepressants or appetite stimulants (15). As the dementia progresses, patients develop swallowing difficulties, often choking on solids as well as liquids. Choking is sometimes managed by thickening of food and liquids, but this strategy may not be effective and can result in under-nutrition and dehydration (16). Providing tube feeding to people with advanced dementia does not increase survival, improve nutritional status, or reduce the prevalence of pressure ulcers. Feeding tubes pose a significant burden and deprive the patient of the taste of food, the pleasure of eating, and contact with caregivers during the feeding process. Foregoing artificial nutrition and hydration in patients with severe dementia who no longer eat or drink is not associated with discomfort because individuals who are dying no longer feel hunger or thirst. Terminal dehydration may actually be beneficial for dying patients because it reduces respiratory secretions (avoiding the need for suctioning), reduces gastrointestinal secretion (decreasing the risk of vomiting and diarrhoea), and increases the secretion of endorphins (possibly decreasing the perception of pain) (17). Thus, tube feeding does not meet any goals of care in advanced dementia.

Antibiotic therapy

In most patients, it is preferable to limit antibiotic therapy to oral preparations, which are at least equally, if not more, effective than parenteral antibiotics. Intravenous therapy can be quite difficult in cognitively impaired individuals if they do not understand the need for it, and intramuscular administration of antibiotics offers a reasonable alternative. The effectiveness of antibiotic therapy may be limited by the recurrent nature of infections in advanced dementia. Antibiotic therapy prolongs survival in very few patients who have terminal stage dementia and, in most cases, just extends the dying process (18). The effectiveness of antibiotic therapy depends on the hydration status of the person, improving survival only in patients who have insufficient water intake (19). Antibiotics might not play a significant role in the maintenance of comfort in demented individuals with pneumonia. The level of discomfort depends on the quality of palliative treatment that is provided for those not receiving antibiotics. Analgesics, antipyretics, and oxygen, if necessary, may provide sufficient comfort in the absence of antibiotics. It should be kept in mind that antibiotic use may cause significant adverse effects—gastrointestinal upset, diarrhoea, allergic reactions, hyperkalaemia, agranulocytosis, and Clostridium difficile infection.

Meaningful activities, psychosocial and spiritual support

People with dementia rarely self-initiate meaningful activities. When not engaged, they often walk around, increasing their risk of falling. When persons with moderate dementia fall and break a hip, they are often poor candidates for rehabilitation and never walk again. Most often when a person with dementia is not engaged in an activity, they sleep, and will wake up in the middle of the night and be given a hypnotic. They may isolate themselves in a room and become depressed, so that an antidepressant is prescribed. An alternative to medication is to engage them throughout the day in meaningful activities.

In order for any activity to be meaningful, the person's leisure interests must be known and all activities must be person-centred. 'It's important to know what disease the person has, but it's more important to know what person the disease has' (20). Most people also want to feel useful, have fun, and be with others. Several programmes have been developed that take into account these very human wishes and needs and three of them are described in Box 19.1.

Box 19.1 Examples of activity programmes for people with dementia

Memory Enhancement Programme. For people with early dementia living in a nursing facility or assisted living community, the Memory Enhancement Programme can engage residents and seems to slow the progression of memory loss. The day begins with residents having breakfast and then joining a small group of others who have mild memory loss. They may start the day with 'volunteer' activities such as cutting coupons for staff or stuffing envelopes with the monthly newsletter for their facility. To lower the anxiety of residents not remembering the names of others in the group, tent name cards are set in front of each resident. They may do word searches that are designed to be 'no fail' for each person. Then, accompanied by the Memory Enhancement Programme staff person, they attend exercises with other residents. Having a staff person assigned to the group lowers their fear that they will not be able to find a bathroom if they need it or may miss lunch and dinner.

The Club. When a person makes the transition to the moderate stage of memory loss, they are usually living in a secured dementia neighbourhood. One programme that has resulted in a lowering of falls and reduced or eliminated the use of antipsychotics is called 'The Club' (21). This programme offers continuous activities during all waking hours. It begins with sorting a variety of items, for Club staff. Residents are thanked for their hard work, helping them to feel useful. This is followed by a routine that is familiar and meets the needs of the group. In many American nursing homes, the daily routine starts with the Pledge of Allegiance to the flag and everyone singing 'God Bless America'. One Club in the United Kingdom begins every day with a discussion based on the 'thought for the day'. Similar to the Memory Enhancement Programme, residents engage in a variety of mental and physical activities throughout the day. The difference between the programmes is that Club residents' activities are less demanding and are

Examples of activity programmes for people with dementia *(continued)*

not integrated with residents outside their neighbourhood. This programme continues after dinner, keeping residents awake until between 8.30 and 9.00 p.m.

Namaste Care™. When residents are in an advanced stage of dementia, they can no longer engage in the type of activities found in The Club. These residents are well cared for physically but are often placed in front of a television where they sleep, are isolated in their rooms, or are placed in front of the nurse's station where they become invisible. The Namaste Care™ programme has been developed for residents with advanced dementia and provides meaningful activities seven days a week, four hours a day (22). The aim is that they live with quality in their lives; they do not simply exist. The programme is offered in a room where distractions are minimized, soft music is playing, and the scent of lavender permeates the air. It is person-centred from the time they are welcomed into the room, with the staff assigned to the room (Namaste Carer) greeting each one in a special way: Grandma receives a hug and Dr. Jones' hand is shaken. They are assessed for pain and placed in a comfortable lounge chair with a blanket tucked around them. Beverages are offered on a continuous basis, which has resulted in a significant lowering of unitary tract infections and skin tears often associated with advanced dementia. Meaningful activities are activities of daily living offered in an unhurried manner with a 'loving touch' approach. The Namaste Carer is talking to the residents as they receive these meaningful activities. While in the room, they are in the presence of other residents, not isolated.

It is important to continue to meet the religious, spiritual, and existential needs of a person with moderate and advanced memory loss. They may not be able to understand or participate in a religious service but they are able to react to items that represent their religion, if they have one. In cases where the person has a specific religious background, objects and rituals associated with it may provide comfort. Quality of life to the end of life is possible for all stages of a dementing illness and, for many people, meaningful activities not only include physical and mental stimulation but also a return to participation in activities that bring them closer to their religious background.

Management of behavioural and psychiatric symptoms of dementia

Problems with communication may be one of the main causes of behavioural symptoms of dementia. Communication becomes more difficult with the progression of dementia. With the development of aphasia, people with dementia may not be able to communicate verbally and their attempts at non-verbal communication may be interpreted as abnormal behaviour. Caregivers need to be careful to exclude environmental (e.g. temperature, noise) and physical (e.g. pain, infection, hunger) causes before they ascribe behavioural changes to the dementing process.

Communication problems may cause a lack of cooperation with care and even rejection of care activities. In most cases, rejection of care happens because the person with dementia does not understand the intention of the caregiver and the need for care and, therefore, resists caregiving efforts. If the caregiver continues with the effort to provide care, the person with dementia may defend him/herself and become combative. Unfortunately, the person with dementia may then be labelled 'aggressive', even though he/she actually considers the caregiver to be the aggressor. Some persons with dementia may in fact be aggressive and strike out without an obvious reason. The best management strategies for rejection of care are to delay the procedure, to distract the person, or to modify the care procedure (e.g. to substitute a bed bath for a shower or tube bath) (23).

Research on behavioural symptoms of dementia and their clinical management is hindered by confusing terminology. Some researchers and clinicians call all behavioural symptoms 'agitation' and do not distinguish behaviours according to the context in which they occur (e.g. whether the person with dementia is solitary or is interacting with others). The term 'agitation' should be reserved for behaviours that occur when the person with dementia is solitary (e.g. restlessness, repetitive physical movements and vocalizations, wandering, and socially inappropriate/disruptive behaviour) (24). It is important to realize that agitated behaviour may communicate unmet needs, very often a lack of engagement with the environment. Therefore, providing appropriate meaningful activities may prevent or decrease agitated behaviours (25).

Psychiatric conditions that lead to behavioural changes include depression and psychotic symptoms, delusions, and hallucinations. There is an overwhelming amount of evidence indicating that depression is one of the most important factors related to the behavioural symptoms of dementia because it increases the risk of both agitation (26) and rejection of care escalating into combative behaviour (27). The relationship between depression and aggressive behaviour is probably due to serotoninergic deficit (28) caused by Alzheimer's disease and possibly by other progressive dementias. Another factor underlining the importance of depression is that it is much more common among residents with dementia than are delusions and hallucinations (29).

Symptoms of depression may be alleviated by non-pharmacological strategies (30). Improvement of dementia symptoms has been found after multimodal therapy that included cognitive stimulation, but a recent review concluded that cognitive stimulation improves cognitive functioning but does not affect mood or problem behaviours (31). Thus, treatment with antidepressants may be needed if non-pharmacological strategies are not sufficient.

Antidepressants are effective in improving behavioural symptoms of dementia if depression is treated effectively. In the DIAD-1 study, sertraline was completely effective in treating depression in only 38% of participants, and behavioural improvement was observed only in participants whose depression improved (32). This is no different from efficacy of antidepressant treatment in cognitively intact individuals, where only one third improve by administration of an antidepressant alone. In most cases, treatment required augmentation of antidepressants.

Unfortunately, even in the absence of psychotic symptoms, antipsychotics are often considered the first line medication for treatment of the behavioural symptoms of dementia (33). They are used despite their limited effectiveness and despite evidence of the possibility of severe side-effects including increased mortality (34). Therefore, antipsychotics should be reserved for persons with dementia who are troubled by delusions and hallucinations or those in whom treatment of depression with antidepressants alone is not effective and requires antidepressant augmentation (35).

Family care and involvement with palliative care for older people with dementia

Establishing a diagnosis of Alzheimer's disease or other progressive degenerative dementia designates other individuals, in most cases family members, as caregivers. These caregivers may experience anticipatory grief—the normal phases of bereavement in advance of the loss of the significant person. They may be grieving, having difficulty in functioning, and be missing the person they once knew. Families need support, from the time of a patient's diagnosis, in making several decisions. The first decision may be about disclosure of the diagnosis to the patient if the health providers did not do it themselves. Reasons for favouring disclosure include a patient's or family member's right to know, the possibility of assistance in coping with and understanding dementia and slowing down the progression of the disease by early treatment, as well as the increased probability of accepting treatment.

The time after diagnosis can be used to involve the person with mild dementia in some decisions about their future medical care, financial arrangements, and their wishes regarding future residence. Caregivers need help from health care providers and lawyers to make appropriate decisions and obtain legal documents. Another difficult decision the caregivers must make is when to stop the person with dementia driving. As dementia progresses, functional dependence, unsafe behaviour, and behavioural symptoms of dementia create a need for constant patient supervision that poses a great burden for the caregivers. There is a high incidence of depression in family caregivers, and even professional staff need support. Since Alzheimer's disease and other progressive dementias last, on average, eight years, caregivers often have to cope with functional impairment and behavioural symptoms for many years. The stress of caregiving also increases the risk of the caregiver developing Alzheimer's disease.

Cognitive impairment of the care recipient is often less stressful for the caregivers than behavioural symptoms of dementia (36). Group-based behavioural interventions reduce distress related to neuropsychiatric symptoms among caregivers of individuals with Alzheimer's disease. Although caregiver distress is related to the direct provision of care for the demented individual, the distress does not cease after the individual is institutionalized. Caregivers often feel that they have failed them by placing them in an institution. Social support for caregivers of institutionalized individuals with dementia is very important because depressive symptoms and anxiety are as high in caregivers after they have institutionalized their relative as when they were in-home caregivers.

Caregivers also need support when making decisions about palliative and hospice care. End-of-life education of caregivers resulted in lower rates of ventilation, intensive care unit admissions, and earlier hospice enrolment. A decision aid increases caregiver knowledge and decreases their decisional conflict regarding long-term tube feeding (37), and watching a video depiction of a patient with advanced dementia, after hearing a verbal description of the condition, resulted in proxies more often selecting comfort care than when listening to a verbal description alone (38). A free decision aid about assisted feeding and tube feeding is available online at <www.med.unc.edu/pcare/resources/feedingoptions> (39).

Cultural and ethnic differences have been reported in the literature with regards to caregiving, end-of-life care (40), and advance care planning (41). In Western culture, emphasis is placed on the patient's autonomy and their independence in decision making about medical care. This is in contrast to Asian culture which places a high value on shared decision making among family members about end-of-life care. The initiation of conversations pertaining to end-of-life care planning triggered much discomfort among Asian families (42) and, thus, implicit non-verbal communication plays a central role when the next of kin attempt to infer a patient's preferences. The family unit fulfils a dominant role in Asian societies, though the right to the patient's autonomy is not revoked. As such, most of the discussions concerning end-of-life care in advanced dementia depend heavily on the family's involvement, which to a certain extent may influence the patient's choices in deciding treatment options or refusal of medical care. In such a situation, health care providers may find themselves involved in family conflicts when there is disagreement between the patient's and family's choice of treatment.

Education of the health care team

Management of dementia requires a cohesive multidisciplinary team working together to provide good-quality care. The team may comprise physicians or dementia specialists, nurses (registered or nursing assistants, advanced nurse practitioners), therapists (physiotherapists, occupational therapists, speech therapists), dieticians, pharmacists, case managers, and social workers. Each member of this team has diverse and varied background knowledge of dementia, thus, in order to deliver quality dementia care, continued education of the health care team is imperative.

Education of the health care team should be at the forefront of many initiatives to improve quality of dementia care. Primary care providers are usually the first point of contact for many older people in the community. Hence, educational interventions for this group of health care providers may improve the detection of dementia (43) and appropriate referrals to dementia specialists for further management. Education also plays a major role in delivering end-of-life care for those with advanced dementia. An educational programme and a booklet on end-of-life care for advanced dementia, provided for staff of a nursing home, was reported to yield higher family satisfaction, which was probably due to the facilitation of communication between staff and family members (44).

There are several educational interventions that can be carried out and they are not just limited to workshops, facilitator-led discussions, or booklets. Online dementia care training in Canada was reported to be successful in improving care for residents in long-term care homes with the application of new knowledge and skills learned by the health care workers (45). Continued innovative ways of educating health care workers may lead to them feeling more empowered, engaged, and confident in caring for this group of vulnerable and frail older people.

Conclusions on palliative care for older people with dementia

Palliative care is an important component of care for people with progressive dementias. It requires recognition that advanced dementia is a terminal condition and includes person-centred care involving the patient's family. Use of palliative care does not exclude curative care for intercurrent conditions in the early stages of dementia. Adoption of palliative care principles requires continuous communication between the patient/family and care providers; the effective use of palliative care for persons with dementia is a challenge for the future.

References

1 World Health Organization. *Dementia: A Public Health Priority*; 2012. Available at: <www.who.int/hiv/topics/palliative/PalliativeCare>. (Accessed September 2013). Ref. type: online source.

2 Alzheimer's Association. *Alzheimer' Disease: Facts and Figures*; 2014. Available at: <http://www.alz.org/alzheimers_disease_facts_and_figures.asp> (Accessed September 2014). Ref. Type: online source.

3 Van der Steen JT, Radbruch L, Hertogh CM, de Boer ME, Hughes JC, Larkin P, et al. White Paper defining optimal palliative care in older people with dementia: a Delphi study and recommendations from the European Association for Palliative Care. *Palliat Med* 2013; **28**(3):197–209.

4 Kitwood T. Toward a theory of dementia care: ethics and interaction. *J Clin Ethics* 1998; **9**:23–34.

5 Brooker D. What is person-centered care in dementia. *Reviews in Clinical Gerontology* 2004; **13**:215–22.

6 Rokstad AMM, Rosvik J, Kirkevold O, Selbaek G, Benth JS, Engedal K. The effect of person-centered dementia care to prevent agitation and other neuropsychiatric symptoms and enhance quality of life in nursing home patients. *Dement Geriatr Cogn Disord* 2013; **36**:340–53.

7 Hartmann CW, Snow LA, Allen RS, Parmelee PA, Palmer JA, Berlowitz D. A conceptual model for culture change evaluation in nursing homes. *Geriatr Nurs* 2013; **34**(5):388–94.

8 Singh I, Ramakrishna S, Williamson K. The Rapid Assessment Interface and Discharge service and its implications for patients with dementia. *Clin Interv Aging* 2013; **8**:1101–8.

9 Mitchell SL, Kiely DK, Hamel MB, Park PS, Morris JN, Fries BE. Estimating prognosis for nursing home residents with advanced dementia. *JAMA* 2004; **291**(22):2734–40.

10 Mitchell SL, Miller SC, Teno JM, Kiely DK, Davis RB, Shaffer ML. Prediction of 6-month survival of nursing home residents with advanced dementia using ADEPT vs hospice eligibility guidelines. *JAMA* 2010; **304**(17):1929–35.

11 Gillick M, Berkman S, Cullen L. A patient-centered approach to advance medical planning in the nursing home. *JAGS* 1999; **47**:227–30.

12 Benkendorf R, Swor RA, Jackson R, Rivera-Rivera EJ, Demrick A. Outcomes of cardiac arrest in the nursing home: destiny or futility? *Prehospital Emergency Care* 1997; **1**:68–72.

13 Hirsch CH, Sommers L, Olsen A, Mullen L, Winograd CH. The natural history of functional morbidity in hospitalized older patients. *JAGS* 1990; **38**(12):1296–303.

14 Fried TR, Gillick MR, Lipsitz LA. Short-term functional outcomes of long-term care residents with pneumonia treated with and without hospital transfer. *JAGS* 1997; **45**(3):302–6.

15 Wilson MM, Philpot C, Morley JE. Anorexia of aging in long term care: is dronabinol an effective appetite stimulant?—a pilot study. *J Nutr Health Aging* 2007; **11**(2):195–8.

16 Campbell-Taylor I. Oropharyngeal dysphagia in long-term care: misperception of treatment efficacy. *JAMDA* 2008; **9**:523–31.

17 Yakovleva T, Marinova Z, Kuzmin A, Seidah NG, Haroutunian V, Terenius L, et al. Dysregulation of dynorphins in Alzheimer disease. *Neurobiol Aging* 2007; **28**(11):1700–8.

18 Van der Steen JT, Lane P, Kowall NW, Knoll DL, Volicer L. Antibiotics and mortality in patients with lower respiratory infection and advanced dementia. *JAMDA* 2012; **13**(2):156–61.

19 Szafara KL, Kruse RL, Mehr DR, Ribbe MW, Van der Steen JT. Mortality following nursing home-acquired lower respiratory infection: LRI severity, antibiotic treatment, and water intake. *JAMDA* 2012; **13**(4):376–83.

20 Hippocrates. *Hippocrates Quotes*. Available at: <http://www.brainyquote.com/quotes/authors/h/hippocrates.html> (Accessed September 2014). Ref. type: online source.

21 Volicer L, Simard J, Pupa JH, Medrek R, Riordan ME. Effects of continuous activity programming on behavioral symptoms of dementia. *JAMDA* 2006; **7**:426–31.

22 Simard J. *The End-of-Life Namaste Program for People with Dementia* (2nd edn). Baltimore, London, Sydney: Health Professions Press; 2013.

23 Sloane PD, Honn VJ, Dwyer SAR, Wieselquist J, Cain C, Meyers S. Bathing the Alzheimer's patient in long term care. Results and recommendations from three studies. *Am J Alzheim Dis* 1995; **10**(4):3–11.

24 Hurley AC, Volicer L, Camberg L, Ashley J, Woods P, Odenheimer G, et al. Measurement of observed agitation in patients with Alzheimer's disease. *J Mental Health Aging* 1999; **5**(2):117–33.

25 Cohen-Mansfield J, Marx MS, Dakheel-Ali M, Regier NG, Thein K, Freedman L. Can agitated behavior of nursing home residents with dementia be prevented with the use of standardized stimuli? *J Am Geriatr Soc* 2010; **58**(8):1459–64.

26 Volicer L, Frijters DH, Van der Steen JT. Relationship between symptoms of depression and agitation in nursing home residents with dementia. *Int J Geriatr Psychiatry* 2012; **27**(7):749–54.

27 Volicer L, Van der Steen JT, Frijters D. Modifiable factors related to abusive behaviors in nursing home residents with dementia. *JAMDA* 2009; **10**:617–22.

28 Lanctot KL, Herrmann N, Eryavec G, van Reekum R, Reed K, Naranjo CA. Central serotonergic activity is related to the aggressive behaviors of Alzheimer's disease. *Neuropsychopharmacology* 2002; **27**(4):646–54.

29 Leonard R, Tinetti ME, Allore HG, Drickamer MA. Potentially modifiable resident characteristics that are associated with physical or verbal aggression among nursing home residents with dementia. *Arch Intern Med* 2006; **166**(12):1295–300.

30 Conn DK, Seitz DP. Advances in the treatment of psychiatric disorders in long-term care homes. *Curr Opin Psychiatry* 2010; **23**(6):516–21.

31 Woods B, Aguirre E, Spector AE, Orrell M. Cognitive stimulation to improve cognitive functioning in people with dementia. *Cochrane Database Syst Rev* 2012 Feb 15; **2**(CD005562).

32 Lyketsos CG, DelCampo L, Steinberg M, Miles Q, Steele CD, Munro C, et al. Treating depression in Alzheimer disease—efficacy and safety of sertraline therapy, and the benefits of depression reduction: the DIADS. *Arch Gen Psychiatry* 2003 Jul; **60**(7):737–46.

33 Cohen-Mansfield J, Jensen B. Assessment and treatment approaches for behavioral disturbances associated with dementia in the nursing home: self-report of physicians' practices. *JAMDA* 2008; **9**:406–13.

34 Ballard C, Creese B, Corbett A, Aarsland D. Atypical antipsychotics for the treatment of behavioral and psychological symptoms in dementia, with a particular focus on longer term outcomes and mortality. *Expert Opin Drug Saf* 2012; **10**(1):35–43.

35 Papakostas GI, Shelton RC, Smith J, Fava M. Augmentation of antidepressants with atypical antipsychotic medications for treatment-resistant major depressive disorder: a meta-analysis. *J Clin Psychiatry* 2007; **68**(6):826–31.

36 Desai AK, Schwartz L, Grossberg GT. Behavioral disturbance in dementia. *Curr Psychiatry Rep* 2012; **14**(4):298–309.

37 Mitchell SL, Tetroe JM, O'Connor AM. A decision aid for long-term tube feeding in cognitively impaired older adults. *JAGS* 2001; **49**(3):313–6.

38 Volandes AE, Lehmann LS, Cook EF, Shaykevich S, Abbo ED, Gillick MR. Using video images of dementia in advance care planning. *Arch Intern Med* 2007; **167**(8):828–33.

39 Hanson LC. Tube feeding versus assisted oral feeding for persons with dementia: using evidence to support decision-making. *Ann Longterm Care* 2013; **21**(1):36–9.

40 Kagawa-Singer M, Blackhall LJ. Negotiating cross-cultural issues at the end of life. *JAMA* 2001; **286**:2993–3001.

41 Carr D. Racial and ethnic differences in advance care planning. *J Aging Health* 2012; **24**:923–47.

42 Sharma RK, Khosla N, Tulsky JA, Carrese JA. Traditional expectations versus US realities. *J Gen Intern Med* 2011; **27**(3):311–7.

43 Perry M, Draskovic I, Lucassen P, Vernooij-Dassen M, van Achterberg T, Rikkert MO. Effects of educational interventions on primary dementia care: a systematic review. *Intern J Geriat Psychiat* 2011; **26**(1):1–11.

44 Arcand M, Brazil K, Nakanishi M, Alix M, Desson JF, Morello R, et al. Educating families about end-of-life care in advanced dementia: acceptability of a Canadian family booklet to nurses from Canada, France, and Japan. *Int J Palliat Nurs* 2013; **19** (2):67–74.

45 Macdonald CJ, Stodel EJ, Casimiro L. Online dementia care training for health care teams in continuing and long-term care homes. *Internat J on E-learning* 2006; **5** (373):399.

Chapter 20

Involvement of family carers in care for older people

Hazel Morbey and Sheila Payne

Introduction to involvement of family carers in care for older people

'Death is now an event of older age, and needs for care and support have become more complex' (1). Moreover, family carers of older people are increasingly aged themselves. They may be caring for spouses or siblings in a same-generation age band, or cross-generationally, where older parents or relatives are cared for by children or other family members who are themselves within an older age group. This is of critical importance and significance to understanding the role, involvement, and experience of family carers of those receiving palliative care, where this is situated in households, neighbourhoods, and community settings. As ageing populations across Europe grow, increasing cohorts of frail older people, often with multiple morbidity and complex needs, require support from family carers. Increasingly, health and social care policies promote palliative care and dying in people's homes. However, this is predicated on the availability and willingness of family members to provide, manage, and sustain support over what can be years of survivorship with long-term, life-limiting illnesses and disease. Essentially, this outlook means that both patients and family carers can coexist in complex health and welfare circumstances, within potentially changeable and reciprocal caring relationships.

Meeting family carer support needs is a central feature of palliative care. Recognizing both experiences *and* needs validates family carers as worthy recipients of support during their provision of palliative care, which includes bereavement support, following the death of their family member. However, many family carers have unmet needs, are unsupported in their roles, and, within home settings, face demands that are less visible. Family carers are often unprepared for the delivery of what can be extensive medical treatments in their homes, managing distressing patient symptoms, and upholding their relative's choices and wishes. While satisfaction and positive caring experiences may be realised in this life phase, ultimately, family carers witness the distress and demise of their family member at the end of their lives.

This chapter reflects on the caring experience as essentially one whereby family carers both give, and also need, care. We discuss family caring as an ageing phenomenon, and we identify the many roles and spheres of care in which family carers support their older relatives, who will often have multiple, complex, and enduring health conditions. Assessment and intervention approaches aimed at addressing needs are discussed before we go on to highlight communication as being of particular importance in ensuring sensitive, timely, and appropriate help is offered by professionals working in this area. We first set the scene with a demographic overview of care provided in the family context.

An overview of contemporary family caring of older people

We promote broad inclusive definitions of family carers that recognize the roles and relations of family caregiving. These move beyond simplistic task and function definitions to place social and emotional bonds of carers and older people as being of equal significance alongside the more practical and physical elements of care work. Inclusive definitions capture a wider range of relationships outside of those that might be assumed the norm in family caring, although some writers draw distinctions between friends or neighbours and related kin (2). Importantly, wider definitions also accommodate inevitable shifts and changes in the nature of family carer experiences during palliative and end-of-life care. The European Association of Palliative Care White Paper on Improving Support for Family Carers in Palliative Care (3) sought to establish the use of family care definitions that encompass the aforementioned factors. Definitions drawn on in the White Paper were developed by the National Institute of Health and Care Excellence in the United Kingdom, and we replicate these for the purposes of our discussion on the involvement of family carers in the care of older people:

> **Carers:** . . . may or may not be family members, are lay people in a close supportive role who share in the illness experience of the patient and who undertake vital care work and emotion management.
>
> **Family:** . . . include[s] those related through committed heterosexual or same sex partnerships, birth and adoption, and others who have strong emotional and social bonds with a patient.

(4:155)

Key to understanding the contemporary landscape of family caring is regarding family carers as both givers and receivers of care (3, 5). While all carers may not need formalized support, they fulfil societal, social, cultural, and lay health support functions, and as such, are worthy recipients of encouragement, help, and services to enable them to fulfil a caring role when needed (6). Many family carers are 'clients' for the purposes of targeted support interventions (7), and within a palliative care context, the competing duality of their giver and receiver status results in the locations of family caring as sites of complex personal and emotional distress, familial and social support, and advanced health care provision. Essentially, this dual experience is marked by the competing demands to attend to their own health and welfare needs while supporting another person with theirs. Indeed, it may be the case, as Payne points out, that 'the needs of carers can exceed those of patients' (3:240).

As ageing populations grow globally, the proportion of aged family carers, usually older spouses or children, supporting older family members in their households, neighbourhoods, and communities, will increase (8, 9). Across Europe and other industrialized countries, demographic projections and trends show tandem growth in ageing populations and family care of increasingly frail older people in the oldest age ranges, with those people of 80 years and over set to triple between 2011 and 2060 (10), and almost quadruple globally (11). Empirical studies reveal especially intense caring relationship scenarios in this context (12, 13), which are inevitable when we consider predominate family carer profiles, with late old-age family carers caring for frail, late old-age dying family members, both of whom may have one or more long-term health condition (14), and where this results in variable and mutual care, in reciprocal caring relationships (12, 15).

Gender particularly characterizes the relations of family caring, which is often noted as a role more commonly assumed by women than men, although proportionally, this varies across age bands, generations, and the family carer/cared-for person's relationship (6, 16–19). In the United Kingdom, women have a 50:50 likelihood of caring by the age of 59 years, while for men, the respective age is 75 years (20). However, while women will primarily continue to fulfil this role, the age differential noted here belies trends in the numbers of men over the age of 65 years who will increasingly become carers (16, 21), with significant growth of older men who care for a family member with dementia, the numbers of whom have almost doubled in the previous 15 years (22).

Further demographic characteristics influence caring relations that were once taken for granted, with changes in generational and family make-up. Increased incidence of divorce, co-habitation, and step and lone parenthood have shifted expectations of who will care for whom, in what may be disparate, disconnected, or confusing familial connections (23). National, internal economic and geographic mobility, and immigration, serve to reconfigure family households, communities, and kinship networks, while employment patterns and family financial imperatives in recessionary circumstances have ramifications for the availability and ability of family carers to support older family members. An increasingly common term in this context refers to a 'sandwich generation' that face caring responsibilities for their younger and older family members (24), while also providing household income through paid employment. Recent Canadian research reveals the high expectations this 'baby boomer' cohort of family carers has of public services to support their role 'as they work to juggle caregiving, work, family, and social commitments' (25:10).

Family carer experiences of caring for an older relative through the palliative phase

The terminal care phase for family carers is multifaceted, complex, and challenging (9). There are diverse combinations of family carer characteristics, with older carers themselves being in poor health, receiving health treatment and/or welfare support and services, together with increasingly frail, older cared-for family members who will die with one or more long-term conditions. In this context, disease trajectories are protracted and uncertain, and care provided at home is complex and demanding. Multiple roles are enacted by family carers, in which they can also experience similar losses to their family member and become almost 'enmeshed with their illness' (26:813). Positive aspects of caring are also reported, whereby family carers find coping strategies that maintain well-being in the face of stressful circumstances (27) and that engender a sense of reward (28), although satisfaction has been found to be greater for older carers, and also for those receiving social support (29).

Palliative care has been largely cancer-focused in many countries (3, 26). However, other life-limiting conditions shape the family carer experience as one that may be characterized by slow progression, prolonged demand, and uncertainty (29, 30). For example, an average 'palliative phase' for Parkinson's disease is 2.2 years (31) and survival with dementia can vary between 3 to 10 years (30).

Family members do not necessarily identify with the 'carer' label or role, with the result that, for many, their experiences and needs are invisible and 'hidden' (32, 33). Furthermore, implicit assumptions are inferred that the position is taken on willingly (23). Many carers may not be prepared for their role, yet the expectation that palliative care is increasingly performed in households and communities by family carers escalates as public services are limited through economic pressures (19).

Older populations have higher risks of developing conditions other than cancers, that necessitate ongoing and rising care needs, often over many years (14). High incidence of diseases such as organ failures, non-malignant lung diseases, neurological diseases, and dementias may be diagnosed, and other long-term, life-limiting conditions (for example, diabetes, arthritis, and osteoporosis) may exist (14, 34). Comorbidity of these health conditions challenges health care systems and clinicians in meeting related treatment and resource overheads. Onerous demands face family carers who support their family member in home environments that, by comparison, are inevitably ill-equipped (23) for the significant care needs that arise from multiple health conditions, and sensory and other infirmities (e.g. mobility), that can be experienced in older age.

The experiences of family carers of heart failure patients illustrate high-level demands where multiple needs exist. These needs demand physical and personal care, management, dispensing, and medication titration, in the context of unpredictable emergency hospital admissions and prognostic and end-of-life uncertainties (29, 35, 36). A recent review of quality of life literature (29) found carers' sense of control to be the strongest indicator of carer burden, with anxiety, poor mental health, and role hostility greater for carers with lower levels of control over the health of their family member.

Depression in family carers is widely reported in the literature (8, 37–39) and is significantly related to the physical symptoms of patients. Mental health assistance has been reported as one of the most important aspects of support services (35). Loss of friends and more limited social activities are shown to have a negative impact, resulting from changes brought about through caring. Depression has also been found to be more frequently experienced by family carers who were abused or neglected by parents in childhood and who take on a caring role for the parent in old age than for non-abused family caregivers (40). Very little is understood about this specific group of carers, with early findings pointing to the need for targeted interventions that assess the quality of relationships in child/parent dyadic caring.

The impact of caring for a family member with dementia is well recognized, with stress and anxiety, emotional strain, social isolation, and prevalence of long-term health conditions for these carers especially high (39, 41). In addition to these negative impacts, Mackenzie et al.'s (39) research shows how carers of family members with palliative phase dementia have impaired attention and memory during periods of chronic stress. Sav et al. (34) also demonstrate the effects of 'treatment burden', with family carers experiencing the consequences of proactive caring in the context of long-term health needs over protracted periods of time where complex treatment regimens are in place.

The role of family carers in palliative care provision for older people

Multiple tasks and roles are undertaken by family carers during the palliative care phase, as shown in Table 20.1 (6). Underpinning all of these roles is an essential emotional element, such that we can describe palliative family carers as conducting 'emotion work', where this is defined as 'the emotional effort made by individuals to manage their own feelings and those of others' (42:537). 'Emotional management' was made explicit in the National Institute of Health and Care Excellence family carer definition (4), and the family carer literature includes many references to emotional elements and impact of the caring role (3, 19, 29, 37, 43).

There is insufficient recognition of the extensive range of tasks and roles taken on by family carers, as the increasingly complex nature of these roles advance with more sophisticated medical treatments permeating the delivery of care in home settings. Medically complex procedures and 'high tec' equipment within the home, such as syringe drivers and oxygen, are all now undertaken and used by family carers (29, 44). These responsibilities run alongside the management, organization, and decision making required by family carers while they experience emotional duress and grief (45), with this intensified near to death (37). Carers who feel more prepared for their role are reported to suffer less distress (46). However, psychological distress and exhaustion, and decline in carers' sense of skill preparedness and quality of life over time, is noted by Grant et al (47), the longer such care is provided. We also see unintended impact on patients and family carers when clinicians step up treatment regimes, which in turn increases 'treatment burden' (34), and where the home is transformed into a clinical care space with equipment, medicines, and staff, such that homes become 'hospices in homes' (17).

With a predominance of long-term degenerative conditions characterizing older age morbidity, the demands borne by family carers may last over many years, with increasing intensity as the palliative phase is reached. Similar patterns in cancer show trends in improved survival rates (48), which will inevitably see family carers managing prolonged and uncertain trajectories to death (49). Specific life-limiting conditions bring challenges particular to each of them, and may confront the carer with uncertainty and unpredictability (29). Dementia may coexist with other significant physical conditions to create

Table 20.1 Spheres, tasks, and roles in palliative family care for older people

Spheres of family caring in palliative care	Care tasks and roles include:
Emotional and psychological	emotional labour of reassurance, comfort, stress relief when relatives experience pain and discomfort, anxiety, depression, and uncertainty.
Familial and social	family mediation; maintaining social and community relationships; access to social events/opportunities; leisure activities.
Financial	multiple finance needs: transport costs to attend health care appointments; welfare benefit claims; costs of special diets, additional heating and washing; employment/sick leave arrangements; pension and insurance payments; charitable funding.
Information and communication	arranging and managing health professional visits; obtaining disease-specific, care-specific, and treatment-specific information; cognitive and memory needs; patient advocacy; symptom reporting; family communicator; hospital or emergency admission; legal information e.g. power of attorney, will making; personal paperwork and bills.
Physical and personal care	symptom and pain management; complex care tasks; medication; handling and lifting; feeding and drinking; shopping, cooking, gardening, pet care; mobility and exercise; equipment and aids; washing/dressing/toilet assistance; household cleaning; wound/infection treatments; disposal of body waste and fluids; night-time supervision/care; sitters or respite care; dying process.
Spiritual/existential	comfort and reassurance; anticipating and planning for dying and death; access to spiritual practitioners; maintain faith practices; observing religious practices.

Reproduced from Sheila Payne and Hazel Morbey, *Supporting family carers: report on the evidence of how to work with and support family carers to inform the work of the Commission into the future of hospice care*, p. 17, Figure 1, Copyright © 2013, Help the Hospices.

exceptionally complex and advanced care needs (30). Dementias bring specific challenging components to care, which Orpin et al. (8) identify as the erosion of patient identity and autonomous functioning. Family carers in these circumstances can face extreme demands whereby they find themselves navigating disrupted 'personas, reputations and relationships built up over a lifetime' and 'moral and social ambiguities around issues of control, authority and responsibility' (8:19).

Assessment and intervention approaches to support family members caring for an older person in the palliative phase

An extensive evidence base exists on carer support interventions and assessment instruments, including those pertaining to palliative and end-of-life care, with several recent systematic reviews (31, 45, 50–54). It is beyond the scope of this chapter to offer a comprehensive overview of this literature, other than to summarize broad intervention categories including: psychological; training/information; positive aspects of a caring role; impact on lifestyle; respite, group, physical, and social support; and palliative and bereavement interventions.

A number of interventions and assessment tools are multidimensional, and there can be crossover in their focus (52, 54). Interventions can be directed specifically at support for carers, or provide benefit through indirect strategies targeted to the cared-for relative's needs. We look at *carer assessment* first, and then discuss *carer interventions*, and propose a *typology of interventions* to capture the range of approaches.

Carer assessment

Most instruments focus on family carer burden, quality of life, needs, and service delivery satisfaction, but there is a notable absence of risk assessment tools for psychosocial problems experienced by family carers (54). Focus within the literature tends to be on the negative impacts of care (e.g. distress and burden), with limited assessment of coping strategies and, specifically, how these are employed by carers of those with advanced conditions (27). Future work should prioritize psychometric testing of existing tools over development of further instruments (54) to ensure they are concise, and to aid their delivery in, and take account of, home settings.

Carer interventions

Key to family carer support in the palliative phase are appropriate interventions for changeable, fluctuating conditions, and also timeliness in implementation. Carer circumstances can match their family member's unpredictable health conditions (9) such that there are limited windows of opportunity for access to, and benefit from, support. Evaluations would be enhanced by examining optimum timing for targeted interventions (6).

Interventions can loosely be classified as those that provide *direct* carer benefit, and interventions targeted at the family member, bringing *indirect* carer benefit. Examples include: a psycho-educational programme that enhanced positive family carer perspectives of their caring role (55); pain management training leading to increased carer self-efficacy (45); and reduced levels of depression for carers of people with Alzheimer's disease through a counselling and support group intervention (41). Sleep, problem solving, telephone, and psycho-educational interventions were all shown to bring benefits, while mixed results were seen for an intervention that promoted self-care (54).

Recent evidence, described in one dyad study for example, combining counselling and rehabilitation skills, involved people with mild to moderate dementia (41). Carers in this study reported less emotional health and relationship strain and lower levels of anxiety and depression. Chai et al. (37) evaluated a web-based support intervention with information, education, and coaching resources for advanced cancer conditions and carer needs. Results reported less negative mood and emotional distress, although physical burden and preparedness were not impacted. Hudson et al. (56) report on a short-term intervention

Table 20.2 Interventions that support adult family carers

Information, training, and education	Supportive activities	Therapeutic activities
• Strategies for safe moving and handling of the patient. • Information resources on disease process, trajectory, and prognosis. • Information on how to provide specific care tasks, equipment, and medication. • Information about the dying process and symptom management in a timely way. • Access to welfare or benefits advice.	• 'Drop in' centre/coffee mornings/lunch clubs. • Self-help groups, virtual or face-to-face. • Walking, exercise, or activity groups. • Volunteers visiting or befriending. • Art-making or creative groups.	• One-to-one or group counselling. • Therapeutic support groups. • Drama, music, or art therapy. • Relaxation, meditation, mindfulness, or yoga classes. • Complementary therapies. • Psychotherapy.

Reproduced from Sheila Payne and Hazel Morbey, *Supporting family carers: report on the evidence of how to work with and support family carers to inform the work of the Commission into the future of hospice care*, p. 23, Figure 2, Copyright © 2013, Help the Hospices.

on carers' sense of preparedness and competency in providing palliative care for patients in their homes. Increased levels in preparedness and competency are shown from support nurse visits, when information and resources, care plans, and additional support are provided. Grande et al. (7) suggest that the competing role of family carers as users *and* providers of support is accounted for during intervention research.

Typology of supportive interventions

We offer a typology of interventions in Table 20.2 that captures potential supportive approaches.

Communication between family carers and professionals providing palliative care for older people

Communication between health professionals and family carers necessitates sensitivity and openness, requiring practitioners to be 'mindful that while caregivers are helping the patient to prepare for dying, they are also trying to prepare themselves for the eventual death of their relative' (53:1).

Health care conversations about end-of-life care topics are challenging for staff, and they need to feel comfortable addressing emotional issues, in addition to undertaking and arranging practical support for patients and family carers (12). Additional challenges can be faced when families have poor relationships that result in emotionally heightened circumstances or avoidance between family members and/or patients. In these situations, health professionals may find their options for providing support are limited (57) or prevent effective communication. For example, Fromme et al. (58) describe greater reticence on the part of male caregivers to openly discuss coping or the strain experienced in their role. Similarly, patient or disease characteristics may present specific challenges, such as with dementia.

Barriers to communication can occur when carers are fatigued, depressed, or fearful. Cherlin et al.'s (59) work supports this mix of factors, where lack of understanding and family carer reluctance lead to ineffective communication. At its extreme, they suggest, this can result in carers hearing, very late in the disease trajectory, that the condition is incurable, and access to hospice care in these circumstances is delayed. This is typically faced in the United States, where 'hospice' provision equates to a programme of home care where curative treatments are foregone.

There is a delicate balance to be found between navigating assessment and support of family carers as 'co-workers' at the same time as creating opportunities for them to have their own needs addressed when their priorities are elsewhere. When difficulties exist in taking end-of-life conversations forward, professionals are rendered unprepared for supporting carers (6). Evidence indicates that end-of-life communication is consistently described as inadequate (43, 57, 60, 61), which results in family carers feeling greater levels of distress (62). Family carers who are enabled to manage symptoms, seek help, and have an understanding of prognosis, are potentially more able to cope with their family member dying (63), transitions in care (1), and subsequent bereavement (64).

Hanratty (1) highlights communication and relationships between multidisciplinary professionals as an important overarching issue for all palliative care settings. Timely communication that crosses care settings is known to be important (57, 59, 61), and there is a limited 'window of opportunity' when interventions and support can be effectively implemented and accessed by carers. There are mutual benefits to optimizing communication and, through paying attention to the lived experience of patients and family members, psychosocial needs can be addressed (43, 60). For example, Hubbard et al. (43) point to enhanced prognostication when 'expert' family carer accounts of symptom presentation inform assessments.

Conclusion and future developments in the involvement of family carers in care for older people

European and national initiatives have largely failed to deliver equitable benefits for family carers whose experiences of supporting dying patients remain unnecessarily challenging, costly, and distressing (1).The considerable health, social, and economic contributions that family carers afford societies are under-recognized and under-recompensed. While there are expressions of esteem encapsulated in family carer policy directives, the care responsibilities they undertake remain hidden, unacknowledged, and poorly valued.

The World Health Organization (65) calls for optimal support and also points to limited evidence of which strategies and interventions provide benefits for family carers. We would propose the following priorities:

- Systematic research of existing family carer assessment tools and support interventions, with a focus on social support, education, and information, that enable family carers to be prepared in their role (66).

- Effective strategies of dissemination of successful interventions to practitioners.

- Family carer assessment should become embedded in routine care, with a range of appropriate direct carer support services that are accessible, timely, and affordable.

- The research agenda should reflect family carer characteristics, previously highlighted, of older, frailer family carers with life-limiting health conditions of their own, providing care for family members with complex, long- term palliative care needs.

References

1 Hanratty B, Lowson E, Grande G, et al. Transitions at the end of life for older adults: patient, carer and professional perspectives. *Health Serv Deliv Res* 2014; **2** (17).

2 Lapierre TA, Keating N. Characteristics and contributions of non-kin carers of older people: a closer look at friends and neighbours. *Ageing & Society* 2013; **33**(8):1442–68.

3 Payne S. White Paper on improving support for family carers in palliative care: Part 1 and 2. Recommendations from the European Association for Palliative Care (EAPC) task force on family carers. *Eur J Pall Care* 2010; **17**(5):238–90.

4 National Institute for Clinical Excellence. *Guidance on cancer services: improving supportive and palliative care for adults with cancer: the manual.* London: NICE; 2004.

5 Payne S, Grande G. Towards better support for family carers: a richer understanding. *Palliat Med* 2013; **27**(7):579–80.

6 Payne S, Morbey H. *Supporting family carers: report on the evidence of how to work with and support family carers to inform the work of the commission into the future of hospice care.* London: Help the Hospices; 2013.

7 Grande G, Stajduhar K, Aoun S, et al. Supporting lay carers in end of life care: current gaps and future priorities. *Palliat Med* 2009; **23**(4):339–44.

8 Orpin P, Stirling C, Hetherington S, Robinson A. Rural dementia carers: formal and informal sources of support. *Ageing & Society* 2012; 32: FirstView:1–24.

9 Wadhwa D, Burman D, Swami N, Rodin G, Lo C, Zimmermann C. Quality of life and mental health in caregivers of outpatients with advanced cancer. *Psycho-Oncology* 2013; **22**(2):403–10.

10 European Commission (EUROSTAT). *Population structure and ageing;* 2014. Available at: <http://epp.eurostat.ec.europa.eu/statistics_explained/index.php/Population_structure_and_ageing#Future_trends_in_population_ageing> (Accessed January 2014). Ref. type: online source.

11 World Health Organization. *Good health adds life to years: global brief for World Health Day* 2012. Switzerland, Geneva: WHO; 2012 [WHO/DCO/WHD/2012.2].

12 Morbey H, Payne S, Froggatt K, Milligan C, Turner M. *Supporting older carers of those nearing the end of life: Lancaster University evaluation of six pilot projects.* FHM, Lancaster University, unpublished report for Age UK; 2013.

13 Payne S, Brearley S, Milligan C, et al. *Unpacking the home: family carers' reflections on dying at home. Marie Curie Cancer Care funded study 2013.* FHM, Lancaster University; 2013.

14 Calanzani N, Higginson IJ, Gomes B. *Current and future needs for hospice care: an evidence-based report*. London: Help the Hospices; 2013.

15 Gott M, Barnes S, Payne S, et al. Patient views of social service provision for older people with advanced heart failure. *Health Soc Care Comm* 2007; **15**(4):333–42.

16 del Río-Lozano M, García-Calvente M, Marcos-Marcos J, Entrena-Durán F, Maroto-Navarro G. Gender identity in informal care: impact on health in Spanish caregivers. *Qual Health Res* 2013; **23**(11):1506–20.

17 Milligan C. *There's no place like home: place and care in an ageing society*. Ashgate, Aldershot; 2009.

18 Pope ND, Kolomer S, Glass AP. How women in late midlife become caregivers for their aging parents. *J Women Aging* 2012; 24(3):242–61.

19 Silverman M. Sighs, smiles, and worried glances: how the body reveals women caregivers' lived experiences of care to older adults. J Aging Stud 2013; **27**(3):288–97.

20 Carers UK. *Facts about carers 2012*. London: Carers UK; 2012.

21 Milligan C, Morbey H. *Understanding the support and support needs of older male care-givers*. FHM, Lancaster University, unpublished report; 2013.

22 Alzheimer's Association. *2013 Alzheimer's disease facts and figures. Alzheimer's Dement* 2013; **9**(2):208–45.

23 Egdell V. Who cares? Managing obligation and responsibility across the changing landscapes of informal dementia care. *Ageing & Society* 2013; 33(05):888–907.

24 Carers UK. *Census data update—May 2013*. London: Carers UK; 2013.

25 Guberman N, Lavoie J-P, Blein L, Olazabal I. Baby boom caregivers: care in the age of individualization. *Gerontologist* 2012; **52**(2):210–8.

26 Boland J, Martin JG, Wells AU, Ross JR. Palliative care for people with non-malignant lung disease: summary of current evidence and future direction. *Palliat Med* 2013; **27**(9):811–6.

27 Roberts D, Appleton L, Calman L, et al. Protocol for a longitudinal qualitative interview study: maintaining psychological well-being in advanced cancer—what can we learn from patients' and carers' own coping strategies? *BMJ* 2013; 3(6):e003046.

28 Nolan M. Positive aspects of caring. In: Payne S, Ellis-Hill C (ed). *Chronic and terminal illness: new perspectives on caring and carers*. Oxford: Oxford University Press; 2001, 22–39.

29 Whittingham K, Barnes S, Gardiner C. Tools to measure quality of life and carer burden in informal carers of heart failure patients: a narrative review. *Palliat Med* 2013; **27**(7):596–607.

30 van der Steen J, Radbruch L, Hertogh C, et al. White Paper defining optimal palliative care in older people with dementia: a Delphi study and recommendations from the European Association for Palliative Care. *Palliat Med* 2013; **28** (3):197–209.

31 Richfield EW, Jones EJS, Alty JE. Palliative care for Parkinson's disease: a summary of the evidence and future directions. *Palliat Med* 2013; **27**(9):805–10.

32 Aoun S, Kristjanson L, Hudson P, Currow D, Rosenberg J. The experience of supporting a dying relative: reflections of caregivers. *Prog Pall Care* 2005; **13**(6):319–25.

33 Burns C, Abernethy A, Dal Grande E, Currow D. Uncovering an invisible network of direct caregivers at the end of life: A population study. *Palliat Med* 2013; **27**(7):608–15.

34 Sav A, Kendall E, McMillan SS, et al. 'You say treatment, I say hard work': treatment burden among people with chronic illness and their carers in Australia. *Health Soc Care Comm* 2013; **21**(6):665–74.

35 Bekelman DB, Nowels CT, Retrum JH, et al. Giving voice to patients' and family caregivers' needs in chronic heart failure: implications for palliative care programs. *J Palliat Med* 2011; **14**(12):1317–24.

36 Gadoud A, Jenkins SM, Hogg KJ. Palliative care for people with heart failure: summary of current evidence and future direction. *Palliat Med* 2013; **27**(9):822–8.

37 Chai H, Guerriere D, Zagorski B, Coyte P. The magnitude, share and determinants of unpaid care costs for home-based palliative care service provision in Toronto, Canada. *Health Soc Care Comm* 2013; **22**(1):30–9.

38 Keesing S, Rosenwax L, McNamara B. 'Doubly deprived': a post-death qualitative study of primary carers of people who died in Western Australia. *Health Soc Care Comm* 2011; **19**(6):636–44.

39 Mackenzie CS, Smith MC, Hasher L, Leach L, Behl P. Cognitive functioning under stress: evidence from informal caregivers of palliative patients. *J Palliat Med* 2007; **10**(3):749–58.

40 Kong J, Moorman SM. Caring for my abuser: childhood maltreatment and caregiver depression. *Gerontologist* 2013:53(S1); doi: 10.1093/geront/gnt136.

41 Judge KS, Yarry SJ, Looman WJ, Bass DM. Improved strain and psychosocial outcomes for caregivers of individuals with dementia: findings from project answers. *Gerontologist* 2013; **53**(2):280–92.

42 Thomas C, Morris SM, Harman JC. Companions through cancer: the care given by informal carers in cancer contexts. *Soc Sci Med* 2002; **54**(4):529–44.

43 Hubbard G, McLachlan K, Forbat L, Munday D. Recognition by family members that relatives with neurodegenerative disease are likely to die within a year: a meta-ethnography. *Palliat Med* 2012; **26**(2):108–22.

44 Moorman SM, Macdonald C. Medically complex home care and caregiver strain. *Gerontologist* 2013; **53**(3):407–17.

45 Hudson P, Remedios C, Thomas K. A systematic review of psychosocial interventions for family carers of palliative care patients. *BMC Palliat Care* 2010; **9**(1):17.

46 Henriksson A, Årestedt K. Exploring factors and caregiver outcomes associated with feelings of preparedness for caregiving in family caregivers in palliative care: a correlational, cross-sectional study. *Palliat Med* 2013; **27**(7):639–46.

47 Grant M, Sun V, Fujinami R, et al. Family caregiver burden, skills preparedness, and quality of life in non-small cell lung cancer. *Oncol Nurs Forum* 2013; **40**(4):337–46.

48 Kim Y, Spillers L, Hall D. Quality of life of family caregivers 5 years after a relative's cancer diagnosis: follow-up of the national quality of life survey for caregivers. *Psycho-oncology* 2012; **21**(3):273–81.

49 Payne S. Survivorship in advanced disease. In: Feuerstein M (ed). *Handbook of cancer survivorship*. New York: Springer; 2007, 429–46.

50 Candy B, Jones L, Williams R, Tookman A, King M. Interventions for supporting informal caregivers of patients in the terminal phase of a disease. *Cochrane Database of Systematic Reviews* 2009; **1**:CD007617.

51 Evans N, Meñaca A, Andrew EVW, et al. Systematic review of the primary research on minority ethnic groups and end-of-life care from the United Kingdom. *J Pain Symptom Manage* 2012; **43**(2):261–86.

52 Gomes B, Higginson IJ. Factors influencing death at home in terminally ill patients with cancer: systematic review. *BMJ* 2006; **332**(7540):515–8.

53 Harding R, List S, Epiphaniou E, Jones H. How can informal caregivers in cancer and palliative care be supported? An updated systematic literature review of interventions and their effectiveness. *Palliat Med* 2012; **26**(1):7–22.

54 Hudson P, Trauer T, Graham S, et al. A systematic review of instruments related to family caregivers of palliative care patients. *Palliat Med* 2010; **24**(7):656–68.

55 Hudson PL, Lobb EA, Thomas K, et al. Psycho-educational group intervention for family caregivers of hospitalized palliative care patients: pilot study. *J Palliat Med* 2012; **15**(3):277–81.

56 Hudson P, Trauer, Kelly B, et al. Reducing the psychological distress of family caregivers of home-based palliative care patients: short-term effects from a randomised controlled trial. *Psycho-oncology* 2013; **22**(9):1987–93.

57 Hudson PL, Aranda S, Kristjanson LJ . Meeting the supportive needs of family caregivers in palliative care: challenges for health professionals. *J Palliat Med* 2004; **7**(1):19–25.

58 Fromme EK, Drach LL, Tolle SW, et al. Men as caregivers at the end of life. *J Palliat Med* 2005; **8**(6):1167–75.

59 Cherlin E, Fried T, Prigerson HG, Schulman-Green D, Johnson-Hurzeler R, Bradley EH. Communication between physicians and family caregivers about care at the end of life: when do discussions occur and what is said? *J Palliat Med* 2005; **8**(6):1176–85.

60 Bajwah S, Higginson IJ, Ross JR, et al. The palliative care needs for fibrotic interstitial lung disease: a qualitative study of patients, informal caregivers and health professionals. *Palliat Med* 2013; **27**(9):869–76.

61 Hebert R, Schulz R, Copeland V, Arnold RM. What questions do family caregivers want to discuss with health care providers in order to prepare for the death of a loved one? An ethnographic study of caregivers of patients at end of life. *J Palliat Med* 2008; **11**(3):476–83.

62 Enguidanos S, Housen P, Penido M, Mejia B, Miller J. Family members' perceptions of inpatient palliative care consult services: a qualitative study. *Palliat Med* 2013; doi: 10.1177/0269216313491620.

63 Benzar E, Hansen L, Kneitel AW, Fromme EK. Discharge planning for palliative care patients: a qualitative analysis. *J Palliat Med* 2011; **14**(1):65–9.

64 Ellington L, Reblin M, Clayton MF, Berry P, Mooney K. Hospice nurse communication with patients with cancer and their family caregivers. *J Palliat Med* 2012; **15**(3):262–8.

65 International Palliative Care Family Carer Research Collaboration. International Palliative Care Family Carer Research Collaboration. Available at: <http://centreforpallcare.org/index.php/research/ipcfcrc/> (Accessed January 2014). Ref. type: online source.

66 Hudson P. Improving support for family carers: key implications for research, policy and practice. *Palliat Med* 2013; **27**(7):581–2.

Chapter 21

Collaboration between professionals as a necessary condition for palliative care

Ruth Piers, Nele Van Den Noortgate, and Andre Vyt

Introduction to collaboration between professionals as a necessary condition for palliative care

Different needs and stimuli have promoted interprofessional collaboration over recent decades, such as the growing belief in the complexity and multidimensionality of health problems, and the increasing specialization of the health care workers involved. Interdisciplinary or interprofessional collaboration provides better service and yields better results. Putting together specialized knowledge from different health care workers leads to a better understanding of patient problems. This is certainly the case for both geriatric and palliative care involving medical, social, psychological, and spiritual aspects. Bringing different health care workers to act together on the same patient situation is crucial in order to fully appreciate the patient's context and to work towards holistic care planning.

In a multi-professional context, the interaction between health care workers may be limited to the exchange of information on demand. However, in order to have a truly interdisciplinary or interprofessional context, the interaction must involve common goal setting, shared decision making, and collaboration on the tasks at hand.

This chapter discusses: (i) the consequences of good interprofessional collaboration for both health care workers and patients; (ii) the strategies for overcoming barriers to interprofessional teamwork; (iii) the required competences and elements for interprofessional collaboration; and, finally, (iv) possible tools for good interprofessional teamwork.

Beneficial outcome of interprofessional collaboration for health care workers and patients

The assets of a well-functioning interprofessional collaboration have been well demonstrated in past decades as making improvement in the effectiveness of care possible. Research in different clinical settings has shown that good interdisciplinary teamwork improves the process of care (1), reduces the incidence of adverse events (2), and is associated with a reduction in length of stay and costs of hospital admission (3–5). Good interdisciplinary teamwork is also positively related to job satisfaction in health care workers and negatively related to burn-out and staff turnover (6–8). A few promising studies in palliative care for older people indicate that good interprofessional collaboration may result in a good outcome for health care workers in this specific setting and, consequently, in the quality of patient care (9–12).

Particular emphasis on matters of ethics is required in caring for vulnerable geriatric patients because they are dependent in many aspects of daily life (13). Additionally, in taking care of frail older people, nurses are often confronted with patients at the end of their lives. Moral distress can arise when health care workers perceive constraints that prevent action in accordance with their moral choice (14). In geriatric nursing care, most moral distress is related to providing care at the end of life that is too aggressive (9). Nurses' self-perception of their own powerlessness is a central theme in moral distress and is related to a lack of collaboration in patient care decision making and a lack of respect for their own knowledge and expertise (14, 15). The considerable moral responsibility conferred on nurses by their unique proximity to the patient and his or her relatives is a strong argument in favour of including nurses in the end-of-life decision-making processes (16, 17). However, problematic interdisciplinary collaboration may inhibit their ability to apply their personal and professional moral reasoning, which can lead, in the long term, to patient avoidance behaviour (18), compassion fatigue (10–19), burn-out (14, 15, 20), and sick leave (9, 20).

As such, promoting interprofessional discussions might be an important strategy to reduce work-related problems (such as moral distress and burn-out) in health care workers (6–9, 11, 20, 21). Integrating the perspectives of all team members leads not only towards improved mutual understanding and fewer conflicts, but also towards better end-of-life decision making and care for patients and their families (21–23).

Barriers to interprofessional collaboration

Interprofessional collaboration has been a focus of worldwide health care policy for a quarter of a century, since the report of a study group of the WHO (World Health Organization) in 1988 (24). Little progress has been noted, however, since then. A follow-up report of the WHO in 2010 (25) concluded that, in order to effectuate this in practice, a synergy is necessary between reforms in higher education, clinical institutions, and political will. Interesting initiatives in interprofessional education in health and social care can lead to highly motivated students embracing the mind-set of collaborative practice, but confrontation between this idealistic attitude on the one hand, and the constraints of the existing methods and regulations in clinical institutions on the other, leads to frustration and the abandoning of interprofessional ideals. More recently, in 2013, the WHO published guidelines for transforming and scaling up health professionals' education and training, in which the concept of interprofessional education is chosen as one of seven major recommendations for training in the coming years.

Following the WHO's Framework for Action, the European Interprofessional Education Network has adopted a charter stating that synergy is *sine qua non* for collaborative practice (26). This charter stipulates the following requirements:[1]

◆ That the professional health and social care bodies explicitly require that the competences necessary for interprofessional collaboration are attained by graduating students.

◆ That educational and clinical institutions designate interprofessional collaborative work as one of the main values in their mission and quality management policies, and support and adhere to bodies and networks that promote and/or supervise interprofessional health and social care.

◆ That educational institutions comply with this need by ensuring that graduates are competent in interprofessional health and social care and that professional body representatives ratify the competence chart of their educational programmes, based on the presence of interprofessional competences.

◆ That clinical institutions comply with this need by ensuring their staff are competent in interprofessional health and social care, by providing continuous training, and by allowing patient representatives and/or representatives from patient organizations to be involved in institutional policy.

◆ That governmental agencies focus on the compliance of clinical and educational institutions with regulations promoting and necessitating interprofessional practice and education, and support the institutions by implementing accreditation and financial mechanisms that foster this practice and education.

◆ That health insurance bodies, patient organizations, and supportive networks explicitly formulate the need for interprofessional collaboration towards clinical and educational institutions, as well as towards governmental agencies.

Correct implementation of interprofessional collaboration needs a change in thinking and in work practice, and specific competences in teamwork and knowledge sharing.

Interprofessional competences

Interprofessional competences are the core of interprofessional teamwork. They play a key role in several dimensions of health care work, such as corresponding and reporting, consulting, goal setting and intervention planning, care management, referral, and follow-up. The umbrella competence of interprofessional collaboration encompasses the communication of ideas from one's own disciplinary framework of reference towards other disciplines, the use of expertise of other disciplines and health care workers, and active and effective involvement in teams. It includes the abilities to harmonize personal ideas and activities with those of others and to cooperate in the planning, follow-up, and evaluation of interdisciplinary care. The interdisciplinary focus of a health care worker becomes evident in their analysis of situations and problems, and in drawing up interventions and care provision.

A team member has to be able to plan activities in accordance with others and to antici-pate problems that may arise for them. A team member needs a mind-set that focuses on the possible role of and information available to other disciplines, while being careful not to draw conclusions on the basis of partial data. An assessment of this competence is not based on depth of knowledge but on the way knowledge is used.

Tools have been developed to assess the quality of interprofessional collaboration (27–29). One of them is the Interprofessional Practice and Education Quality Scales (27), to be used with the PROSE Online Diagnostics and Documenting System. It is a team-oriented self-assessment toolbox using a validated 60-item questionnaire consisting of three sub-scales (20 items each) on aspects of interprofessional teamwork. The first sub-scale covers the conditions for interdisciplinary collaboration; the second covers specific aspects relating to the interdisciplinary work processes; and the third covers the individual interdisciplinary competences and mind-set of the health workers. Each item is rated on a five-point Likert scale and, optionally, respondents can also make comments about the item. The system generates performance indexes based on summations of item scores.

Tools are also available for assessing interprofessional competence (i.e. competences that are especially important for effective interprofessional collaboration). An interna-tional collection of tools is generated by the American National Center for Interprofes-sional Practice and Education (<www.nexusipe.org>). Several competence frameworks have been developed in the United Kingdom (e.g. Assessment and Learning in Practice Settings (ALPS)—<www.alps-cetl.ac.uk>), and training packages have been deployed in higher education to develop the skills in graduating students (e.g. the InterDis learning trajectory) (30–32). An exploration of these in respect of quality assurance of interprofes-sional training has been carried out in a European project of the European Interprofes-sional Practice and Education Network (33).

The European Association for Palliative Care also recognizes the inherent value of in-stitutional collaboration and shared learning across disciplines. In a recent paper, it has outlined core competences for health and social professionals in palliative care (34, 35). Comprehensive care coordination and interdisciplinary teamwork is brought forward as one of the ten core competences for palliative care workers. The paper describes how to provide interdisciplinary learning in palliative care, incorporating both shared and discipline-specific learning (35). Interprofessional learning in a clinical environment, with real patients, has been shown to be suited to demonstrating and learning about interprofessional practice. In the United Kingdom, undergraduate students from differ-ent disciplines positively evaluated a hospice-based interprofessional practice placement, reporting an increased understanding of both their own roles and those of other profes-sionals in the team (36).

Elements and tools for effective interprofessional teamwork

Interprofessional collaboration depends largely on elements such as the management structure, the methods used for decision making, and patient records management, but also on the interprofessional competences of the staff. Key elements for successful team-work are as follows: shared goal planning placing the patient's needs at the forefront, shared complementary responsibility among all team members, effective leadership stimulating openness and self-reflection, and effective coordination. These key elements are further elaborated in the following paragraphs.

Interprofessional teamwork exists when health care professionals not only make appropriate referrals to each other, and consult each other when needed, but also jointly contribute to setting up interventions and care planning. It involves shared goal setting, the commonality of a shared reference framework, swift interplay between team members, and the common ethical principle of placing the patient's (and family's) needs, desires, and limitations to the fore (1, 30, 34–38).

A team should consist of members who take up complementary roles. They should have knowledge of, and respect for, the competences and contributions of other professionals in the team. It also implies the abandonment of stereotyped roles and role perceptions, hierarchical relationships, and professional jargon. The social worker and the nurse are not the only ones focusing on the social well-being of the patient, and the physician does not always knows best about physical discomfort and pain diagnostics (1, 21, 25, 30, 34–38).

A well-functioning team needs effective leadership stimulating openness and self-reflection (1, 37, 38). All team members should be aware that their judgement of what constitutes appropriate care is a personal issue related to their worldview and is, therefore, coloured by their own emotions, attitudes, backgrounds, and beliefs. Becoming aware of one's own emotions/attitudes is a key condition for providing good-quality care adapted to the needs and preferences of the patient (14, 16, 20). Realizing that there are different ways of thinking about moral issues can help health care workers to understand their own process of decision making and to tolerate differences in the moral reasoning and decision making of others (16, 20, 34, 35).

To achieve effective interprofessional collaboration, health care workers need specific tools and working methods. Efficient communication and information management is a major issue. Although modern information technology can enable us to take great steps forward, it cannot guarantee efficient collaboration and open communication. Regular close communication between team members and team management are essential components to achieving this (12, 33, 40).

Interdisciplinary meetings foster collaboration between different disciplines. Creating opportunities for formal and informal dialogue between health care workers is important in improving interdisciplinary collaboration, given the creation of a safe atmosphere. A safe atmosphere will, for instance, make open and honest communication about difficult ethical issues possible, thereby increasing feelings of autonomy and empowerment regarding daily patient care (9, 11, 12, 20, 41).

Previous patient situations may be used as a tool to improve future patient care decisions or to address policies and practices that create distressing patient care situations. Structured moral case deliberations stimulate health care workers to share their feelings and to go beyond their emotions. Also, regular debriefings and interdisciplinary intervision

(Balint groups) are effective in reducing moral distress, improving the ethical environment, and, consequently, optimizing the quality of patient care (9, 11, 12, 20, 42, 43).

For interprofessional teamwork, we need shared complementary responsibility, effective team coaching, and coordination of care planning. The quality of team meetings—a core aspect of teamwork—can be enhanced by elements such as the preparation of documents, the presence of key persons, the availability of information through instruments such as shared electronic patient files, and the management of the meeting process (32, 39, 40). The team coach should structure the meeting in such a way that enough time is devoted to a shared problem definition, with exploration and analysis, before constructing an intervention strategy. Finally, a meeting should end with a clear follow-up of goals and tasks.

One important tool for promoting interprofessional teamwork is the shared care plan (40, 44) (see Table 21.1). The actively contributing health care workers are identified on a matrix, by the team, for each goal for which one person takes responsibility, while another takes responsibility for coordinating the shared care. The joint use of this matrix is aimed at better involvement of team members. Further study is needed on the implementation of this tool, and cultural sensitivity and country differences with regard to professionals' roles and competences need to be taken into account in its interpretation.

A shared care planning tool

Effective goal setting and care planning is frequently hindered by a mind-set in which health care workers are focused on their own professional identity and qualifications rather than on common goals for the patient or client system. This mind-set also limits the quality of interprofessional collaboration and shared care. To counter this, a planning tool can help by making a clear differentiation between goals and actions and by clearly identifying shared goals, responsibilities, task differentiation, and collaboration (40, 44). This is illustrated by the following case:

A man, 86 years of age, was brought to the hospital by his son after he had fallen in his house and could not get up by himself. Luckily, he had been able to drag himself to his telephone and call his son. There is a bleeding wound on his forehead.

The patient's wife died two years ago. Since then he has lived alone in his house. His son came to visit him regularly. Although the son interpreted the back pain as a sign of normal ageing, the aggravating back pain impeded the patient from going outside for shopping. The patient, who used to have good contact with his nephew, did not have the energy any more to go and visit him.

Three years ago, treatment was started for mild prostate cancer. This seemed to be well under control until some months ago, he started to suffer severe back pain. The blood test showed a high increase in markers indicative of prostate cancer, and bone imaging showed multiple lumbar fractures based on bone metastases.

The classical care plan, with action points, would look like Table 21.1: Part A. In this plan, the actions of the health care workers, as individuals, are at the forefront. However, taking the perspective of the patient himself, as the main entrance to deal with all health and social care issues, would result in a different care plan. In this case, the main concerns of the patient were 'not to be a burden to family members' and 'dying without suffering too much pain'.

Table 21.1 Shared care matrix

Part A. A classical multidisciplinary care plan with action points

ACTIONS	Physician	Nurse	Physiotherapist / occupational therapist	Social worker	Psychologist
Treat prostate cancer/cancer pain	X				
Treat depressive mood	X				X
Reduce falls/install a mobility aid			X		
Wound care		X			
Plan discharge to home setting				X	

Part B. An interdisciplinary care plan focusing on joint/shared/common goals of care

GOALS OF CARE	Physician	Nurse	Physiotherapist / occupational therapist	Social worker	Psychologist
Patient does not suffer severe pain, by installing adequate (holistic)pain treatment	**X**	X	X	X	X
Patient regains psychosocial well-being, by health care workers treating depression and breaking social isolation	X	**X**		X	X
Patient is more active at home and has a reduced fear of falling, by health care workers promoting and sustaining his mobility	X	X	**X**	X	

Legend: The responsible health care worker for each shared goal is indicated in bold.

During the hospital stay, the health care professionals and the core social network were true partners in laying out the hallmarks of a strategy in which the wish, the needs, and the limitations of the patient were combined with the desires and limitations of the family. A nurse from the in-hospital palliative support team called to explain about palliative home care teams or palliative units, in case his suffering could not be alleviated by normal measures in the future.

In order to honour his wish not to burden his family, professional home care was installed; when his son called, they could spend quality time together. Also, a service of voluntary drivers was contacted so he was able to visit his nephew again.

The shared care matrix for this patient would then look like Table 21.1: Part B.

Conclusion on collaboration between professionals as a necessary condition for palliative care

Good interprofessional teamwork is crucial to providing holistic patient-centred care, which is the core goal of palliative and geriatric medicine. Integrating perspectives of all team members does not only lead towards mutually improved understanding and less moral distress, but also towards better end-of-life decision making and care adapted to the needs of the patient and family members. For interprofessional teamwork, we need shared goal planning, a shared complementary responsibility, effective team coaching, and co-ordination of care planning. Frequent interdisciplinary meetings are needed to safeguard effective interprofessional collaboration. Shared care plans, such as the one presented here, are efficient tools to promote interprofessional teamwork by making a clear differentiation between goals and actions and by clearly identifying shared goals, responsibilities, task differentiation, and collaboration.

Although the objectives of interprofessional practice are obviously appropriate, the recent WHO guidelines document (2013) stresses the need for further research evidence. There are studies demonstrating the effectiveness of interprofessional practice, though their numbers remain low. Several reasons account for this. As an increase in effectiveness and cost effectiveness of health care is increasingly determined by a complex variety of contextual factors, complex research designs are required, making it difficult to generate corroborating and easy-to-publish evidence. As long as every profession creates its own professional code, without including a common deontology as a health care worker, it will be hard to overcome the traditional siloing between professions. Care for older patients, and especially palliative care, is one of the sectors in health and social care where different professions need to collaborate in order to maintain or increase the quality of life and the quality of dying. Politicians, educational leaders, clinical institutions, and researchers need to work together on implementing this interprofessional collaboration.

Note

1 (Adapted from the *Charter for IPE in Europe* © 2014, EIPEN)

References

1 Mickan, SM, Rodger SA. Effective health care teams: a model of six characteristics developed from shared perceptions. *J Interprof Care* 2005; **19**(4):358–70.

2 Sargeant J, Loney E, Murphy G. Effective interprofessional teams: 'contact ss not enough' to build a team. *J Contin Educ Health Prof* 2008; **28**(4):228–34.

3 Zwarenstein M, Goldman J, Reeves S. Interprofessional collaboration: effects of practice-based interventions on professional practice and health care outcomes. *Cochrane Database Syst Rev* 2009; **3**:CD000072.

4 Zwarenstein M, Reeves S, Barr H, Hammick M, Koppel I, Atkins J. Interprofessional education: effects on professional practice and health care outcomes. *Cochrane Database of Systematic Reviews* 2000; **3**: doi:10.1002/14651858.CD002213.

5 Risser DT, Simon R, Rice MM, Salisbury ML. A structured teamwork system to reduce clinical errors. In: Spath PL (ed). *Error reduction in health care: a system approach to improving patient safety.* Chicago: AHA; 297–334.

6 Curley, C, Mc Eachern, JE, Speroff, T. A firm trial of inter-disciplinary rounds on the inpatient medical wards: an intervention using continuous quality improvement. *Med Care* 1998; **36**:AS4–12.

7 Rice K, Zwarenstein M, Conn LS, Kenaszchuk C, Russell A, Reeves S. An intervention to improve interprofessional collaboration and communication: a qualitative study. *J Interprof Care* 2010; **24**(4):350–61.

8 Deneckere S, Euwema M, Lodewijckx C, et al. Better interprofessional teamwork, higher level of organized care, and lower risk of burnout in acute health care teams using care pathways: a cluster randomized controlled trial. *Med Care* 2013; **51**(1):99–107.

9 Piers RD, Van den Eynde M, Steeman E, Vlerick P, Benoit DD, Van Den Noortgate NJ. End-of-life care of the geriatric patient and nurses' moral distress. *JAMDA* 2012; **13**(1):80.e7–13.

10 Slocum-Gori S, et al. Understanding compassion satisfaction, compassion fatigue and burnout: a survey of the hospice palliative care workforce. *Pall Med* 2011; **27**(2):172–8.

11 Swetz KM, Harrington SE, Matsuyama RK, et al. Strategies for avoiding burnout in hospice and palliative medicine: peer advice for physicians on achieving longevity and fulfilment. *J Pall Med* 2009; **12**(9):773–7.

12 Jünger S, Pestinger M, Elsner F, et al. Criteria for successful multiprofessional cooperation in palliative care teams. *Pall Med* 2007; **21**(4):347–54.

13 Rees J, King L, Schmitz K. Nurses' perceptions of ethical issues in the care of older people. *Nurs Ethics* 2009; **16**(4):436–52.

14 Mobley MJ, Rady MY, Verheijde JL, et al. The relationship between moral distress and perception of futile care in the critical care unit. *Intensive Crit Care Nurs* 2007; **23**:256–63

15 Kompanje EJ, Piers RD, Benoit DD. Causes and consequences of disproportionate care in intensive care medicine. *Curr Opin Crit Care* 2013; **19**(6):630–5.

16 Rushton CH. Defining and addressing moral distress: tools for critical care nursing leaders. *AACN Adv Crit Care* 2006; **17**(2):161–8.

17 Peter E, Lunardi VL, Macfarlane A. Nursing resistance as ethical action: literature review. *J Adv Nurs* 2004; **46**(4):403–16.

18 De Villers MJ, DeVon HA. Moral distress and avoidance behaviour in nurses working in critical care and noncritical care units. *Nurs Ethics* 2013; **20** (5):589–603.

19 Figley CR (ed). *Compassion fatigue*. New York, London: Routledge; 1995.

20 Piers RD, Azoulay E, Ricou B, et al. Perceptions of appropriateness of care among European and Israeli intensive care unit nurses and physicians. *JAMA* 2011; **306**(24):2694–703.

21 Puntillo KA, McAdam JL. Communication between physicians and nurses as a target for improving end-of-life care in the intensive care unit: challenges and opportunities for moving forward. *Crit Care Med* 2006; **34**(11):S332–S340.

22 Boorsma M, Frijters DH, Knol DL, et al. Effects of multidisciplinary integrated care on quality of care in residential care facilities for elderly people: a cluster randomized trial. *CMAJ* 2011; **183**(11):E724–32.

23 Bern-Klug M, Gessert CE, Crenner CW, et al. 'Getting everyone on the same page': nursing home physicians' perspectives on end-of-life care. *J Palliat Med* 2004; **7**(4):533–44.

24 World Health Organization. *Learning together to work together for health*. Technical Report Series No. 769. Geneva: World Health Organization; 1988.

25 World Health Organization Study Group on Interprofessional Education and Collaborative Practice. *Framework for ACTION on interprofessional education and collaborative practice*. Geneva: World Health Organization; 2010.

26 European Interprofessional Practice and Education Network (EIPEN). *Charter for IPE in Europe*. Available at: <http://eipen.eu/doc/Charter_for_IPE_in_Europe.pdf>. Ref. type: online source.

27 Vyt A. *Interprofessional Practice and Education Quality Scales (IPEQS). A tool for self-assessment*. Antwerp: Garant; 2015.

28 Batorowicz B, Shepherd TA. Measuring the quality of transdisciplinary teams. *J Interprof Care* 2008; **22**(6):612–20.

29 Kenaszchuk C, Reeves S, Nicholas D, Zwarenstein M. Validity and reliability of a multiple-group measurement scale for interprofessional collaboration. *BMC Health Serv Res* 2010; **10**:83.

30 Vyt A. Interprofessional education and collaborative practice in health and social care: the need for transdisciplinary mindsets, instruments and mechanisms. In: Gibbs P (ed). *Transdisciplinary professional learning and practice* . Berlin/Zug: Springer; 2015; 69–88.

31 Walsh C, Gordon F, Marshall M, Wilson F, Hunt T. Interprofessional capability: a developing framework for interprofessional education. *Nurs Educ Pract* 2005; 5(4):230–7.

32 Wilcock P, Headrick L. Interprofessional learning for the improvement of health care: why bother? *J Interprof Care* 2005; 19:111–7.

33 Vyt A. *Exploring quality assurance for interprofessional education from a European perspective.* Antwerp: Garant; 2009.

34 Gamondi C, Larkin P, Payne S. Core competencies in palliative care: an EAPC White Paper on palliative care education—part 1. *Eur J Pall Care* 2013; 20(2):86–91.

35 Gamondi C, Larkin P, Payne S. Core competencies in palliative care: an EAPC White Paper on palliative care education—part 2. *Eur JPall Care* 2013; 20(3):140–4.

36 Dando N, d'Avray L, Colman J, Hoy A, Todd J. Evaluation of an interprofessional practice placement in a UK in-patient palliative care unit. *Palliat Med* 2012; 26(2):178–84.

37 Headrick LA, Wilcock PM, Batalden PB. Interprofessional working and continuing medical education. *BMJ* 1998; 316:771–4.

38 McPherson K, Headric L, Moss F. Working and learning together: good quality care depends on it, but how can we achieve it? *Qual Health Care* 2001; 10 (Suppl II):46–53.

39 Vyt A. Interprofessional and transdisciplinary teamwork in health care. *Diabetes Metababol Res Rev* 2008; 24:106–9.

40 Vyt A. *Interprofessioneel en interdisciplinair samenwerken in gezondheid en welzijn.* Antwerp; Garant; 2012.

41 Ten Have ECM, Nap RE, Tulleken JE. Quality of interdisciplinary rounds by leadership training based on essential quality indicators of the Interdisciplinary Rounds Assessment Scale. *Intensive Care Med* 2013; 39(10):1800–7.

42 Kjeldmand D, Holmström I. Balint groups as a means to increase job satisfaction and prevent burnout among general practitioners. *Ann Fam Med* 2008; 6:138–45.

43 Benson J, Magraith K. Compassion fatigue and burnout: the role of Balint groups. *Aust Fam Physician* 2005; 34:497–8.

44 Vyt A, Brocatus N, Vandaele B. *A practical framework to enhance collaborative practice: interprofessional shared care planning through the use of a matrix planning tool and the integrative approach of ICF.* (Poster presentation) VIIth All Together Better Health Conference, Pittsburgh, 6–8 June 2014. Available at: <http://www.atbh7.pitt.edu/files/Proceedings.%20pdf>.

Chapter 22

Communication and advance care planning for older people

Kristian Pollock and Jane Seymour

Introduction to communication and advance care planning for older people

This chapter provides an overview of the research evidence about communication and advance care planning (ACP) for older people. It considers the barriers and facilitators of ACP as a process of communication about difficult issues which may be distressing to all participants and highlights the need for more research about the content of ACP discussions in naturalistic settings and participants' experiences of taking part in these. The chapter also considers the wider social efforts which have been undertaken to change public attitudes to death and dying and increase awareness of the need to talk about, and actively plan for, care at the end of life.

Palliative care involves a commitment to support patients through the experience of life-limiting and terminal conditions and, ultimately, to realize personal goals for 'dying well'. This requires excellent control of symptoms and also that there be open awareness and communication about prognosis. Awareness of dying enables the patient to 'live well' while preparing for an experience of dying shaped by personal preferences for care. ACP is seen as central to the achievement of such goals and has become a core component of the end-of-life care policy in many countries throughout the developed world, particularly the United States, Canada, Australia, and Europe (1, 2).

Over the last century, an epidemiological transition has increased life expectancy, particularly among populations of the developed world. Most deaths now follow an extended period of ageing with progressive degenerative co-morbid conditions and progressive frailty. Increasingly, older people experience conditions such as advanced dementia, in which loss of mental capacity may be anticipated. Fifteen percent of the populations of OECD countries (country members of the Organisation for Economic Co-operation and Development) are aged 65 or over, and this figure is projected to nearly double, reaching 27%, by 2050. On average, the percentage of the population aged 80 or over will increase during this period from 4% to 10% (3). Most resource-poor countries exhibit similar trends, with the fastest growth in older populations now taking place in Asia. Average life expectancy in the United Kingdom has reached 78.7 years for men and 82.6

years for women, with the modal age being 85 and 89, respectively (4). The rising trend for dying in advanced old age means, effectively, that ACP predominantly involves older adults (5).

From documentation to discussion in advance care planning

In recent years, the focus of anticipatory planning has shifted from controlling interventions and outcomes through legally authorized and documented advance directives to refuse treatment (also called living wills), to a more informal process of discussion and reflection about goals of care (2, 6, 7). Advance directives to refuse treatment have proved hard to interpret in the complexities of real-world settings and, in practice, have been widely disregarded (7–10). Moreover, the focus on documentation of preferences does not enhance communication (11), and it is evident that skilled communication is critical to the success of ACP (12). A widely cited definition of ACP in England states this to be:

> . . . a voluntary process of discussion and review to help an individual who has capacity to anticipate how their condition may affect them in the future and, if they wish, set on record: choices about their care and treatment and/or an advance decision to refuse a treatment in specific circumstances, so that these can be referred to by those responsible for their care or treatment (whether professional staff or family carers) in the event that they lose capacity to decide once their illness progresses. (13)

An association between discussion of patient preferences and improved end-of-life care outcomes has been reported (14, 15). However, reported inadequacies in communication about end-of-life care are frequent (16, 17), especially in hospitals (18). Good and timely ACP is widely regarded as key to avoiding futile, costly, and invasive treatment and enabling death in the preferred place of home (19, 20).

The promise of advance care planning

ACP has become a key component of end-of-life care policy in many countries of the developed world (2, 10). In Britain, the End-of-life Care Strategy (21) places particular focus on initiating ACP for all patients entering the last year of life. Programmes such as Respecting Choices in the United States and Australia (22), and social marketing enterprises such as the Dying Matters Coalition in the United Kingdom (<http://dyingmatters.org/>) encourage people to undertake ACP while relatively young and well, and to revisit choices regularly throughout their lives. The situation is more variable across Europe, ranging from euthanasia as a legal option in Belgium and the Netherlands, to the absence of any statutory framework for advance decisions in Greece (10).

Despite being heavily promoted as a means of improving end-of-life care, evidence for the effectiveness of ACP remains limited and patchy (23). Evaluation is difficult because of the wide range of study quality and methods. Some studies report positive outcomes (12, 24). A recent randomized controlled trial of a facilitated ACP intervention among older patients in Australia found that end-of-life care preferences were much more likely to be known and followed in the intervention group. Patients and their relatives reported greater satisfaction with care, and families felt significantly less stress, anxiety, and depression (15). However, qualitative findings of real-world settings suggest that ACP is rare and that older patients' preferences and responses to ACP are variable, complex, and frequently ambivalent (25–29). The most successfully reported method of implementing ACP is through structured interventions, such as the Respecting Choices programmes, which use dedicated facilitators and effective methods of documenting and transferring information across services (2, 22); (see Chapter 25).

Whole systems programmes require a prolonged and substantial input of resources and professional motivation which has been rarely sustained in real-world settings and, overall, ACP remains uncommon (30–36). A survey performed by the British National Centre for Social Research found that while the majority of respondents indicated feeling comfortable talking about death and dying, only 5% had completed any form of ACP. Less than half had discussed their wishes for end-of-life care, including 23% of those aged over 75 (33). Those who declare themselves comfortable in discussing death as a hypothetical topic may view things differently when later confronting their own mortality (25, 27, 28, 37, 38). Empirical findings about communication in ACP reveal considerable variability across studies but, overall, the gap between policy and practice is substantial (29, 32, 38). Good communication is key to ACP. However, the reported quality of communication is often poor (10, 12, 39).

Barriers to good communication in advance care planning

Patient perceptions of professional communication skills strongly influence willingness to discuss end-of-life care (12). ACP can be undertaken by a range of professionals, in hospital and community settings, and so the generalization of advanced communication skills to non-specialist practitioners is challenging. The complexity of modern health care systems, the diversity of services involved in individual cases, and the number and turnover of professionals providing patient care militates against the achievement of continuity and sustained relationships which could support ACP as a process of ongoing discussion and review. Practical considerations, such as lack of time or a suitable and private location to hold discussions which may be difficult and lengthy, are additional constraints (32, 40, 41). Evidence suggests there is a continuing and widespread professional reluctance and discomfort to engage in ACP (29, 32, 42, 43).

The difficulty of prognostication is an important barrier to professional initiation of ACP, particularly in relation to patients with conditions such as heart failure and chronic obstructive pulmonary disease, characterized by prolonged frailty and dwindling (32, 44, 45). Professionals are cautious about anticipating how long patients may live, from a reluctance to destroy hope or to be proved wrong (46). This makes it difficult to identify the 'right' time to broach the topic (6, 40, 47). Professionals are also wary of raising false expectations about care which may prove impossible to meet. While the policy rhetoric emphasizes choice, in practice, both professionals and patients know that options may be limited or illusory, and depend on resources being available to support preferred death in a hospice or at home (42, 48, 49).

Professional responses to advance care planning

Even when health professionals accept the desirability of ACP in principle, ambivalence and reluctance are frequently encountered (32, 40, 47, 50, 51). Professionals report uncertainty about recognizing appropriate opportunities to initiate ACP and are anxious not to cause distress. This leads to avoidance and procrastination (32, 42). Professionals fear jeopardizing relationships with patients who do not want, or are not ready, to consider ACP (26, 43). Initiating the discussion is easier if patients take the lead but patients often expect professionals to take responsibility for doing this. Consequently, ACP may not happen, or be considered too late, when options are restricted (29, 34, 52). Professional caution may be sound in protecting the considerable minority of patients who do not wish, or are not yet ready, to engage in ACP. However, it deprives patients who would welcome such a discussion of the opportunity to have one. The knowledge that patients are likely to change their preferences as their illness progresses may call in question the value of formulating plans in advance. In practice, ACP tends to happen, if at all, at a late stage of the patient's illness, and often in response to critical events (34).

Patient responses to advance care planning

Advocates of ACP view anticipatory planning as intrinsically beneficial. However, little is known about patient and public perspectives or experience of ACP or their preferences for communication (53, 54). Some studies report benefits and patient willingness to engage in ACP discussion (15, 36, 55, 56). However, qualitative evidence suggests that a substantial minority of older patients find the discussion of death and dying uncomfortable and distressing and do not wish to engage in ACP, or certainly not before their prognosis has become clearly limited (26, 53, 57, 58). This applies particularly to older patients affected by chronic degenerative diseases such as chronic obstructive pulmonary disease or heart failure, who view their illness as a fact of life rather than a terminal condition, and do not see the relevance of discussing death and dying (12, 25). Patients may find it difficult to make decisions or anticipate their responses to a hypothetical future that is beyond imagination (41). Some patients may opt for denial as a positive coping strategy (7, 53).

Rather than plan for an uncertain future, some older patients, confronted with their imminent mortality, reportedly prefer to live in the present, and take 'each day as it comes'. Acknowledgement of death and dying is resisted because it threatens to undermine the quality of remaining life lived in the present (27, 28, 53). In a study of older British patients with advanced heart failure, Gott et al. (25) found that patients did not want an open awareness of dying, or a precise prognosis. Nor did they value personal autonomy or choice or control over dying, preferring instead to delegate the burden of decision making to trusted (professional and family) others. Far from being dysfunctional, these authors acknowledge the value of denial as a positive coping strategy for patients in their management of chronic and debilitating illness. In another British study of well older people's views of ACP, Samsi et al. (27) found that rather than engage in anticipatory planning, respondents preferred to confront future difficulties when they arose and to delegate decision making to others. Similar findings are reported by Carrese et al. (28) in a study of chronically ill older patients in the United States. These findings suggest that many older people, regardless of their current state of health, may not be receptive to the offer of an ACP discussion.

The role of carers in advance care planning

ACP aims to enable patients to shape the experience of death and dying in accordance with their personal goals and preferences. The focus is on the patient as an autonomous agent. However, it is consistently reported that a key motivator for ACP is patients' desire to relieve family members of the burden of care and responsibility for making difficult decisions (25, 33, 41, 53, 54, 59). ACP is a professional construct and tends to be framed as an intervention requiring professional mediation. Little is known about the extent or nature of discussions about end-of-life issues that may go on within families, though some studies report patients may look to relatives as well as, and possibly instead of, professionals for this purpose (59). The availability and willingness of family carers to provide care is critical to enabling patients to die at home (41). However, carers' entitlement to information about prognosis and their role in decision making and future planning is frequently unclear, and carers assess professional communication about end-of-life care often to be inadequate (12).

The nature of advance care planning discussions

Despite considerable promotion of ACP as a means of improving end-of-life care, there is little evidence about how it is carried out, or the communication practices necessary to support successful discussion of patients' future preferences and goals (6, 40). However, studies reporting accounts of such interactions describe similar communicative strategies and devices to those found in studies exploring how professionals deliver a poor prognosis or other forms of 'bad news'. This literature has been drawn on in the following discussion.

Enabling patients to have time and space to raise issues and explore concerns is an important aspect of the ACP process. However, evidence suggests that professional agendas tend to dominate discussions, focused on negative portrayals of life-sustaining treatments, and patient goals and values are rarely explored in detail (7, 60). McDonagh (39) found that health professionals directed the discussion in family conferences about critically ill patients, and that carer satisfaction was related to the length of time they themselves were able to speak. Rather than reflecting established preferences, it is through the process of reflection and discussion, involving co-construction between patient and professional, that choices for end-of-life care are established (43). Preferences emerge and change through time. In this process, patients are likely to be influenced by professional views and expectations, and to be directed towards what are seen to be 'appropriate' choices (dying at home, having a 'Do Not Resuscitate' order in place, and, in some cases, opting to refuse further hospitalization). Several studies comment on patient apprehension about feeling coerced into formulating preferences for future care, or that advance care statements might be abused, introducing euthanasia 'by the back door' (35, 41). Munday (43) reports professional awareness of this risk.

Many studies describe the caution and circumspection that professionals employ when seeking cues of patient receptivity to ACP (29, 40, 43, 61). Open questions may be used as opportunities, or 'offers', which patients may elect to take up or ignore, and the use of 'hypothetical' questions and scenarios may soften the impact of confronting difficult issues directly (60, 62). Vague and indeterminate language, allusion, and euphemism are employed by professionals as well as patients (43, 51, 60, 62). Ambiguity sustains multiple interpretations which may avoid distress but perpetuate misunderstanding and, in particular, encourages each party to assume agreement where none exists (29). Indeterminate language prompts professional inference and assumptions about patient preferences which steer choices in the direction of approved or professionally preferred options (43).

Patients and professionals may promote a common interest in maintaining 'false optimism'. Reluctance to destroy hope is a common reason for professionals to avoid end-of-life discussions, and there is evidence that patients strive to balance understanding of their situation with the maintenance of hope (47, 58). A normative commitment to full and open disclosure of their illness and prognosis may run alongside a preference for vagueness and uncertainty: individuals may assert a desire to know, but not too much (63–65). Professional caution seems well founded in the face of widespread ambivalence among patients towards acknowledgement of poor prognosis and planning for the future. Unwanted information can be destructive and patients may be unprepared for the impact of disclosure even when it confirms what was expected (63). Several studies describe a process of collusion between patients and professionals in deflecting talk about a bad prognosis and limited life expectancy (38, 47, 51). However, as The (51) notes, if patients remain unaware of their prognosis, they cannot plan. In her study, lung cancer patients who insisted on maintaining a 'recovery story' eventually confronted a difficult situation and found themselves unable to adjust or prepare for their impending death.

Documentation and advance care planning

Somewhat paradoxically, as the focus of anticipatory planning moves from the formality of Advance Directives to Refuse Treatment to the informality of ACP, a plethora of templates, documents, and resources has developed to encourage the recording of patients' end-of-life care preferences and to support professional and patient discussion (e.g. Gold Standards Framework[1], End-of-Life Care Pathway[2], Five Wishes[3], Respecting Choices[4]). Documents, templates, and tools may be useful for professionals lacking confidence in carrying out ACP discussions, and for facilitating the process and sharing of information between services and professionals. However, documentation is itself an agent in communication, shaping and confining the nature and scope of the discussion. There is a danger that overreliance on such documents will serve to simplify and reduce the process of ACP to a prescriptive, task-oriented, tick-box exercise and that documentation becomes an end, rather than the means, to supporting ACP (23, 42). Documentation may capture aspects of future care which can be easily identified and measured, but at the expense of open reflection and discussion. Documented ACP supports professional planning and resource management, but may constrain effective communication about patient goals by too rigidly structuring the process and outcomes of discussion. The bureaucratization of ACP has intensified as professionals come under increasing pressure to meet quality assurance targets linked to financial incentives (48). There is a risk that professional pressure to engage in, and record, ACP discussions may encourage coercion of patients to confront issues that they find unwelcome and distressing.

Advance care planning and cultural diversity

ACP has developed within a particular cultural and professional ideology which stresses the value of individual autonomy and personal choice on the one hand and a culture of practice promoting a particular vision of 'the good death' on the other. This paradigm does not accommodate cultural diversity and it is clear that ACP poses challenges for older patients and professionals from diverse cultural backgrounds. There has been little consideration of the views and preferences of populations from non-Western backgrounds regarding ACP, or how best to communicate these (9, 66–68). Seymour et al. (69) report that Chinese older people considered talk of death to be inauspicious, and dying at home to be contaminating. These respondents expressed a preference for death in hospital rather than at home.

Non-Western cultures do not share Western preoccupations about autonomy and choice. Responsibility for communicating and decision making about illness may vest collectively within the family group rather than the individual patient (68, 70, 71). Direct disclosure of a poor prognosis may be considered burdensome and inappropriate. Cultural and religious beliefs have considerable impact in shaping diverse attitudes towards ACP and preferences for care among the populations of complex societies. Difficulty in communication between health professionals and patients from Black and Minority Ethnic (BAME) communities has been a frequent finding associated with a poor experience of care (67).

Advance care planning within the public health agenda

Increasing demand and rising costs of end-of-life care throughout the developed world call for radical changes to public understanding and anticipation of death and dying. ACP has been promoted as a means of raising patient and public awareness and engagement, as well as of improving the quality of end-of-life care. It is also aimed at contributing to strategies for social change. The English End-of-life Care Pathway Strategy views greater public openness and willingness to communicate about these issues as key to improving end-of-life care. Public reluctance to talk about death and dying is widely assumed (21). However, there has been little research internationally which specifically explores this question (72), although several sources suggest that the public may be more receptive than is often thought (33, 54).

Policy efforts to position ACP within a more open culture of communication and death awareness have met with variable success. Some national schemes involving social marketing models have attempted to change public awareness of death and dying and promote increased understanding and acceptance of ACP. In the United States, these include philanthropically funded projects (Last Acts, Death in America, Kokua Mau) (9). In the United Kingdom, a national initiative, hosted by the Dying Matters Coalition, has been established with the aim of changing public knowledge and attitudes towards death and dying and of normalizing the topic by encouraging people to talk about their wishes and to share experiences of dying and bereavement (<http://dyingmatters.org/>). It is too early to evaluate the impact of this campaign, though the effect of the American schemes is considered to be small (9). The most successful model for increasing acceptance and uptake of ACP at a community level has been the whole systems, integrated approach developed by Respecting Choices in Wisconsin (22) and discussed in Chapter 25.

As a professional project to 'empower' patients and a policy initiative to improve health care, ACP has been largely directed by clinicians. An alternative approach has proposed the vision of 'compassionate communities' in which the population takes back responsibility and control of death and dying through awareness and commitment to organizing local community support for dying patients and their families (73); (see Chapter 18).

At a micro level, an example of the potential for changing public attitudes to talking about, and planning for, death and dying is the model of peer education undertaken by Seymour and colleagues (74). Older lay volunteers were recruited to develop and then use training materials to support community-based peer education for ACP and associated end-of-life care issues. This project highlights the potential of peer education to build on lay understanding and perspectives in developing policy and extending public understanding and discussion of ACP.

Conclusion on communication and advance care planning for older people

ACP has been established as a policy driver to improve the quality of end-of-life care and the experience of dying. Skilled and sensitive communication about patient understanding of prognosis in formulating goals of care is fundamental throughout this process. However, little is known about how professionals initiate ACP, or the content of these discussions. ACP is well established in countries with a developed palliative care infrastructure such as the United States, Canada, Australia, and much of Europe. It is reported to be most successful when embedded within a whole systems approach, engaging trained facilitators and integrating health and social services as well as wider community resources within a specific locality, as in the Respecting Choices programme in Wisconsin. More generally, however, take up and implementation of ACP is not routine, and the majority of dying patients have not discussed their preferences or completed written plans. There is evidently a considerable gap between policy and practice.

ACP remains largely a professional project. However, wariness about causing distress and uncertainty about the appropriate time discourage professionals from initiating discussion. When ACP occurs, it tends to be oriented to a professional agenda and frequently characterized by vague and indeterminate language. Patients and professionals may collude to maintain false optimism. There are concerns that the documentation developed to support ACP may have the effect of simplifying and over-structuring discussion, reducing the content to a list of tasks.

ACP has developed in the absence of strong evidence or consultation about public preferences and perspectives. However, patient goals regarding the 'good death' may often differ from those of ACP, particularly among patients from different cultures and minority ethnic groups. A substantial minority does not wish to engage in planning future care, preferring instead to focus on the present. Professional caution seems well founded in the face of widespread ambivalence among patients towards acknowledgement of poor prognosis and planning an uncertain future. Many patients are strongly motivated to undertake ACP to avoid burdening their families with the responsibility for difficult decisions about their care. However, people strive to maintain personal integrity through the maintenance of social roles and obligations, rather than the exertion of precedent autonomy.

The social, personal, and economic consequences of the demographic transition towards death in great old age constitute a major issue for public health. ACP is promoted as a means of developing a radical change to public understanding and anticipation of death and dying. However, in the face of limited take up within formal health care provision, alternative models of community care and communication 'from the ground up' have been proposed as more democratic models of engagement based on public goals and values for communication about end-of-life care.

Notes

1 <http://www.goldstandardsframework.org.uk/>
2 <http://www.nottslandd.nhs.uk/attachments/article/74/1.%20Nottinghamshire%20EOLC%20
Pathway%20for%20all%20Diagnoses.pdf>
3 <http://www.agingwithdignity.org/catalog/product_info.php?products_id=28
4 <http://www.gundersenhealth.org/respecting-choices>

References

1 **Andorno R, Biller-Andorno N, Brauer S.** Advance health directives: towards a coordinated European policy? *EJHL* 2009; **16**(3):207–27.
2 **Thomas K, Lobo B.** *ACP in End of Life Care.* Oxford: Oxford University Press; 2011.
3 Organisation for Economic Co-operations and Development. *Ageing Societies OECD (2009), "Ageing societies", in OECD Factbook, 2009: Economic, Environmental and Social Statistics.* Paris: OECD Publishing; <http://dx.doi.org/10.1787/factbook-2009-3-en>; 2009.
4 Office for National Statistics. *Mortality in England and Wales: Average Life Span, 2010.* London: Office for National Statistics; 2010.
5 **Seymour J.** Looking back, looking forward: the evolution of palliative and end-of-life care in England. *Mortality* 2012; **17**(1):1–17.

6 Horne G, Seymour J, Payne S. ACP: evidence and implications for practice. *End of Life Care* 2009; **3**(1):58–64.

7 Davison SN, Holley JL, Seymour J. ACP in patients with end-stage renal disease. In: Chambers EJ, Brown E, Germain M (eds). *Supportive Care for the Renal Patient*. Oxford: Oxford University Press; 2010, 49–74.

8 Thompson T, Barbour RS, SchwArtz LJ. Adherence to advance directives in critical care decision making: vignette study. *BMJ* 2003; **327**(1011):1–7.

9 Wilkinson A, Wenger N, Shugarman LR. *Literature Review on Advance Directives*. Washington, DC: Rand Corporation; 2007.

10 Meeussen K, Van den Block L, Deliens L. ACP: international perspectives. In: Gott M, Ingleton C (eds). *Living with Ageing and Dying, Palliative and End of Life Care for Older People*. Oxford: Oxford University Press; 2011, 102–15.

11 Prendergast TJ, Puntillo K. Withdrawal of life support: intensive caring at the end of life. *JAMA* 2002; **288**(21):2732–40.

12 Janssen DJA, Engelberg RA, Wouters EFM, Curtis JR. ACP for patients with COPD: past, present and future. *Patient Educ Couns* 2012; **86**:19–24.

13 National End of Life Care Programme. *Capacity, Care Planning and ACP: A Guide for Health and Social Care Staff*. Leicester: National End of Life Care Programme; 2011.

14 Zhang B, Wright AA, Huskamp HA, Nilsson ME, Maciejewski ML, Earle CC, et al. Health care costs in the last week of life: associations with end of life conversations. *Arch Intern Med* 2009; **169**(5):480–8.

15 Detering KM, Hancock AD, Reade MC, Silvester W. The impact of ACP on end of life care in elderly patients: randomised controlled trial. *BMJ* 2010; **340**:c1345.

16 Russ AJ, Kaufman SR. Family perceptions of prognosis, silence and the 'suddenness' of death. *Cult Med Psychiatry* 2005; **29**(1):102–23.

17 Gott M, Ingleton C, Bennet MI, Gardiner C. Transitions to palliative care in acute hospitals in England: qualitative study. *BMJ* 2011; **324**(d1773).

18 Health care Commission. *Spotlight on Complaints. A Report on Second Stage Complaints About the NHS in England*. London: Commission for Health care Audit and Inspection; 2007.

19 Higginson IJ, Sen-Gupta GJA. Place of care in advanced cancer: a qualitative systematic literature review of patient preferences. *J of Palliat Med* 2000; **3**(3):287–300.

20 NHS Confederation. Improving end-of-life care. *Leading Edge* 2005; **3**(12):1–8.

21 Department of Health. *End of Life Care Strategy—Promoting High Quality Care for All Adults at the End of Life*. London: Department of Health; 2008.

22 Hammes B, Rooney B. Death and end-of-life planning in one Midwestern community. *Arch Intern Med* 1998; **158**:383–90.

23 Mullick A, Martin J, Sallnow L. An introduction to ACP in practice. *BMJ* 2013; **347**:f6064.

24 Wright AA, Zhang B, Ray A, Mack JW, Trice E, Balboni T, et al. Associations between end-of-life discussions, patient mental health, medical care near death, and caregiver bereavement adjustment. *JAMA* 2008; **300**(14):1665–73.

25 Gott M, Small N, Barnes S, Payne S, Seamark D. Older people's views of a good death in heart failure: implications for palliative care provision. *Soc Sci Med* 2008; **67**:1113–21.

26 Horne G, Seymour J, Shepherd K. ACP for patients with inoperable lung cancer. *Int J Palliat Nurs* 2006; **12**(4):172–9.

27 Samsi K, Manthorpe J. 'I live for today': a qualitative study investigating older people's attitudes to advance planning. *Health Soc Care Comm* 2010; **19**(1):52–9.

28 Carrese JA, Mullaney JL, Faden RR, Finucane TE. Planning for death but not serious illness: qualitative study of housebound elderly patients. *BMJ* 2002; **325**:125.

29 Barclay S, Momen N, Case-Upton S, Kuhn I, Smith E. End-of-life care conversations with heart failure patients: a systematic literature review and narrative synthesis. *Brit J Gen Pract* 2011; **61**(582):e49–62.

30 NHS Public Health North East. *A Good Death Consultation: Full Research Findings*. NHS Public Health North East; 2010.

31 Exley C, Bamford C, Hughes J, Robinson L. ACP: an opportunity for person-centred care for people living with dementia. *Dementia* 2009; **8**(3):419.

32 Momen N, Barclay S. Addressing 'the elephant on the table': barriers to end of life care conversations in heart failure—a literature review and narrative synthesis. *Curr Opin Support Palliat Care* 2011; **5**(4):312–6.

33 Shucksmith J, Carlebach S, Whittaker V. *Dying*. London: National Centre for Social Research; 2012.

34 Gott M, Gardiner C, Small N, Payne S, Seamark D, Barnes S. Barriers to ACP in chronic obstructive pulmonary disease. *Palliat Med* 2009; **23**(7):642–8.

35 Sahm S, Will R, Hommel G. Attitudes towards and barriers to writing advance directives amongst cancer patients, healthy controls, and medical staff. *J Med Ethics* 2005; **31**(8):437–40.

36 Conroy S. *ACP, National Guideline*. London: Royal College of Physicians; 2009.

37 Fried TR, Drickamer M. Garnering support for ACP. *JAMA* 2010; **303**(3):269–70.

38 Richards N, Ingleton C, Gardiner C, Gott M. Awareness contexts revisited: indeterminacy in initiating discussions at the end-of-life. *J Adv Nurs* 2013; **69**(12):2654–64.

39 McDonagh JR, Elliott TB, Engelberg RA, Treece PD, Shannon SE, Rubenfeld GD, et al. Family satisfaction with family conferences about end-of-life care in the intensive care unit: increased proportion of family speech is associated with increased satisfaction. *Crit Care Med* 2004; **32**(7):1484–8.

40 Almack K, Cox K, Moghaddam N, Pollock K, Seymour J. After you: conversations between patients and health care professionals in planning for end of life care. *BMC Palliat Care* 2012; **11**:15.

41 Seymour J, Gott M, Bellamy G, Ahmedzai SH, Clark D. Planning for the end of life: the views of older people about advance care statements. *Soc SciMed* 2004; **59**(1):57–68.

42 Seymour J, Almack K, Kennedy S. Implementing ACP: a qualitative study of community nurses' views and experiences. *BMC Palliat Care* 2010; **9**(4):1–29.

43 Munday D, Petrova M, Dale J. Exploring preferences for place of death with terminally ill patients: qualitative study of experiences of general practitioners and community nurses in England. *BMJ* 2009; **338**:b2391:1–9.

44 Murray SA, Kendall M, Boyd K, Sheikh A. Illness trajectories and palliative care. *BMJ* 2005; **330**(7498):1007–11.

45 Finucane TE. How gravely ill becomes dying: a key to end-of-life care. *JAMA* 1999; **282**(17):1670–2.

46 Christakis NA. *Death Foretold, Prophecy and Prognosis in Medical Care*. Chicago: University of Chicago Press; 1999.

47 Broom A, Kirby E, Good P, Wootton J, Adams J. The troubles of telling: managing communication about the end of life. *Qual Health Res* 2014; **24**(2):151–62.

48 Munday D, Dale J, Murray SA. Choice and place of death: individual preferences, uncertainty, and the availability of care. *J R Soc Medicine* 2007; **100**:211–7.

49 Gott M, Ingleton C (eds). *Living with Ageing and Dying. Palliative and End of Life Care for Older People*. Oxford: Oxford University Press; 2011.

50 McNamara B. Good enough death: autonomy and choice in Australian palliative care. *Soc Sci Medicine* 2004; **58**:929–38.

51 Thé BAM, Hak A, Koeter GH, van der Wal G. Collusion in doctor-patient communication about imminent death: an ethnographic study. *West J Medicine* 2001; **174**:247–53.

52 Momen N, Hadfield P, Kuhn I, Smith E, Barclay S. Discussing an uncertain future: end-of-life care conversations in chronic obstructive pulmonary disease. A systematic literature review and narrative synthesis. *Thorax* 2012; **67**(9):777–80.

53 Horne G, Seymour J, Payne S. Maintaining integrity in the face of death: a grounded theory to explain the perspectives of people affected by lung cancer about the expression of wishes for end of life care. *Int J Nurs Stud* 2012; **49**:718–26.

54 Clarke A, Seymour J. 'At the foot of a very long ladder': discussing the end of life with older people and informal caregivers. *J Pain and Symptom Manage* 2010; **40**(6):857–69.

55 Steinhauser KE, Christakis NA, Clipp E, McNeilly M, Grambow S, Parker J, et al. Preparing for the end of life: preferences of patients, families, physicians, and other care providers. *J Pain Symptom Manage* 2001; **22**(3):727–37.

56 Ratner E, Norlander L, McSteen K. Death at home following a targeted ACP process at home: the kitchen table discussion. *JAGS* 2001; **49**:778–81.

57 Sanders C, Rogers A, Gately C, Kennedy A. Planning for end of life care within lay-led chronic illness self-management training: the significance of 'death awareness' and biographical context in participants accounts. *Soc Sci Med* 2008; **66**:982–93.

58 Davison S, Simpson C. Hope and ACP in patients with end stage renal disease. *BMJ* 2006; **333**(7574):886–90.

59 Singer PA, Martin DK, Lavery JV, Theil EC, Kelner M, Mendelssohn DC Reconceptualizing ACP from the patient's perspective. *Arch Int Med* 1998; **158**(8):879–84.

60 Tulsky J, Fischer GS, Rose MR, Arnold RM. Opening the black box: how do physicians communicate about advance directives? *Ann Int Med* 1998; **129**(6):441–9.

61 Cox K, Moghaddam N, Almack K, Pollock K, Seymour J. Is it recorded in the notes? Documentation of end-of-life care and preferred place to die discussions in the final weeks of life. *BMC Palliat Care* 2011; **10**(18):1–9.

62 Lutfey K, Maynard DW. Bad news in oncology: how physician and patient talk about death and dying without using those words. *Soc Psych Q* 1998, **61**(4):321–41.

63 Innes S, Payne S. Advanced cancer patients' prognostic information preferences: a review. *Palliat Med* 2009; **23**(1):29–39.

64 Leydon GM, Boulton M, Moynihan C, Jones A, Mossman J, Boudioni M, et al. Cancer patients' information needs and information seeking behaviour: in depth interview study. *BMJ* 2000; **320**(7239):909–13.

65 Curtis JR, Engelberg RA, Young JP, Vig LK, Reinke LF, Wenrich MD, et al. An approach to understanding the interaction of hope and desire for explicit prognostic information among individuals with severe chronic obstructive pulmonary disease or advanced cancer. *JPalliat Med* 2008; **11**(4):610–20.

66 Kai J, Beavan J, Faull C, Dodson L, Gill P, Beighton A. Professional uncertainty and disempowerment responding to ethnic diversity in health care: a qualitative study. *PLoS Med* 2007; **4**(11):e323.

67 Calanzani N, Koffman J, Higginson IJ. *Palliative Care and End of Life Care for Black, Asian and Minority Ethnic Groups in the UK*. London: King's College, 2013.

68 Kwak J, Ko E, Kramer BJ. Facilitating ACP with ethically diverse groups of frail, low-income elders in the USA: perspectives of care managers on challenges and recommendations. *Health Soc Care Comm* 2014; **22**(2):169–77.

69 Seymour J, Payne S, Chapman A, Holloway M. Hospice or home? Expectations of end-of-life care among white and Chinese older people in the UK. *Sociol Health Illn* 2007; **29**(6):872–90.

70 **Doorenbos AZ, Nies MA.** The use of advance directives in a population of Asian Indian Hindus. *J Transcult Nurs* 2003; **14**(7):17–24.

71 **Searight HR, Gafford J.** Cultural diversity at the end of life: issues and guidelines for family physicians. *Am Family Physician* 2005; **71**(3):515–22.

72 **Cox K, Bird L, Arthur A, Kennedy S, Pollock K, Kumar A, et al.** Public attitudes to death and dying in the UK: a review of published literature. *BMJ Support Palliat Care* 2013; **3**(1):37–45.

73 **Kellahear A.** *Compassionate Cities.* London: Routledge; 2005.

74 **Seymour J, Almack K, Kennedy S, Froggatt K.** Peer education for ACP: volunteers' perspectives on training and community engagement activities. *Health Expectations.* 2011; **16**(1):43–55.

Part V

Innovations in palliative care for older people

Chapter 23

EU civil society initiatives to protect the right to live and die in dignity

Anne-Sophie Parent

Introduction to EU civil society initiatives to protect the right to live and die in dignity

For more than a decade now, European civil society organizations representing older people have battled hard to promote the right to live and die in dignity. Various initiatives and projects have been launched to raise awareness of elder abuse and encourage policy makers to take measures to promote better quality elder care, including palliative care.

A marked example is the campaign launched by AGE Platform Europe in 2007 to convince the EU institutions, the United Nations, and the Council of Europe of the need to take action to protect older people from elder abuse and guarantee their right to enjoy a dignified life, free from unnecessary pain, discomfort, or distress until death. This priority was triggered by feedback from AGE Platform Europe's members and research published in various countries that showed that the living and caring conditions of the very old and frail are sometimes far from optimal and that elder abuse is a widespread phenomenon that affects a significant number of very old people across the EU. Elder abuse is a single or repeated act or lack of appropriate action that causes harm or distress to an older person or violates their human and civil rights. Failure to provide adequate palliative care to older people is, therefore, a form of elder abuse.

An EU-wide campaign on the issue of elder abuse

Based on its members' request, AGE action started with a wide campaign to put the issue of elder abuse onto the EU agenda. Their objective was to convince EU institutions and member states to commit to combating elder abuse in the framework of their discussions on the need to reform health and long-term care services across the EU to limit the impact of demographic ageing on their public budgets. For AGE's members, it was essential that these difficult debates, which were starting in all EU countries, should not focus exclusively on the financial sustainability of national health and long-term care systems but should also seek to improve the quality of health and long-term care from the perspective of the care recipient, i.e. should offer innovative and evidence-based quality services for present and future generations of patients, including palliative care, to better respond to the needs and expectations of Europe's ageing population.

In November 2007, supporting AGE's call in its communication on services of general interest, the European Commission emphasized the role of high-quality social services as of general interest for the fulfilment of EU's core values and objectives. It proposed a strategy aimed at promoting the quality of social services. The Commission announced, at the time, that it would not propose EU legislation but rather promote the development of EU 'voluntary quality guidelines' for social services, including elder care. This was done in cooperation with the Social Protection Committee—the EU advisory policy committee composed of representatives of national ministries—who published the voluntary European Quality Framework for social services in 2009 (1).

In February 2008, the European Commission published a special Eurobarometer report on health and long-term care in the European Union which stated that 47% of Europeans were of the view that poor treatment, neglect, and abuse of dependent older people are widespread occurrences in their country (2). A month later, the Commission published a study on elder abuse and organized an EU conference to discuss how it can be largely prevented by promoting high-quality long-term care for older people.

At the same time, following AGE recommendations, the European Parliament adopted a resolution on the demographic future of Europe which included an article calling on the European Commission and member states to take action to combat elder abuse, improve the quality of elder care, and draw up a comprehensive strategy for a large-scale information and action campaign in this field to include training of care workers, definition of quality standards, and penalties for maltreatment (3).

This showed that thanks to AGE's campaign, in the last decade, the fight against elder abuse and the improvement of the life and care quality of older people have gained importance at international and European level, with the support of several EU Presidencies, the European Parliament, and the European Commission. Although still taboo in most countries, these issues are increasingly being identified as a serious infringement of older people's human rights which can be found in all countries and in all care settings (i.e. at home, in the community, and in institutional care). The campaign has also triggered a change of paradigm from fighting elder abuse to promoting the well-being and dignity of older people, raising the importance of palliative care as an essential element of the quality care path.

In the framework of EU treaties, the responsibility for organizing, funding, and providing health and long-term care lies with national or local public authorities. However thanks to its campaign, AGE had managed to get the support of the European Parliament and the European Commission to foster a debate on elder abuse as a violation of older people's human rights which should be combated notably by improving the quality of health, long-term care, and palliative care.

European Charter of the rights and responsibilities of older people in need of long-term care and assistance

In parallel to this, AGE seized the opportunity of a call for proposals from the European DAPHNE III Programme, managed by Directorate General Justice and Home Affairs of the European Commission, and, together with a group of partners from 11 EU countries, launched a project called **European Strategy to combat Elder Abuse against Older Women (EUSTACEA)**, aimed at developing a European Charter of the rights and responsibilities of older people requiring assistance and long-term care. Through this project, the EUSTACEA partners endeavoured to launch a discussion, across the EU, on how best to recognize and affirm the rights of the most vulnerable older people. Their objective was to give a voice to older people and ensure that they are heard by the relevant decision makers.

Building on existing national initiatives such as the Charter of the rights of people with dependency, adopted in 2007 by the German Government, and the French Charter of the rights of people in need of long-term care and assistance, after 18 months of intense discussion and consultation, with grass-root actors to take on board cultural diversity, the project partners agreed on a common text for the first-ever European Charter stating the rights and responsibilities of older people who are dependent on others for their well-being.

The EUSTACEA Charter was officially launched at the European Parliament in November 2010 and since has become a reference document, not only in the partner countries but also in new countries, and at EU level (4). For example, it was disseminated to all local social centres in France by Union nationale des centres communaux d'action sociale (UNCCAS), the umbrella organization of local social centres. Overall, the EUSTACEA Charter has helped build consensus among a wide range of stakeholders on the need to take concrete action to fight elder abuse and promote quality palliative care. Article 8 of the Charter states the right to palliative care and support, and to respect and dignity in dying and in death in the following terms:

> **You have the right to die with dignity, in circumstances that accord with your wishes and within the limits of the national legislation of your country of residence.**

8.1 You have the right to compassionate help and palliative care when you reach the end of your life and until you die. You have the right to measures to relieve pain and other distressing symptoms.

8.2 You have the right to expect that everything possible should be done to make the process of dying dignified and tolerable. Those treating and accompanying you at this time should respect your wishes and uphold them wherever possible.

8.3 You have the right to expect that the medical and care professionals involved in your end-of-life care should include and offer support to those close to you or other trusted persons, according to your wishes. Your right to exclude certain people should also be respected.

8.4 You have the right to determine whether and to what extent treatment, including life-prolonging measures, should be initiated or continued. Your advance instructions should be respected if you are no longer assessed as being mentally competent.

8.5 Nobody may take any measures that would systematically lead to your death, except if they are authorised by the national legislation of your country of residence and you have explicitly given such instructions.

8.6 In the event that you are not able to express yourself, your advance instructions concerning decisions about your end-of-life care must be fulfilled within the limits of the national legislation of your country of residence.

8.7 You have the right to respect and observance of your religious beliefs and any wishes expressed during your lifetime about the arrangements for care and treatment of your body after your death.

Reproduced from DAPHNE —EUSTACEA, European Charter of the rights and responsibilities of older people in need of long-term care and assistance, Article 8.

The WeDO project to promote the well-being and dignity of older people

AGE's next goal was to move from fighting elder abuse to promoting the well-being and dignity of older people. Building on the EUSTACEA project, AGE and partners from 12 countries—many of whom had been involved in the EUSTACEA project—launched the Well-being and Dignity of Older People (WeDO) project to encourage a shift of paradigm from combating mistreatment to fostering good treatment in elder care. The project's key objective was to develop a European Quality Framework for long-term care based on the European Charter. This two-year project was co-financed by Directorate General Employment and Social Affairs of the European Commission, under a call for proposals for a pilot project on preventing elder abuse requested by the European Parliament. The WeDO project, which ended in December 2012, developed practical tools that are now used in several countries at grass roots and national level and include sections on palliative care and end-of-life care.

For example, the WeDO Quality Framework calls for

an integrated response to care and assistance needs [that] covers very different types of care: all healthcare; social services targeting older people in need of care and assistance; care for cognitive diseases; palliative and end-of-life care; services delivered at home, in the community or in a residential care home; public or private-funded; and informal care or care by volunteers. (5)

The Quality Framework also calls for continuous care, which means that

services for older people in need of care and assistance should be organised so as to ensure continuity of service delivery as long as it is needed and, particularly when responding to long-term needs, according to a life-cycle approach. This enables older people to rely on a continuous, uninterrupted range of services, from early intervention, care and support, to palliative care, while not disrupting the service. Care providers should work together to facilitate transitions between different care services and settings as needs evolve. (6)

Since it was launched, the European Quality Framework has inspired several national initiatives across the EU, including legislative work, and has encouraged stakeholders from other countries to join the WeDO community.

WeDO2—supporting good practice in delivering long-term care services

WeDO2 aims at pursuing the work done by the WeDO project through supporting the exchange of learning experiences and good practices between organizations working in the field of formal, non-formal, or informal adult education (older people and/or informal carers' organizations, universities, training centres, service providers) to improve their ability to train senior people and informal and formal carers to cooperate in planning and delivering long-term care services and so improve the quality of life for older people in need of care and assistance. Coordinated by the Vrije Universiteit Brussel (Belgium) and supported by AGE, the project started in September 2013 and will last two years. A concrete achievement of WeDO2 is the endorsement of the European Quality Framework by the relevant Ministers of Flanders, Wallonia, and Brussels regions in February 2014.

International impact of the European Charter and Quality Framework

The EUSTACEA Charter and WeDO Quality Framework both gained visibility at international level when AGE was invited to present its work in the field of human rights at the 4th Meeting of the United Nations Open Ended Working Group on the Rights of Older People and at the Council of Europe Drafting Group on the Rights of the Elderly, in 2012. Both the Charter and the Quality Framework were well received in these international fora because they had been developed with considerable civil society consultation, building a consensus on the human rights challenges of older people in long-term care.

As demonstrated in the European Commission staff working document entitled 'Long-term care in ageing societies—challenges and policy options', published in 2013, there is an increasing interest among EU policy makers in working together on improving long-term care to help member states cope with the expected growing numbers of dependent older people. The Social Protection Committee Working Group on Ageing (SPC WG AGE) has released, in June 2014, a report on long-term care in Europe. International organizations such as the Organisation for Economic Co-operation and Development (OECD), the United Nations, the World Health Organization, and the Council of Europe are also increasingly working on this issue.

Next steps in improving quality of long-term care

Improving the quality of long-term care as a means to protect older people's rights to live and die in dignity remains a key priority of the AGE campaign for a society for all ages, i.e. a society where everyone is valued and empowered to participate in the community regardless of their age. AGE seized the opportunity of the launch of the European Innovation Partnership on Active and Healthy Ageing (EIP AHA) to press for work to start on age-friendly environments, in cooperation with the World Health Organization, promoting a holistic vision of active and healthy ageing as being 'the process of optimizing opportunities for physical, social and mental health to enable older people to take an active part in society without discrimination and to enjoy an independent and good quality of life' (7). AGE's call was heard by the European Commission and supported by the EIP AHA Steering Group. This is how Action Group D4 was created, bringing together all stakeholders interested in working cooperatively on the promotion of age-friendly environments in a broader sense.

In 2013, together with a large consortium of stakeholders representing regions, cities, research centres, and civil society organizations from 16 countries, AGE applied for EU funding to set up an EU thematic network on age-friendly environments and launch an EU Covenant on Demographic Change. This project, called AFE-INNOVNET, was selected for funding by the European Commission and started its work on 1 February 2014. The project is setting up a large EU-wide community of local and regional authorities and other relevant stakeholders across the EU who want to work together to find smart and innovative evidence-based solutions to support active and healthy ageing and develop age-friendly environments. The project will also pay particular attention to the specific needs of the growing number of older people with dementia and their carers.

This work is being done in close cooperation with WHO, which provides technical expertise and documents to support the EU network on age-friendly environments. The ultimate aim of the project is to develop a strong movement across the EU for the promotion of age-friendly environments, using the relevant EU policy processes and funding instruments to share experience and pool resources, and to become the WHO Global Network of Age-Friendly Cities and Communities programme for the EU area.

Conclusion

Developing age-friendly environments in Europe will require coordinated efforts to adapt our everyday living and working environments to the needs of Europe's ageing population in order to empower people to age in better physical and mental health, to promote their social inclusion and active participation, and to help them maintain their autonomy and a good quality of life in their old age, including those who need care and assistance. Age-friendly environments therefore also imply the development of quality integrated health and long-term care that cover the needs of our ageing population from a life-course perspective, i.e. that coordinates preventive, curative, palliative, and end-of-life care in an approach that is patient-centred, respectful of the patient's right to self-determination and dignity, and empowering for those who need support and for their informal carers.

References

1 Social Protection Committee. *Voluntary European Quality Framework for Social Services*; European Commission, 2009.

2 European Commission. *Euro-barometer on Health and Long-term Care in the European Union*; Eurostat, 2008.

3 European Parliament. Resolution of 21 February 2008 on the demographic future of Europe [2007/2156 (INI)].

4 AGE Platform Europe, EUSTACEA project, European Charter of the rights and responsibilities of older people in need of care and assistance, 2010.

5 WeDO project, European Quality Framework for long-term care services, 2012, p. 10.

6 WeDO project, European Quality Framework for long-term care services, 2012, p. 17.

7 World Health Organization website, Ageing and Life Course, "what is active ageing", 2014.

Chapter 24

Care pathways for older people in need of palliative care

Clare Gardiner, Tony Ryan, Merryn Gott, and Christine Ingleton

Introduction to care pathways for older people in need of palliative care

Alongside the rise of palliative medicine as a medical specialty, the introduction of care pathways has been one solution to improving care and dignity at the end of life. Care pathways first appeared in the United States in the 1970s (1, 2), and since then usage has become internationally widespread (3). Definitions of what constitutes a care pathway lack consistency, however within Europe, the European Pathway Association has been established in order to support consistent development, implementation, and evaluation of care pathways. They provided a consensus definition of care pathways: multi-component interventions intended to facilitate decision making and organization of care for a well-defined group of patients over a well-defined period (4). Within the field of palliative care, a number of key drivers, including concerns about hospital-based care and issues addressing the needs of older people, have prompted the development of systematic approaches towards end-of-life care (5, 6).

This chapter provides an overview of existing care pathways in palliative care, including both those which focus on the dying phase and those intended to provide care over a longer trajectory. We then consider the specific needs of older people with dementia and examine issues relating to the development of care pathways for older people. An analysis of the evidence base is provided, and recommendations are made for future development and implementation.

Overview of existing care pathways in palliative and end-of-life care

In this section, we will address particular aspects, strengths, and weaknesses of some of the most influential care pathways within the field of palliative and end-of-life care. Box 24.1 first provides the characteristics of care pathways in palliative and end-of-life care to highlight what we see as the common features of those pathways included in this chapter.

Box 24.1 Characteristics of care pathways in palliative and end-of-life care

- **Training and education**: Within pathways, these can be used at the beginning, or indeed throughout, the patient experience. Educational activities are shown to relate to the needs of family members in helping them to locate their loved one's experience in the illness trajectory. Training is included to help in the preparation of clinical staff in the use of guidelines or, more generally, around end-of-life issues.

- **Assessment**: All care pathways include a significant emphasis upon initial and on-going assessment. Initial assessment includes methods to indicate prognosis or palliative care need. In some cases, assessment is used to highlight particular issues which may have a significant bearing on care planning, such as mental capacity. On-going assessment focuses on physical, psychological, and spiritual needs.

- **Advance care planning**: This may include the preparation and completion of preferences and also the facilitation of advance care planning processes. In some care pathways, this specifically includes guidance on the convening of meetings with patients and carers and the skilful elicitation of preferences.

- **Recording activity**: Some pathways are more focused on this aspect of their guidance. The recording of care interventions, alongside medication, is of course consistent with standard clinical practice, but pathways of this nature also include reference to the importance of recording information exchanges, preferences, and, in some cases, variances from plans.

- **Interdisciplinary communication**: All pathways within the palliative and supportive care field view communication across the team as being essential in maintaining care plans and strategies which might promote high-quality care and the fidelity of patient preferences and plans. Some include specific tools to facilitate good communication.

One of the earliest examples of a care pathway for end-of-life care was developed as part of the Study to Understand Prognoses and Preferences for Outcomes and Risks of Treatment (SUPPORT) study, which was aimed at improving end-of-life care for patients in hospitals in the United States. The SUPPORT intervention involved a specially trained nurse eliciting patient preferences, improving understanding of outcomes, improving pain control, and facilitating advance care planning (7). Despite its evidence-based development, a controlled trial of SUPPORT was unable to demonstrate any improvements in care or patient outcomes as a result of its implementation. One of the conclusions was that such pathways may be more successful with physician leaders rather than nurse leaders as implementers (7). More recently, a physician-led Inpatient Comfort Care Pathway was developed to implement the perceived best practices of American hospice care in an inpatient setting (8). A before–after intervention trial of an Inpatient Comfort Care Pathway indicated increased documentation of symptoms and improved processes of care after implementation. However, the authors were keen to highlight that paradigm shifts in hospital culture were necessary to assure successful implementation (7, 8).

Care pathways for older people with dementia

People with dementia have been shown to experience multiple co-morbidities at the end of life (9, 10) and to receive sub-optimal care during this period. There is overwhelming evidence that people with dementia experience interventions which seek to prolong life at the expense of palliation, indicating poor transition to palliative regimes of care (11). A number of innovations, in the form of pathways, have been developed to overcome these difficulties. In the United States, the Palliative Excellence in Alzheimer's Care Efforts (PEACE) (12) programme is notable in that it seeks to bring together advanced planning, family support, and a palliative emphasis from diagnosis to the end of life. Based within the community, it has demonstrated some evidence of acceptability and improved outcome in that two thirds of the people with dementia included in the original evaluation died in their own homes. Aminoff (2008) developed Relief of Suffering Units for people in the last month of life, with the aim of providing intensive palliative and supportive care to enable people with dementia to die with dignity (13). Although this approach is not defined as a pathway, its intention is to support those patients meeting specific mini mental state examination (MMSE) criteria and to provide patient-centred care. A recent study identified the need to move beyond task-focused approaches to enhance person-centred care approaches, as well as enriched relationships with families, as the key cornerstones to improving end-of-life care for people with dementia (14). Unlike other pathways and interventions, the evidence of effectiveness for such ways of working within a dementia context is limited.

Palliative care pathways

The majority of palliative and end-of-life care pathways focus on patients in the dying phase, yet there is significant potential for improving and standardizing care for patients who have palliative care needs but who are not imminently dying. A number of recent interventions from the United Kingdom have attempted to fulfil this potential. The Gold Standards Framework is a quality improvement training programme and framework to enable frontline generalist care providers to deliver a 'gold standard' of care for people nearing the end of life (15). Whilst a range of evidence has been published in support of the Gold Standards Framework, including demonstrated reductions in hospital admissions and improved quality of care, there have been some criticisms over the variable quality of the evidence to support its wider implementation (16).

The Assessment Management Best practice Engagement Recovery uncertain (AMBER) Care Bundle is a more recent development which aims to provide a systematic approach to managing the care of hospital patients who are facing an uncertain recovery and who are at risk of dying in the next one to two months (17). The 'bundle' concept is different from a care pathway in that it combines a small number of specific components or actions to improve care. Early pilot work has indicated positive outcomes (18), and formal prospective evaluation is now required to support widespread implementation (19).

The Route to Success for End-of-life Care in Care Homes was developed in the United Kingdom by the National End-of-life Care Programme in 2010. It specifically addresses the needs of patients in care homes, and aims to enhance the quality of care provided at the end of life. The six-step approach aims to reduce unplanned admissions and ensure residents' wishes and preferences are met wherever possible (20). The principles of Route to Success are clearly underpinned by best practice guidance. However, the extent to which this has translated to improved patient care is unclear without robust research evidence.

The Liverpool Care Pathway for the Dying

By far the most influential and widely adopted end-of-life care pathway, internationally, is the Liverpool Care Pathway for the Dying (LCP) (21). The LCP was developed in the United Kingdom in the 1990s and was designed to transfer the high standard of palliative care established in hospices to other clinical settings, in particular the acute hospital. It provides guidelines for best practice focusing on symptom control, frequent reassessment, appropriate discontinuation of active treatments, and psychological, social, and spiritual care of patients in the last three days of life (22). Following its development, the LCP was widely adopted across the United Kingdom under the backing of the End-of-life Care Programme (23). It has since been translated into many languages and adopted across Europe, with adapted versions being utilized internationally, including in the United States (24), New Zealand (25), and Australia (26).

Although widely adopted and presenting strong face validity, a British media campaign which claimed the LCP was a 'pathway to euthanasia' (22) led to an independent review of the LCP in 2013 (27). Whilst noting the worthy principles which underpin the LCP, the review recommended that it be discontinued and replaced with individual care plans backed up with disease-specific guidance (27). Concerns were not with the LCP itself, but rather with the fact that it was not being implemented properly in all cases. Of particular concern was the treatment of older patients: evidence in the review suggested that age discrimination, assumed mental incapacity, and variability of care in nursing homes were in evidence. Underpinning the recommendations of the review was the lack of an evidence base for the LCP (27). More recently, a landmark Italian study reported the results of the first cluster randomized trial of the LCP. The findings showed that after implementation of the LCP programme in an Italian hospital, no significant difference was noted in the overall quality of care scores between the LCP wards and the control wards (28). Further studies on the effectiveness of the LCP, with careful consideration of implementation issues, are being conducted in several other countries.

Care pathways for older people

That older people have specific needs at the end of life is now well established. However, concerns have been raised as to whether traditional models of palliative care are appropriate for an older population (29, 30). Although the Route to Success has been developed for use in care homes where mainly older people reside, none of the other pathways described here provide specific guidance on how they should be implemented with an older population and if, or how, they should be modified to be appropriate for older people.

In a recent systematic review which aimed to synthesize evidence relating to the efficacy of care pathways, it was found that they are more effective in contexts where care is specific to a diagnostic group and, therefore, predictable (31). Clearly in the context of palliative care for older people, 'diagnosing dying' and providing appropriate care is less than predictable. Therefore, to date, care pathways have mainly been limited to monitoring older people with a specific and discrete diagnosis or disease. Additionally, care pathways have been generally aimed at short-term care patients, requiring high service volumes or expensive procedures, or those who are at high risk of complications (32). However, the uncertainty and unpredictability of dying trajectories in late old age and for those with co-morbidities means that individuals may experience a number of episodes where they may be perceived to be dying, but survive. This calls for the development and maintenance of cross-boundary care pathways that are easily accessible, with systems which allow information linking and sharing, using common templates, across multiple agencies and across a diversity of care settings. This presents difficult challenges for clinicians, health care managers, and policy makers.

The evidence base for care pathways

Crucial to the successful implementation of care pathways is robust evidence on effectiveness and acceptability to patients, families, and professionals. Early care pathways reported mixed results with regard to clinical effectiveness (7, 8). Various suggestions have been made as to why these pathways have only been able to demonstrate limited success. One key issue is a perceived lack of individual and collective commitment to achieving the goals of improved end-of-life care (7, 8). Issues with staff engagement, a death-denying or cure culture, and a lack of commitment to the goals of palliative care are well recognized as barriers to the provision of optimum palliative care, especially with relation to the care of older people (6). Addressing these complex issues requires a whole-systems approach and innovative methods for engaging staff.

A number of recent systematic reviews provide further evidence regarding the efficacy and effectiveness of care pathways for end-of-life care. The majority of review evidence focuses on the LCP or variants, and whilst most studies support the utility of care pathways, the lack of robust comparative evidence precludes any definitive recommendations (1, 33, 34). Whilst care pathways may well offer potential to enhance end-of-life care, the state of knowledge regarding end-of-life care pathways is still in its infancy.

Driven in part by lessons learned from the review of the LCP, a number of suggestions have been made for the implementation of any future palliative care pathways. These include improved awareness of the vulnerability to misinterpretation; addressing the challenges to the prevailing culture of medicine; a greater need for intensive and ongoing training; ensuring interventions are patient-centred; and removing financial incentives (20). Ultimately, an integrated multi-professional approach and an open, flexible, and participative culture is required, otherwise they may be viewed as a 'paper exercise' and merely another type of clinical audit tool—an approach to care that does not seem to resonate with the philosophical statements about the individuality of patient care needs at the end of life.

Conclusion on care pathways for older people in need of palliative care

A wide range of care pathways have been developed and implemented over the years but none have been developed specifically for older people. Since the evidence base for effectiveness is generally weak, the field of palliative care needs to respond by ensuring interventions are developed, implemented, and, most importantly, evaluated in line with the best possible evidence.

Some of the evidence suggests that the issue is not with care pathways per se, but with their appropriate implementation. This highlights a need to focus not only on pathway development, but also on ways to ensure continued engagement and pathway facilitation in order to achieve pathway aims. Therefore, pathway development needs to consider the full range of requirements and include supporting infrastructure and communication tools, if pathways are to be successfully implemented (32).

For older people in particular, the high prevalence of chronic conditions, dementia, and frailty, together with long and unpredictable trajectories, means that care pathways are hard to deliver. Cross-boundary care pathways are required which are accessible, practical, and well supported, in order to allow information sharing across multiple agencies in multiple care settings. Pathways should engage not only with the clinical staff who are delivering the intervention, but also with the wider public and media, in order to avoid criticisms of the kind directed at the LCP. There is still much to recommend care pathways for older people at the end of life, but it is the implementation, communication, and evaluation that need closer attention as we move forward.

References

1 **Parry R, Seymour J, Whittaker B, Bird L, Cox K.** *Rapid Evidence Review: Pathways Focused on the Dying phase in End-of-life Care and Their Key Components.* London, UK: National End of Life Care Programme; 2013.

2 **Coffey RJ, Richards JS, Remmert CS, LeRoy SS, Schoville RR, Baldwin PJ.** An introduction to critical pathways. *QMHC* 2005; **14**(1):46–55.

3 **Vanhaecht K, Ovretveit J, Ellot MJ, Sermeus W, Ellershaw J, Panella M.** Have we drawn the wrong conclusions about the value of care pathways? Is a Cochrane Review appropriate? *EHP* 2012; **35**(1):28–42.

4 **European Pathway Association.** *Clinical/Care Pathways*; 2007. Available at: <http://www.e-p-a.org/clinical---care-pathways/index.html> (Accessed May 2014). Ref. type: online source.

5 **Gardiner C, Cobb M, Gott M, Ingleton C.** Barriers to the provision of palliative care for older people in acute hospitals. *Age & Ageing* 2011; **40**:233–8.

6 Connors AF, Jr, Dawson NV, Desbiens NA, et al. A controlled trial to improve care for seriously ill hospitalized patients: the Study to Understand Prognoses and Preferences for Outcomes and Risks of Treatments (SUPPORT). *JAMA* 1995; **274**(20):1591–8.

7 Bailey FA, Burgio KL, Woodby LL, Williams BR, Redden DT, Kovac SH, et al. Improving processes of hospital care during the last hours of life. *Arch Intern Med* 2005; **165**(22):1722–7.

8 Ryan T, Ingleton C, Gardiner C, Parker, Gott M, Noble B. Symptom burden, palliative care need and predictors of physical and psychological discomfort in two UK hospitals. *BMC Palliat Care*, 2013; **12**:11.

9 Sampson E, Burns A, Richards M. Improving end-of-life care for people with dementia. *Br J Psychiatry* 2011; **199**:357–9.

10 Ryan T, Gardiner C, Bellamy G, Gott M, Ingleton C, and nursing staff. Barriers and facilitators to the receipt of palliative care for people with dementia: the views of medical and nursing staff. *Palliat Med* 2012; **26**(7):879–86.

11 Shega JW, Levin A, Hougham GW, Cox-Hayley D, Luchins D, Hanrahan P, et al. Palliative Excellence in Alzheimer Care Efforts (PEACE): a program description. *J Palliat Med* 2003; **6**(2):315–20.

12 Aminoff BZ. End-stage dementia: Aminoff Suffering Syndrome and Relief of Suffering Units. *Open Geriatr Med J*; 2008, **1**:29–32.

13 Lawrence V, Samsi K, Murray J, Harari D, Banerjee S. Dying well with dementia: qualitative examination of end-of-life care. *Br J Psychiatry* 2011; **199**:417–2.

14 Ellershaw J, Ward C. Care of the dying: the last hours or days of life. *BMJ* 2003; **326**:30–4.

15 Beeston L. *Gold Standards Framework Literature Search Part A—Tabulated Account of Reviewed Published Articles*; 2013. Available at: <http://www.goldstandardsframework.org.uk/cd-content/uploads/files/Part%20A%20%20GSF%20Lit%20search%20-%20%20Tabulated%20account%20of%20reviewed%20published%20articles%20Sept%202013.pdf> (Accessed February 2014). Ref. type: online source.

16 Carey I, Hopper A, Morris M. A care bundle to improve end-of-life care in hospitals. *BMJ* 2010; **340**:c3231.

17 National End of Life Care Programme (NEOLCP). *Newsletter*. Leicester, UK: NEOLCP; July 2011.

18 Currow DC, Higginson I. Time for a prospective study to evaluate the Amber Care Bundle. *BMJ Support Palliat Care* 2013; **3**(4):376–7.

19 The End of Life Care Programme. *Route to Success in End of Life Care—Achieving Quality in Care Homes*. London, UK: Department of Health; 2010.

20 Boockvar KS, Meier DE. Palliative care for frail older adults: 'there are things I can't do anymore that I wish I could'. *JAMA* 2006; **296**(18):2245–53.

21 Barclay S. The Liverpool Care Pathway for the dying: what went wrong? *Br J Gen Pract* 2013; **63**(615):509–10.

22 Department of Health. *End of Life Care Strategy for England*. London, UK: Department of Health; 2008.

23 Billings JA, Block SD. The demise of the Liverpool Care Pathway? A cautionary tale for palliative care. *J Palliat Med* 2013; **16**(12):1492–5.

24 Royal Australian College of General Practitioners. *Medical Care of Older Persons in Residential Aged Care Facilities (Silver Book)*; 2013. Available at: <http://www.racgp.org.au/your-practice/guidelines/silverbook/general-approach-to-medical-care-of-residents/palliative-and-end-of-life-care/> (Accessed May 2014). Ref. type: online source.

25 New Zealand Ministry of Health. *The New Zealand Palliative Care Strategy*.Wellington, New Zealand: Ministry of Health; 2001.

26 Neuberger J, Guthrie C, Aaronovitch D, Hameed K, Bonser T, Harries R, et al. *'More Care Less Pathway': An Independent Review of the Liverpool Care Pathway*; 2013. https://www.gov.uk/government/publications/review-of-liverpool-care-pathway-for-dying-patients.

27 Costantini M, Romoli V, Di Leo S, Beccaro M, Bono L, Pilastri P, et al. Liverpool Care Pathway for patients with cancer in hospital: a cluster randomised trial. *Lancet* 2014; **383**(9913):226–37.

28 Thomas K. The Gold Standards Framework in community palliative care. *Eur J Palliat Care* 2003; **10**(3):113–5.

29 Fried LP, Tangen CM, Walston A, Newman AB, Hirsch C, Gottdiener J, et al. Frailty in older adults: evidence for a phenotype. *J Gerontology* 2001; **56**(3):M145–56.

30 Allen D, Gillen E, Rixson L. The effectiveness of ICPs for adults and children in health care settings: a systematic review. *JBI Reports* 2009; **7**:80–129.

31 Dubuc N, Bonin L, Tourigny A, Mathieu L, Couturier Y, Tousignant M, et al. Development of integrated care pathways: toward a care management system to meet the needs of frail and disabled community-dwelling older people. *Int J Integr Care* 2013; **13**:e017.

32 Phillips JL, Halcomb EJ, Davidson PM. End-of-life care pathways in acute and hospice care: an integrative review. *J Pain Symptom Manage* 2011; **41**(5):940–55.

33 Watts T. End-of-life care pathways and nursing: a literature review. *J Nurs Manag* 2013; **21**(1):47–57.

34 Chan R, Webster J. End-of-life care pathways for improving outcomes in caring for the dying. *Cochrane Database of Systematic Reviews* 2010; **1**(CD008006).

Chapter 25

A programme for advance care planning for older people: Respecting Patient Choices

William Silvester and Karen Detering

Introduction to the Respecting Patient Choices programme

The Respecting Patient Choices® programme (1) is a leading advance care planning (ACP) programme in Australia. Based at the Austin Hospital in Melbourne, it began in 2002 as a pilot programme, with the assistance of the Respecting Choices® programme in La Crosse, Wisconsin, United States. Through funding from the Australian federal government and various Australian state and territorial governments, it has extended to numerous other hospitals and residential aged care facilities throughout Australia. Although there is different legislation on ACP and end-of-life care in each Australian state and territory, the Respecting Patient Choices programme was implemented throughout Australia by relying on the legislative and common law respect for autonomy and advance care directives (1, 2). The common law in Australia also supports respect for patient control over their end-of-life care (3, 4). Support for ACP and end-of-life care is now enshrined in specific legislation in each state and territory, except New South Wales (1).

This chapter will describe the evolution of Respecting Patient Choices, including implementation of advance care planning in hospitals and the community, and the research supporting the benefits of advance care planning and delivery to older people, both in hospitals and aged care homes.

Components of the Respecting Patient Choices programme

The Respecting Patient Choices programme (1) promotes a model of coordinated ACP, whereby trained non-medical facilitators, in collaboration with treating doctors, assist patients and their families to reflect on the patient's goals, values, and beliefs, and to discuss and document their future choices about health care. In this approach, patients are encouraged to appoint a substitute decision maker and to clearly document their treatment preferences and minimal acceptable outcomes in an advance care directive. Patients are also encouraged to include their family, particularly the nominated substitute decision maker, in their discussions, so that others can hear firsthand what the person's wishes are, and how they have arrived at these decisions. Once completed, copies of the advance care directive are distributed to relevant family members and to treating doctors and hospitals, so that they can easily be retrieved in the future. Further essential components of the Respecting Patient Choices® programme include systematic education of doctors, a systems approach to physical and electronic storage of the advance care directive in a patient's medical record, and programme evaluation and quality improvement.

A randomized controlled trial of coordinated advance care planning

In 2010, a randomized controlled trial, assessing the impact of coordinated ACP on end-of-life care in older patients, was published in the British Medical Journal (5). In this study of 304 legally-competent medical in-patients aged at least 80 years, half received coordinated ACP using the Respecting Patient Choices model. The ACP conversation included the following elements:

+ Clarifying the patient's understanding of their illness and treatment options.
+ Identifying (and appointing) their preferred substitute decision maker.
+ Discussing their goals and values, in relation to their illness and future.
+ Identifying their views regarding an acceptable outcome from treatment.
+ Considering particular treatments that they would *not* want.

This conversation took a median of 60 minutes over one to three meetings. For those study patients who died, the end-of-life wishes were known and respected in 86% of the patients in the intervention group and only 30% of the control group (p < 0.001).

This study also showed that ACP improves end-of-life-care, patient and family satisfaction with care, and family satisfaction with the quality of their family member's death. Furthermore, it showed that ACP significantly reduced the incidence of clinically significant symptoms of anxiety, depression, and post-traumatic stress disorder in surviving relatives of patients who died. This was thought to occur because the family were involved in the ACP discussion, were aware of their family member's wishes, felt less burdened by decision making, played a role in ensuring that the doctors were aware of and complied with those wishes, and were satisfied with the end-of-life care.

New developments in Respecting Patient Choices

Since 2010, the predominant provision of ACP by Respecting Patient Choices has been by non-medical facilitators, with accumulated experience of providing ACP to more than 5000 patients. Although old patients and those with poor prognoses are targeted, including those with cancer, frailty, and chronic illness, the service is available to all patients, including those undergoing surgery. In the British Medical Journal study (5) only English-speaking competent patients were included. Subsequently, in consideration of the cultural diversity of the Australian population (27% of the current population was born overseas), ACP has been successfully delivered to patients from a variety of ethnic backgrounds who speak a range of languages. ACP is also successfully delivered to non-competent patients, such as those with dementia. In such cases, although the non-competent person is included in the discussion to the best of their ability, the person's family and substitute decision maker play the active role in the ACP discussion and completion of an advance care directive specifically designed for those who are no longer competent. The research confirms that, for non-English speaking and non-competent people, ACP can be undertaken just as effectively, and it emphasizes the importance of including the person's family in the discussions. This is crucial because the person, particularly the older one, turns to the family for guidance and support in such personal and intimate discussions and because the family needs to be aware of the older person's deliberations, decisions, and reasons as they, the family, will be the people contacted by the health professionals when important decisions need to be made.

In 2004 and 2005, the Respecting Patient Choices model of ACP was piloted in 17 aged care homes located in close proximity to the Austin Hospital (6). An important element of this model in these homes comprised engagement with senior management in each aged care home to ensure support for the required system changes and staff training. The system changes included:

a) writing of ACP policies and procedures,

b) involvement of general practitioners in the discussions and completion of advance care directives, and

c) appropriate filing of the advance care directives, completed by the competent residents or by the families on behalf of the non-competent residents, so that they were prominent and easily found when required.

Training was delivered to senior nurses who would normally be involved with overseeing the nursing care of the residents. The two-day training experiential workshop included:

a) teaching on the theory and legalities of ACP,

b) small group discussions about the more difficult aspects of end-of-life care in residential aged care, and

c) role plays to practise the ACP discussion and completion of advance care directives.

Of more than one thousand of the residents in these 17 facilities, just over half were introduced to ACP by the facility staff. Of all those introduced, only 2% refused further discussion, which defies those critics of ACP who purport that older people, and their families, do not want to have a say about their future health care. Indeed, the majority of those who curtailed discussions were the family members of non-competent residents who were clearly struggling to contemplate the mortality of their old parents.

Of those introduced to ACP, more than half completed advance care directives, with the majority being completed by families of residents who had lost capacity to make decisions. The most common request in the advance care directives was for no life-prolonging measures in the event of illness and good symptom and pain management, with only one in five requesting hospital transfer in the event of deterioration.

Nearly 90% of the residents who died had advance care directives and the wishes of all but a few were respected at the end of life. Importantly, of those who did not participate in ACP, nearly 50% were transferred to hospital to die, compared to less than one in five of those who had participated in ACP. Furthermore, interviews revealed that there was a high level of satisfaction regarding ACP with the residents, family, staff, and general practitioners who participated.

The Respecting Patient Choices model has also been successfully applied to chronic disease (chronic obstructive pulmonary disease, chronic heart failure, chronic renal failure), oncology, and surgical patients.

Training on Respecting Patient Choices

Care for older people around the world, including Australia (7), is replete with examples of people receiving medical treatment that they did not want and was not in their best interests. This is particularly relevant to older residents of residential aged care facilities, the majority of whom have dementia, chronic illnesses, or significant frailty. The most common barriers to providing good end-of-life care in aged care are: uncertainty about what the old person would want; family guilt or paralysis about making difficult decisions; lack of skills or comfort of the aged care staff in discussing end-of-life care and the need to make timely and appropriate decisions for the old person; and the absence of a systematic approach to identifying and managing the dying resident. Furthermore, the staff may be impeded by the lack of support from the person's family doctor who also lacks the skills on how to handle decisions at the end of life and who may have difficulty distinguishing between a new condition, that warrants treatment, and a deterioration, which heralds the fact that the patient is dying and should be kept comfortable and be allowed to die in a dignified way. All of these barriers can be addressed by adequate systems to support and encourage ACP and by up-skilling the aged care providers and the general practitioners in the delivery of ACP and end-of-life care in the aged care setting (7).

Hundreds of aged care staff have been trained, in many states of Australia. Over time, changes have been made to the training to improve the sustainability of the ACP practice. These have included:

a) development of an aged care-specific advance care directive (8),

b) separation of the two days of the workshop by several weeks to give the participants time to practise their ACP discussion skills before returning to share their experience and learn from their colleagues, and

c) the need for the participants to complete 'homework', including formulation of ACP policies for their aged care facilities, engagement with local general practitioners, and meetings with other participants to encourage peer support and build supportive networks.

Sustainability is also supported by ensuring that the provision of ACP and palliative care is built into the accreditation of aged care facilities. Satisfying certain accreditation criteria to meet minimum standards has raised the profile of, and interest in, ACP and led to many requests for information and training.

The Respecting Patient Choices training programme for all health care staff (predominantly nurses, but inclusive of doctors and allied health staff) was originally a 16-hour interactive workshop over two sequential days. Although the workshop was very well received, about 10 years ago, the theory and didactic teaching of ACP (including ethics and law, video clips, and on-line testing) were inserted into an e-learning module, followed by a one-day experiential workshop which consists of facilitated discussions and role play and focuses primarily on 'how to have the conversation'. During the workshop, all participants are expected to actively engage in role play as the facilitator, complete a full ACP discussion, and document the outcome of this discussion in an advance care directive. A major benefit of this change is that the participants can learn the theory at their own pace and at their own convenience and at times suitable for their employers.

The evaluated outcomes of this training have shown that the education programme is extremely valuable in helping staff develop confidence and competence to facilitate ACP conversations. Regular evaluation enables ongoing development and improvement of the training.

The Respecting Patient Choices model of ACP education also includes guidance for health care services to introduce the system changes required for successful organization-wide implementation of ACP, and to conduct their own facilitator training programmes, thereby encouraging future sustainability of ACP implementation (1). The Respecting Patient Choices model also encourages ACP facilitator mentoring, whereby 'new' ACP facilitators can observe experienced facilitators conducting ACP discussions.

The most recent innovation has been the production of an interactive multimodality training programme specifically designed for junior doctors and general practitioners to build their confidence and ability to conduct ACP discussions with their patients. The training package comprises pre-reading materials on ACP theory, a DVD, an interactive e-simulation, and a 2–3 hour experiential workshop with an accompanying workshop facilitator manual. The DVD contains scenarios showing real general practitioners discussing ACP with actor patients, with both 'good' and 'bad' ACP conversations, accompanied by expert commentary. There are also recorded ACP discussions between hospital doctors and actual patients. The educational package follows an evidence-based, stepwise approach to ACP. It demonstrates improvement in doctors' confidence in undertaking ACP discussions with patients, and improved their performance on the patient e-simulation. The materials were rated highly and acceptable to the participants (9).

Large-scale implementation of the Respecting Patient Choices programme

In 2013, the Australian federal government funded Respecting Patient Choices to lead a consortium of eight organizations in a Aus$15 million, three-year project to improve the delivery of end-of-life care to older Australians receiving aged care in aged care homes or within their own homes (through 'home care packages'). The Decision Assist Programme (10) comprises:

a) a 24/7 telephone advisory service to health professionals on palliative care,

b) an 'office hours' telephone advisory service to health professionals for ACP,

c) workshops on ACP and palliative care to aged care nurses,

d) education for general practitioners on ACP and palliative care for older people,

e) innovative ways of building linkages between aged care and palliative care, and

f) information technology resources including a website and a smart phone app.

There is a strong interest in such training from aged care nurses, reflecting their commitment to high quality of care to older people and their recognition that improving the provision of such care assists the aged care providers to meet the accreditation standards set by the Australian federal government.

There is much enthusiasm in the health industry for this initiative, with the overall aim of improving end-of-life care for older people and enabling them to receive this care in their normal abode, if that is their choice. By recognizing the time pressures on general practitioners in their daily work, and by giving the aged care nursing staff the skills, the comfort, and the authorization to talk to older people about what they want (and do not want) near the end of life and then to meet those wishes when the time comes, this injection of funds, into a hitherto neglected area of health care, is a welcome and exciting opportunity.

Having observed, in the hospital setting, with the increasing illness acuity and reducing length of stay of patients, that nurses and allied health staff struggle to include ACP in their normal daily workload, the majority of ACP is conducted by trained nurses who are specifically employed to complete this task. For example, in the renal unit, a nurse who works in the dialysis unit three days per week is paid to deliver ACP to the dialysis-dependent patients two days per week. This same arrangement is in place in other clinical units such as cardiology, respiratory, aged care, and general medicine. The benefits of this model are that the funded ACP facilitators are protected from other clinical work, become expert at ACP discussions and completion of advance care directives, are seen as a resource by other hospital staff, and have the confidence of the medical staff to engage with their patients on such crucial elements of care as patient-initiated treatment limitation.

Conclusion on the Respecting Patient Choices programme

The Respecting Patient Choices programme, established in 2002, has succeeded in implementing ACP in both the acute sector and in aged care and, also, in building the evidence for the benefits of ACP and in the feasibility of delivering ACP in different settings, populations, and disease groups. The recognition of the benefits of ACP for the burgeoning older population is reflected in the government funding to support ACP being undertaken in the community, specifically with general practitioners and in aged care settings. The secret to gaining funding is to:

a) start small and demonstrate success,

b) work with health departments and policy makers to develop national, state, and local policy,

c) gain the attention of the politicians by emphasizing the quality imperative,

d) conduct rigorous publishable research, and

e) engage the media to sell your 'good news' story.

It is also essential to work with doctors who are crucial to the acceptance of ACP.

References

1 Advance Care Planning Australia. Available at: <http://advancecareplanning.org.au/> (Accessed June 2014]. Ref. type: online source.

2 National Advance Care Directives Working Group. *A National Framework for Advance Care Directives*; September 2011. Available at: <http://www.ahmac.gov.au/cms_documents/AdvanceCareDirectives2011.pdf> (Accessed June 2014). Ref. type: online source.

3 The Supreme Court of Western Australia. *Bright Water Care Group (Inc) v Rossiter.* Available at: <http://www.supremecourt.wa.gov.au/_files/proceedings.pdf> (Accessed June 2014). Ref. type: online source.

4 Ellis G. *The right of self-determination: Brightwater Care Group (Inc) v Rossiter. The University of Notre Dame Australia Law Review 209.* UNDAULawRw 9; 2010, 12. Available at: <http://www.austlii.edu.au/au/journals/UNDAULawRw/2010/9.pdf> (Accessed June 2014). Ref. type: online source.

5 Detering KM, Hancock AD, Reade MC, Silvester W. The impact of advance care planning on end of life care in elderly patients: randomised controlled trial. *BMJ* 2010; **340**:c1345.

6 Austin Health. *Final Evaluation of the Community Implementation of the Respecting Patient Choices Program.* Austin Health; Melbourne, 2006.

7 Scott IA, Mitchell GK, Reymond EJ, Daly MP. Difficult but necessary conversations—the case for advance care planning. *Med J Aust* 2013; **199**(10):662–6.

8 Silvester W, Parslow RA, Lewis VJ, Fullam RS, Sjanta R, Jackson L, et al. Development and evaluation of an aged care specific advance care plan. *BMJ Support Palliat Care* 2013; **3**(2):188–95.

9 Detering K, Silvester W, Corke C, Milnes S, Fullam R, Lewis V, et al. Teaching general practitioners and doctors-in-training to discuss advance care planning: evaluation of a brief multimodality education programme. *BMJ Support Palliat Care* 2014; **4**(3):313–21.

10 Palliative Care Australia. Available at: <http://www.palliativecare.org.au/DecisionAssist.aspx> (Accessed 15 June 2014). Ref. type: online source.

Part VI

Conclusion: what does a public health approach to improving palliative care for older people look like?

Chapter 26

A public health approach to improving palliative care for older people

Sandra Martins Pereira, Gwenda Albers, Roeline Pasman, Bregje Onwuteaka-Philipsen, Luc Deliens, and Lieve Van den Block

Introduction to a public health approach to improving palliative care for older people

This book provides a wide range of information to help societies to plan, organize, and provide appropriate care for the growing numbers of older people living and dying with multiple chronic diseases. Many authors from different countries and several continents around the world have made valuable contributions, helping us to provide insights into the current state of policy work, research, and innovations in the field of public health and palliative care for older people. The attention given to palliative care is increasing and, with the ageing of populations, the recognition of palliative care as a public health priority is expanding. In the beginning of 2014, a ground-breaking resolution on the need for strengthening palliative care as a component of integrated treatment within the continuum of care was adopted by the World Health Assembly of the World Health Organization (WHO), defining broad recommendations to member states and the Director-General of the World Health Organization (1).

In this final chapter, we will elaborate on the growing evidence supporting a public health approach to palliative care for older people and build on and specify some of the WHO recommendations, using the contributions of the different authors brought together in this book. We first reflect on what and how palliative care can complement care for older people and summarize policy developments in palliative care before we formulate specific recommendations for policy and decision makers at international and national level in the field of palliative care for older people. These recommendations can support policy and decision makers at many levels; as described in Chapter 3, key drivers influencing change and development can be identified at individual, group/team, organizational, regional/network, and national levels.

Palliative care can strengthen and complement care for older people

With the ageing of populations, a growing number of people suffer from comorbidities and die from diseases other than cancer. Although palliative care has traditionally been focused on cancer patients, throughout this book, the contributors refer to the evidence that is emerging for the effectiveness of palliative care interventions in diseases other than cancer and the added value of its early introduction (2–9). Evidence has shown that a palliative care approach is highly effective in managing pain and physical symptoms, and can maintain quality of life and reduce the utilization of more costly health services (Chapters 9, 12, 17). In fact, although older people often experience high needs and symptom burden, as do their family members, they commonly miss out on the benefits of palliative care including social and spiritual support, advance care planning, and effective pain and symptom management throughout the trajectory preceding death (Chapters 12, 16, 22). The authors have stressed that further research on the needs for care and solutions specific to older people is important; however, the more pressing issue is to implement existing knowledge and to sustain changes in palliative care practice throughout health care systems. Although there has been quite a lot written about integrating palliative care into services and settings, as well as throughout health care systems (Chapter 4) (10), this has not yet been operationalized very far, nor implemented sufficiently, due probably to the complexity of integration at many different levels.

It can be argued that providing all older people with life-limiting illnesses with access to specialist palliative care or hospice services is not a sustainable or affordable health care model. In Chapter 17, Quill and Carroll elaborate on a generalist plus specialist palliative care model to ensure the efficient and effective provision of palliative care for all patients in need, including older people, a model that is considered to be sustainable in the long run. According to this model, all health care professionals need to develop and maintain basic palliative care skill sets and specialist palliative care is only used in complex situations. In this book, programmes such as the Liverpool Care Pathway, the Gold Standards Framework, the Route-to-Success, the AMBER Care Bundle, the Palliative Excellence in Alzheimer's Care Efforts (PEACE) (all described in Chapter 24), and the Respecting Patient Choices programme (presented in Chapter 25) are examples of how a palliative care approach can be integrated into care for older people.

Such a general plus specialist palliative care model is also in line with what, in 2003, the Council of Europe (11) recommended on the organization of palliative care, namely that all health care professionals should be familiar with the essential principles of palliative care and must apply these principles appropriately in their practice. Building this model requires effective educational interventions to establish first a minimum generalist palliative care level of competence among all health care professionals. Educational interventions to provide all health care providers with a minimum level of generalist palliative care competency may improve the detection of palliative care needs and increase appropriate referrals to palliative care specialists. This can facilitate further management and appropriate care provision for older people.

In addition, while palliative care can strengthen care for older people as just described, it could also be that palliative care specialists can learn more about caring for older people with several comorbid conditions including dementia and frailty. Palliative care specialists and members of specialist palliative care teams have been mostly involved and trained in caring for cancer patients. Therefore, these professionals may need continuing education on how to provide palliative care for older people who may have multiple conditions, cognitive deterioration, and experience prolonged illness trajectories. This has also been stressed by other researchers, such as in the field of neurology (12), in which the need for palliative care teams to receive specialist training for managing neurology patients is advocated. Both these neurology researchers and the American Geriatric Society (13) have also highlighted the potential for synergy and need for collaboration between their specialty and palliative care. Consequently, multidisciplinary collaboration (Chapter 21) between professionals and disciplines will be essential in future medicine, care, and education.

To integrate existing and new models of palliative care into health and social care systems, and to promote the development of palliative care in long-term care settings, governments need to address it within their policy-making structures in order to encourage regional and local bodies to develop and implement adequate policies on quality of and access to palliative care.

Palliative care for older people: policy developments

There are great differences across continents and countries in the state of development of palliative care policies in general, and in palliative care for older people in particular (Chapters 5 to 10). While national policies in Australia (Chapter 7), for example, continue to reflect demographic changes with the 2012 federally funded 'Living Longer—Living Better' aged care reform, including the development of palliative aged care advisory services to build capacity among care providers, in other regions of the world (e.g. Africa, Latin America, and the Caribbean), ageing has had a relatively low priority among national policy makers and palliative care provision remains poor. In other areas (e.g. Asia), country variations, from isolated provision to advanced integration of palliative care, are evident despite the overall sweeping demographic changes caused by falling mortality and rising life expectancy. Similar variations also exist between European countries. In this context, completely diverse health and social care systems coexist, challenging the configuration of a common strategy for guaranteeing coordination between health and social care services to diminish inequalities among (older) European citizens in regard to access to palliative care.

These differences, however, are not only affected by the demographic and epidemiological conditions of these countries, but also by, among other things, their socio-economic level of development and their cultural roots, posing diverse challenges to health and social care systems. In Asian countries, populations are ageing more rapidly than in many other countries, and care for older people is provided mainly by family members and domestic workers. Similar cultural patterns are described for regions such as Spain and other southern-European countries, where social models of care are highly affected by strong family ties. In addition, traditional medicine and healing activities in Africa often play an important role in end-of-life practices in this region.

As is the case in palliative care practice, policies on palliative care have also mainly focused on cancer patients and, much less often, on people suffering from other diseases or on older people. This is illustrated in all chapters about policy (except Chapter 5, which discusses how palliative care in Africa primarily focuses on patients suffering from HIV/AIDS). This is probably the reason why, in some regions (e.g. Asia), policies and palliative care programmes are rooted in cancer programmes. Policies on care for older people are often mainly focused on preventing diseases, promoting healthy and active ageing, and on rehabilitation, rather than on palliative care or improving the quality of life towards its end. EU actions (Chapter 23) to develop age-friendly environments in Europe put their main focus on empowering older people and promoting their social inclusion and active participation. However, recently, palliative care is starting to be included in policies on ageing. This will probably increase in the future, as recent EU collaborations among existing ageing platforms and palliative care research groups and organizations have begun (e.g. the EU-funded project PACE, comparing the effectiveness of palliative care for older people across Europe; see <www.eupace.eu>).

Another important observation from Chapters 5 to 10 on palliative care policies worldwide is that in certain countries, such as those in North America, access to hospice care, as a specialist palliative care service, is restricted to people with a limited diagnosis and prognosis. Consequently, older people, who often suffer simultaneously from several pathologies and comorbidities, including cognitive deterioration and frailty, for a long period of time, are less likely to receive hospice care. Accordingly, since palliative care teams have developed mainly within hospitals, to care for advanced cancer patients (North America, Europe, and Asia) or for people who fulfil criteria of limited life expectancy (e.g. less than three to six months), accessibility for older people appears to be hindered, resulting in inequalities of access to this type of care. If policies on palliative care were to focus more on people's needs rather than their life expectancy or diagnosis, inequalities in accessing palliative care could be tackled more efficiently.

As was mentioned by the WHO (1), our book also reports that stringent and restrictive laws and regulations on opioid consumption (as in Asia, Latin America, and the Caribbean) interfere negatively in the development of palliative care by restricting the appropriate prescription, administration, and dispensing required to assess and treat pain and other symptoms among older people. Moreover, one of the largest barriers to the provision of good-quality care is the lack of training of health and social care workers on pain and symptom control.

A common element across all chapters focused on policy making is the important role played by non-governmental organizations advocating the development of palliative care. Non-governmental organizations were described as being of considerable importance in providing active support, initiating palliative care services (e.g. in African countries), providing advice to policy makers on including palliative care as an inherent part of national health care programmes (e.g. in Asia), and playing a dynamic and scientific role in creating specific taskforces and working groups to develop guidance documents and influence policy makers (e.g. in Europe, Australia, the United States, and Canada). Non-governmental organizations can, therefore, also play an important role in improving the quality of and access to palliative care for older people.

Finally, since the societal challenges of ageing populations have been recognized, the relevance of community involvement and the active participation of citizens are seen as making a valuable contribution to the development of palliative care. This trend in citizenship behaviour can be enhanced not only by supporting local, regional, national, and international initiatives, but also by creating awareness and challenging governments to develop the policies required to respond to growing needs. In Chapter 18, compassionate communities were described as networks that could encourage people to take some active responsibility for care and to recognize that ageing and dying, death and bereavement are part of everyday life and happen to everyone. It is recognized that these networks could enhance the health and well-being of older people at the end of life.

The way forward: policy recommendations towards improving the quality of and access to palliative care for older people

Although attention to palliative care is increasing, further developments are needed both at a professional and a policy level in order to improve access to and quality of palliative care for older people. In this final part of the book, we provide a set of recommendations for policy and decision makers at organizational, regional, national, and international level. This could support the wider integration and further development of palliative care for older people. Based on the contributions of the authors in this book, we highlight and reflect on the themes that emerge consistently throughout the different chapters and are summarized in Box 26.1.

Integrating palliative care for older people: multiple approaches at multiple levels

In this book, the integration of palliative care into general health care for older people is an overarching central concept. It is also stressed in the WHO resolution 'Strengthening of palliative care as a component of integrated treatment within the continuum of care' (1) that palliative care should be an integral component of health systems worldwide. Integration is a concept that can be defined in many different ways and there are various perspectives on it; hence, it requires multiple approaches at multiple levels to be implemented.

Integrating access to palliative care services into national and international health care policies

For palliative care to reach its full potential, all people with palliative care needs, regardless of their age, diagnosis, life expectancy, and whether or not they are receiving potentially

Box 26.1 Policy recommendations towards improving quality of and access to palliative care for older people

1 Integrating palliative care for older people: multiple approaches at multiple levels

- Integrating access to palliative care services into national and international health care policies
- Promoting a paradigm shift in medicine towards basic palliative care knowledge and skills for all health care professionals
- Supporting inter-professional collaboration
- Including palliative care in national and international policies on ageing and dementia
- Promoting community-level approaches

2 Ensuring education in palliative care at multiple levels

3 Clarifying the concept of palliative care for older people

4 Evaluating and monitoring the quality of and access to palliative care

5 Promoting research towards evidence-based palliative care for older people

curative or life-sustaining treatments, should be able to receive care according to the palliative care philosophy or to access specialist palliative care services when general palliative care is insufficient, in whichever setting they are (e.g. home, hospital, nursing home). This can only be attained when policies are developed—at international as well as national, regional, and organizational levels—that take into account differing national health care systems and cultures. To widely implement new models and innovative interventions as outlined in Chapters 17 (generalist plus specialist palliative care), 22 and 25 (communication and advance care planning), and 24 (care pathways for older people), national health care policies need to ensure that palliative care services are included and to establish mechanisms to access those services throughout the whole health care system. As was pointed out by the WHO (1), a policy concerning drugs should be an integral part of each national policy, to ensure that all relevant drugs are available across all levels of care. This includes the drugs essential for health care professionals to manage symptoms such as pain and psychological distress, and, in particular, opioid analgesics to alleviate pain and respiratory distress. This recommendation is especially important for older people as evidence suggests that they tend to be underserved in relation to palliative care services and drugs for symptom control (Chapter 12).

Promoting a paradigm shift in medicine towards basic palliative care knowledge and skills for all health care professionals

While access to specialist palliative care services is a prerequisite for high-quality palliative care, not all people need specialist palliative care, but would benefit from receiving compassionate and patient-centred family-focused care—which is palliative care by definition—from their general physician and other health care professionals. To fully achieve this, a paradigm shift in medicine is needed. Curing diseases and saving lives has been considered as the main purpose of medicine, leading to doctors aiming to keep people alive as long as possible, sometimes using aggressive or invasive treatments. As a consequence, doctors are evaluated (and evaluate themselves) on how many lives they have saved instead of how they support their patients to die comfortably and with dignity. All health care professionals, as well as policy and decision makers in the field of medicine, need to keep in mind that some conditions simply cannot be cured and some patients will die from their illness no matter how hard they try to prevent this. The principles of palliative care need to be embedded in standard medical practice; this is probably one of the most important prerequisites to achieving the integration of palliative care into the whole health care system. This requires that practicing health care professionals receive education in palliative care competences and that the core curricula for those who will become health care professionals include palliative care as a central component of the learning objectives. The important role of education and training will be further discussed in the following paragraph.

The paradigm shift (i.e. the shift in thinking towards patient-centred, family-focused, coordinated care concentrating on improving quality of life and not only the length of life) is an approach that has also been advocated by others such as primary care health professionals. As described in Chapter 4, 'integrated care' is a concept that is increasingly used to refer to care that is focused and organized around the health care needs of people and communities rather than on specific diseases, which is of particular interest in the context of older people who often suffer from multiple diseases. As such, the Chronic Care Model is adopted by the WHO in its global strategy to work towards high-quality, people-centred, and integrated care (10) for people with chronic conditions.

Supporting inter-professional collaboration

Another essential part of integration involves inter-professional collaboration and the provision of holistic multidisciplinary care, as is stressed in Chapters 16 and 21. Providing holistic, patient-centred, family-focused care, addressing the complex needs of the patient and their family in the physical, psychological, social, and spiritual domains, cannot be done by one profession or professional solely. In addition, teamwork is relevant not only for patients and families, but also for the support and beneficial well-being it provides to professionals. Regular interdisciplinary meetings need to be part of work schedules and included in organizational and institutional policies to stimulate more collaboration, communication, and exchange of knowledge between professionals from different disciplines. Moreover, interdisciplinary collaboration at policy level is also important. Palliative care clearly has overlapping interests with primary care and, in the context of older people, with geriatric medicine, neurology, and other medical specialties, which makes joint working between different disciplines and sectors highly valuable. Interdisciplinary working groups, special interest groups, or task forces could be established and serve as a platform to drive communication and initiatives for collaboration and to advocate for international and national policy making.

Including palliative care in national and international policies on ageing and dementia

Further development and rethinking of existing international policies could have important potential for integrating palliative care as a fundamental component into policies on ageing and dementia. Ageing and dementia are high on policy agendas around the world (as demonstrated by the recent actions of the European Commission, Council of Europe, WHO, Organisation for Economic Co-operation and Development, United Nations, G8 Dementia Summit, and EU summit on chronic diseases organized by the European Commission).

It is remarkable that current policies focus extensively on healthy ageing and the prevention of disease, whereas death is inevitable for everyone and is often preceded by a relatively long period of gradual decline and potentially complex symptoms and problems. Accordingly, a review analysing dementia strategies from seven countries (14) found that most, or possibly all, national strategies adequately address earlier transitions in the trajectory (e.g. symptom recognition to diagnoses, or home to hospital and back) but far fewer address the later transitions like those from home to residential care or to palliative or end-of-life care. The review concluded that the next generation of national dementia strategies needs to focus on more aspects, such as later transitions, and use person-centred outcomes, evaluating the effectiveness of the implementation and dissemination of the strategy (14).

Policy makers need to become aware of the importance and added value of palliative care for older people with chronic and life-threatening diseases, and palliative care associations could be more involved in policy work on ageing and dementia (15). This means that at a national and international level, palliative care associations can best intensify their dialogue with policy and decision makers in actions related to healthy and active ageing, chronic diseases, dementia, long-term care, or integrated care.

While palliative care needs to be included in policies on ageing and dementia, reconsidering the existing palliative care policies, that usually have a main focus on cancer patients, could also be a way to improve access to and quality of palliative care for older people. The next generation palliative care policies could benefit from including a focus on non-cancer patients and older people and developing referral criteria based on needs rather than age, prognosis, or estimated life expectancy. Palliative care policies can also learn from the expertise and knowledge available in existing policy work on ageing and dementia and how to effectively implement them. The same holds true for current clinical guidelines within the field of palliative care that have often been developed from within oncology.

Promoting community-level approaches

To increase the likelihood that people who need palliative care reach the right services, it is crucial for the general public to understand what palliative care is, who should be referred to services, what those services are, and how patients and families may benefit from palliative care programmes. Palliative care is commonly mistaken for 'giving-up treatment' and associated with the expectation of death. As illustrated in Chapter 18, community approaches could stimulate the general public to take some responsibility (e.g. by volunteering to help teams of health care professionals) and can, therefore, be an important part of integration of palliative care for older people. The media need to be involved in disseminating reliable information of educational value and in raising awareness.

Community-level approaches are needed to make people aware of the fact that ageing, death, dying, and bereavement are part of everyday life, to make it less of a taboo topic, and to stimulate individuals and communities to support each other. Dementia-friendly cities (Chapter 18) can be considered as a good practice example, successfully creating awareness and understanding of dementia.

Ensuring education in palliative care at multiple levels

Education is key to improving access to quality palliative care. Therefore, palliative care should be an integral component of the on-going education and training offered to all health care professionals who should be familiar with the essential principles of palliative care and must apply these principles appropriately in their practice (11). This need for education in palliative care has been highlighted by several international entities and legal bodies such as the WHO (1) and the Worldwide Palliative Care Alliance (16), as well as in many of the chapters in this book (Chapters 3, 12, 14, 18, 20, 21, amongst others).

In a White Paper on education published by the European Association for Palliative Care (17), it was recognized that health and social care professionals involved in palliative care at any level should possess a set of core competences enabling them to provide proper care and share a common language for palliative care practice and education. Although complex to define, these competences refer to demonstrable and measurable attitudes (knowledge, skills, and behaviours) that can be expected of certain professionals during and after an education or training programme, for example, in palliative care. According to the European Association for Palliative Care, the core competences in palliative care are:

- applying the core constituents of palliative care in any setting where patients and families are based;
- enhancing patient's comfort and meeting their psychosocial and spiritual needs;
- responding to the needs of family caregivers;
- responding to the challenges of clinical and ethical decision making in palliative care;
- practicing comprehensive care coordination and interdisciplinary teamwork across all settings;
- developing interpersonal and communication skills appropriate to palliative care; practicing self-awareness and undergoing continuing professional development (17).

Different levels of education need to be promoted for professionals to obtain specific knowledge and develop a set of generalist and specialist competences in palliative care. On the one hand, general education on palliative care should be established at an undergraduate level for all students undertaking their primary education in any health care discipline, as well as in public health education. However, evidence has shown that the inclusion of palliative and end-of-life care in medical and nursing undergraduate curricula, although gaining more relevance, is still below optimal (18–23), and that within public health education, little is taught on palliative care (24). On the other hand, a postgraduate level of palliative care should be promoted for those health care professionals who are providing, or will provide, a specialist level of palliative care and for those who have, or will have, palliative care as a main focus of their work. In these cases, diverse levels of education may be implemented: for a generalist provision of palliative care, education at an undergraduate level may suffice, together with continuum education for existing practitioners; for specialist palliative care provision, postgraduated education in palliative care is required (17).

In a first attempt to map palliative medicine specialties in Europe, a recent publication has shown that only 7 countries (out of 53) have a specialty or sub-specialty in palliative medicine (25). This highlights the need of further investment in postgraduate education in palliative care among physicians, as the specialist education and recognition of physicians with expertise in palliative medicine is one of the cornerstones of ensuring that patients have access to high-quality care throughout their disease trajectory and during the dying phase (26).

To summarize, as advocated by several international organizations (e.g. the WHO, Worldwide Palliative Care Alliance, European Association for Palliative Care), palliative care should be included as a regular, mandatory, routine element of all health and social professionals' undergraduate education. Moreover, it should be established as part of the in-service and continuum education of all caregivers who are expected to provide care to people with palliative care needs (e.g. at the primary care level, in hospitals, in long-term care facilities).

One of the elements that could improve palliative care education is to further develop standards and norms, as well as learning objectives and curricula, and establish optimal ways to teach and evaluate to what extent competences in the delivery of palliative care are mastered. Further developments are needed, not only to help professionals develop and improve their core competences to provide palliative care across all settings, but also on the best educational strategies to promote those competences.

Requiring interdisciplinary teamwork, palliative care also calls for an interdisciplinary approach in the implementation of educational programmes. National and international policies can advocate the establishment of common and shared curricula, and professional organizations in health and social sciences can come together to develop standards and curricula where shared core competences can be developed and learning objectives and educational strategies can be commonly defined. This is even more relevant for the development of palliative care for older people where, due to the diversity and complementary nature of the many disciplines involved, collaboration is needed to promote synergies.

Importantly, not only should all health and social care professionals receive education in palliative care and develop their competences, professionals working in specialist palliative care should also have a set of core knowledge and skills in other areas relevant to the care of older people, such as geriatrics, internal medicine, neurology, psychiatry, or other medical specialties. Specific knowledge about different diseases and their progression and trajectories, together with the development of specific skills to better approach, communicate with, and care for older, frail people should be promoted among all professionals who might care for patients in need of palliative care. Sharing discipline-specific skills among professionals belonging to different fields, and having the willingness to learn with and from each other, are paramount to the improvement and better development of palliative care (17).

Not only professional carers but also family and other informal carers need to receive education and training in several dimensions of care provision, both to be able to provide better care as well as to be capable of better managing the burden caused by being an informal caregiver. Specific education for family carers about strategies for safe moving and handling of the patient; information about disease processes, trajectory, prognosis, dying process, and symptom management; about how to deliver tangible care, equipment, and medication; and also about how to access welfare and social and health care benefits is, therefore, needed (Chapter 20).

Finally, citizens need to be able to talk about life, ageing, and the process of living with life-threatening diseases, dying, and death. Increasing societal awareness about living at older ages, palliative care, dying, and death through community learning approaches and activities might also contribute to the integration of palliative care as an inherent component of care for older people.

Clarifying the concept of palliative care for older people

While reading through the various chapters in this book, it can be observed that, despite the existence of the WHO definition, different definitions of palliative care are used and palliative care is interpreted in different ways. Palliative care is often presented alongside other concepts such as hospice care, supportive care, terminal care, end-of-life care, comfort care, and compassionate care. In addition, several practice innovations in this field—such as the Route to Success programme in nursing homes and the Respecting Patient Choices programme on advance care planning (Chapters 22, 25)—are explicit in not using the term 'palliative care'. Such programmes aim to implement a palliative care approach or the principles of palliative care, but have chosen not to include palliative care in their titles, probably to avoid associations with dying and death.

Moreover, in this book, we see that the way health care systems are organized might influence the way palliative care is defined and implemented in practice. This is the case, for example, in the United States, where palliative care is defined as specialized medical care and distinguished from hospice care (Chapter 9). In contrast, different definitions might represent diverse views on what palliative care is and how it should be organized in practice, influencing the organization and delivery of services. Therefore, conceptual work on palliative care might lead to more clarification, which in turn might lead to more effective cross-national and cross-cultural comparisons of health care systems, contributing to the improvement of palliative care services.

Often major questions arise on what palliative care actually is and how it relates to other already existing types of care. Chapters 12 and 19 show that older people often suffer from multiple symptoms and complex needs which are difficult to assess and manage. This situation might be made worse by the lack of clarity and consensus among professionals on what palliative care needs are, leading to the need for better definition, so that professionals become better able to identify patients who might benefit from palliative care.

Palliative care must be defined in a way that is clear for all stakeholders (e.g. people in policy, people in practice, and people who may use it). This is an essential discussion and policy can help in bringing people together, advocating them to cooperate more and better.

Another specific concept that might benefit from further conceptual work is the one of 'early palliative care'. The 'early' introduction of palliative care in the disease trajectory is commonly advocated in the field of palliative care, as evidence has shown the benefits of such an approach (2–9, 27) (Chapters 12, 13, 17, and 19). Nonetheless, most of this evidence is based on research conducted in oncology settings with cancer patients, whose disease trajectories, as Chapter 12 shows, are more clearly defined and established. When it comes to non-cancer patients and to older and frail people, multi-morbidities and less clear disease patterns emerge, together with difficulties in making an accurate prognosis. This challenges the meaning of 'early' introduction, raising the need to further study and clarify this concept.

Furthermore, according to the European Association for Palliative Care (28), there is no exact point in any disease trajectory signposting the transition from curative to palliative care. In some cases, patients might benefit from palliative care at the moment they are diagnosed with an incurable disease, while in others, palliative care might only be needed at an advanced stage of disease development. This scenario gets more complex when considering older people with multiple diseases, comorbidities, and frailty, for whom signposting a specific moment of transition between care structures and approaches might be problematic. Therefore, additional difficulties may occur in defining when the 'right' moment to refer an older patient to a palliative care specialist is.

In summary, clarification of what 'early' palliative care means for older people is needed, together with clarification of whether there can be a 'right' time identified to introduce palliative care. Moreover, optimal referral criteria to specialist palliative care for older people need to be defined to guide professionals in their decisions. In fact, although several guidelines concerning referrals to palliative care coexist, there is no clear concept of what an optimal referral actually is.

Evaluating and monitoring the quality of and access to palliative care

Evaluation is an integral part of policy, programme development, and service planning, in order to determine the impact and effectiveness of a particular intervention or service. Monitoring, referring to routine data collection, and reporting, is needed to provide feedback to suggest incremental adjustments in the organization and development of health and social care systems over time and, as such, for palliative care. Both evaluation and monitoring are essential to informing decision making at policy level as well as at operational levels (29).

To monitor palliative care systematically at national and global level, a good-quality information system should be available to support data collection, reporting, and information exchange, as is raised in Chapters 2 and 10. Besides an adequate technical system, it is important to appoint a national and/or regional coordinating body responsible for overseeing all palliative care activities and for the collection of the monitoring data. The Australian Palliative Care Outcomes Collaboration (PCOC), measuring the quality and outcomes of palliative care on a routine basis, has demonstrated a way to support improved outcomes and care processes, and allows for benchmarking between services. Although not mentioned in this book, another interesting example of an assessment system is the interRAI, International Resident Assessment Instrument, which has been shown to provide insights into the service needs, quality of care, and impact of policy choices on vulnerable persons across the continuum of care, and is used in several OECD countries (<http://www.interrai.org/assets/files/par-i-chapter-3-old-age.pdf>). Operational person-level data could be an important source of evidence for decision makers, from those at the bedside through to their counterparts in national governments.

The use of patient-reported outcome measures and the need to adjust them to be used with older people is discussed in Chapter 12. Further, the use of assessment instruments should become an integral part of normal clinical and social care practice. The information could also be of interest to patients and health care professionals as they can review their own care and compare quality of care across care providers, which would make people feel more engaged.

From a public health perspective, it is essential to monitor palliative care across all settings and beyond the specialist services. Therefore, monitoring tools should be appropriate to use both at a specialist as well as at a generalist palliative care level, across all levels of the health care system. To develop a basic information system to collect the necessary data on a regular basis for monitoring and evaluation, decisions first need to be made on what the core indicators are, and on their respective standards. There are several initiatives aiming to develop a core set of quality indicators for palliative care across settings (30–32). While it is beyond the scope of this book to summarize all of these initiatives, one important quality indicator, that was highlighted in Chapter 11, concerns place of death. Although there are important international place-of-death analyses ongoing, death certificate data only provide insights into age, gender, cause of death, and place of death, and are often coded in a way that palliative care units or hospices cannot be identified. Hence, policy makers might benefit from including more basic end-of-life parameters in their death certificates, such as the use of specialist palliative care services, or evaluations by the physicians signing the death certificates of the quality of dying or quality of end-of-life care delivered.

Promoting research towards evidence-based palliative care for older people

Research is essential to obtain strong evidence and is crucial to moving forward. Most of the existing evidence about palliative care has been developed based on a specific diagnosis and/or on looking at a certain period of the disease trajectory (e.g. terminal phase, last days of life), raising the need for research on older people's trajectories and their needs for care. In addition, research is needed to update and develop evidence-based guidelines and tools on palliative care, focusing specifically on older people and people with dementia. Such research is multidisciplinary by principle and would preferably include multiple disciplines and professions.

Another relevant issue in this field that could benefit from research is the needs of family caregivers. In Chapters 2 and 20, it is highlighted that most family caregivers of older people are themselves in older age groups, suggesting that assuming the role of an informal caregiver may cause additional burdens. More evidence on how to help these family caregivers to cope with their own suffering and needs, and how to improve their own quality of life, is therefore needed.

Further, research on the implementation, evaluation, and cost effectiveness of palliative care models is needed, with a special focus on older people and taking into account cultural and economic factors, in order to assess what might be more effective in low- and mid-income countries and to identify specific referral criteria for specialist palliative care and complex interventions. This may be done by further studying existing models or innovative practices in this field, taking the best practices into consideration.

Since the majority of interventions in palliative care aim to improve the quality of care and quality of life of the patient and his or her family, quality indicators and tools are needed to adequately identify palliative care needs and assess quality of care (Chapter 12). Research should evaluate quality of care processes and outcomes to help policy makers and health care managers understand what is needed. Concrete examples of such types of tools were provided in Chapter 12—namely, patient-reported outcome measurements including several elements, of which some are specific to older people. In addition to these, cost-effective studies of different models of care are needed to better show the benefits of integrated palliative care provision for older people.

Implementing research on palliative care for older people is marked by several challenges, and ethical issues may arise: due to their frailty, older people, especially when nearing the end of their lives, are in a more vulnerable condition; also, cognitive impairment may limit the possibility of older people being included and participating in studies. However, it is necessary to include the perspectives of patients and families when conducting research among older people and/or people with dementia. While it is recommended to use already existing databases (e.g. documental analysis of patients' records) as much as possible, it is also important to optimize careful inclusion of older people themselves, as they often welcome the opportunity to contribute to creating new knowledge (33).

Finally, research funding in the past has been focused on cancer research, which has led to enormous breakthroughs, making cancer often a chronic disease with many survivors. A similar type of focus has occurred in promoting research on HIV/AIDS and dementia, although to a lesser extent than in cancer. This has contributed to longer life expectancies and better quality of life for these patients. However, as this book shows, older people often have multiple problems and frailties, meaning that a disease-oriented structure and model of research funding is not applicable. As a consequence, and because older people might not fit easily into existing disease-oriented research designs, they are more at risk of being left out of some relevant research projects. Hence, more funding is needed for palliative care research, especially including older people and not necessarily for disease-oriented projects. In fact, international and national funding policies are urged to provide more funding in order to support quality research focusing on the needs and problems of all people, regardless of their age or disease.

Conclusion on a public health approach to improving palliative care for older people

In this chapter, recommendations were developed based on the existing evidence on palliative care for older people from a public health perspective (see Box 26.1). Considering palliative care as a dynamic, evolving concept and an inherent part of every health care system, this set of recommendations has been structured in several major dimensions (integration, education clarification of concepts, monitoring, and research), aiming to contribute to the development of palliative care especially focusing on older people. Regional, national, ethical, and culturally sensitive approaches should be taken into consideration when implementing these recommendations, as they need to be adjusted to each specific reality. Moreover, while one recommendation might already contribute to the development of palliative care for older people, several recommendations should be combined and integrated to achieve the goal that palliative care reaches all older people who are in need of it.

These recommendations have been made possible thanks to the contributions of the authors, whose geographic distribution, interdisciplinary backgrounds, and multiple perspectives and experiences provide us with a broad, global public health perspective on the subject. We hope that the reader enjoyed and learned as much from these contributions as we, the editors, did, and that this book will inspire policy and decision makers, as well as academics, health care managers, professionals, and many others, to improve palliative care for older people.

References

1 World Health Organization. *Strengthening of palliative care as a component of integrated treatment throughout the life course.* EB134/28. 134th session; 2013.

2 Bakitas M, Lyons KD, Hegel MT, Balan S, Brokaw FC, Seville J, et al. Effects of a palliative care intervention on clinical outcomes in patients with advanced cancer: the Project ENABLE II randomized controlled trial. *JAMA* 2009; **302**(7):741–9.

3 Temel JS, Greer JA, Muzikansky A, Gallagher ER, Admane S, Jackson VA, et al. Early palliative care for patients with metastatic non-small-cell lung cancer. *NEJM* 2010; **363**(8):733–42.

4 Hall S, Kolliakou A, Petkova H, Froggatt K, Higginson IJ. Interventions for improving palliative care for older people living in nursing care homes. *Cochrane Database Syst Rev* 2011; **3**:CD007132.

5 Reyes-Ortiz CA, Williams C, Westphal C. Comparison of early versus late palliative care consultation in end-of-life care for the hospitalized frail elderly patients. *Am J Hosp Palliat Care* 2014; **8**:1–5.

6 Zimmermann C, Swami N, Krzyzanowska M, Hannon B, Leighl N, Oza A, et al. Early palliative care for patients with advanced cancer: a cluster-randomised controlled trial. *Lancet* 2014; **383**(9930):1721–30.

7 Morrison RS, Dietrich J, Ladwig S, Quill T, Sacco J, Tangeman J, et al. Palliative care consultation teams cut hospital costs for Medicaid beneficiaries. *Health Aff (Millwood)* 2011; **30**(3):454–63.

8 Edmonds P, Hart S, Gao W, Vivat B, Burman R, Silber E, et al. Palliative care for people severely affected by multiple sclerosis: evaluation of a novel palliative care service. *Mult Scler* 2010; **16**:627–36.

9 Higginson IJ, McCrone P, Hart SR, Burman R, Silber E, Edmonds PM. Is short-term palliative care cost-effective in multiple sclerosis? A randomized Phase II trial. *J Pain Symptom Manage*, 2009; **38**:816–26.

10 World Health Organization Regional Office for Europe. *Strengthening people-centred health systems in the WHO European region. A framework for action towards coordinated/integrated health services delivery (CIHSD)*. Copenhagen: World Health Organization; 2013.

11 Council of Europe. *Recommendation Rec (2003) 24 of the Committee of Ministers to member states on the organisation of palliative care.* <http://www.eapcnet.eu/LinkClick.aspx?fileticket=3KJ5U3BQLVY%3d&tabid=1709>.

12 Boersma I, Miyasaki J, Kutner J, Kluger B. Palliative care and neurology: time for a paradigm shift. *Neurology* 2014; **83**(6):561–7.

13 McCormick WC, on behalf of American Geriatrics Society, American Association for Hospice and Palliative Medicine, and John A Hartford Foundation. Report of the Geriatrics–Hospice and Palliative Medicine Work Group: American Geriatrics Society and American Academy of Hospice and Palliative Medicine leadership collaboration. *JAGS* 2012; **60**(3):583–7.

14 Fortinsky RH, Downs M. Optimizing person-centered transitions in the dementia journey: a comparison of national dementia strategies. *Health Aff (Millwood)* 2014; **33**(4):566–73.

15 Van den Block L. The need for integrating palliative care in ageing and dementia policies. *Eur J Public Health* 2014; **4**:1–2.

16 World Palliative Care Alliance. *Global atlas of palliative care at the end of life*. Geneva: World Health Organization and Worldwide Palliative Care Alliance; 2014.

17 Gadamondi C, Larkin P, Payne S. Core competencies in palliative care: an EAPC White Paper on palliative care education. Eur J Pall Care 2013; 20(2):86–91.

18 Cheng DR, Teh A. Palliative care in Australian medical student education. *Med Teach* 2014; **36**(1):82–3.

19 Oneschuk D, Moloughney B, Jones-McLean E, Challis A. The status of undergraduate palliative medicine education in Canada: a 2001 survey. *J Palliat Care* 2004; **20**(1):32–7.

20 Sullivan AM, Lakoma MD, Block SD. The status of medical education in end-of-life care: a national report. *J Gen Intern Med* 2003; **18**(9):685–95.

21 Dickinson GE. End-of-life and palliative care issues in medical and nursing schools in the United States. *Death Stud* 2007; **31**(8):713–26.

22 Wilson DM, Goodwin BL, Hewitt JA. An examination of palliative or end-of-life care education in introductory nursing programs across Canada. *Nurs Res Pract* 2011; **907172**:1–5.

23 Pereira S. Formação sobre cuidados paliativos no ensino pré-graduado em enfermagem. In: Carvalho AS, Osswald W (Coords). *Ensaios de Bioética Nº 2*. Porto: Instituto de Bioética da Universidade Católica Portuguesa; 2011, 203--216..

24 Lupu D, Deneszczuk C, Leystra T, McKinnon R, Seng V. Few U.S. public health schools offer courses on palliative and end-of-life care policy. *J Palliat Med* 2013; **16**(12):1582–7.

25 Bolognesi B, Centeno C, Biasco G. *Specialisation in palliative medicine for physicians in Europe 2014—a supplement of the EAPC atlas of palliative care in Europe*. Milan: EAPC Press; 2014.

26 **Payne S.** Preface. In: Bolognesi B, Centeno C, Biasco G. *Specialisation in palliative medicine for physicians in Europe 2014—a supplement of the EAPC atlas of palliative care in Europe.* Milan: EAPC Press; 2014, 11.

27 **Hui D, Kim SH, Roquemore J, Dev R, Chisholm G, Bruera E.** Impact of timing and setting of palliative care referral on quality of end-of-life care in cancer patients. *Cancer* 2014; **120**(11):1743–9.

28 **Radbruch L, Payne S, Board of Directors of the European Association for Palliative Care.** White Paper on standards and norms for hospice and palliative care in Europe. Recommendations from the European Association for Palliative Care. *Eur J Pall Care* 2009; **16**(6):278–89.

29 **Eagar K, Cranny C, Fildes D.** *Evaluation and palliative care: a guide to the evaluation of palliative care services and programs.* Centre for Health Service Development, University of Wollongong; 2004.

30 **Leemans K, Cohen J, Francke AL, Vander Stichele R, Claessen SJ, Van den Block L, et al.** Towards a standardized method of developing quality indicators for palliative care: protocol of the quality indicators for palliative care (Q-PAC) study. *BMC Pall Care* 2013; **12**:6.

31 **De Roo ML, Leeman K, Claessen SJ, Cohen J, Pasman HR, Deliens L, et al.,** on behalf of Euro-IMPACT. Quality indicators for palliative care: update of a systematic review. *J Pain Symptom Manage* 2013; **46**(4):556–72.

32 **Woitha K, Van Beek K, Ahmen N, Jaspers B, Mollard JM, Ahmedzai SH, et al.** Validation of quality indicators for the organization of palliative care: a modified RAND Delphi study in seven European countries (the Europall project). *Palliat Med* 2014; **28**(2):121–9.

33 **Alzheimer Europe.** *Involving people with dementia. Ethics of dementia research.* Available at: <http://www.alzheimer-europe.org/Ethics/Ethical-issues-in-practice/Ethics-of-dementia-research/Involving-people-with-dementia#fragment-1> (Accessed August 2014). Ref. type: online source.

Index